Nutritional Health Bible

About the author

Linda Lazarides is widely recognized as one of Britain's top nutritional therapists, and is one of the few in her profession who has worked for the National Health Service. She is director of the Society for the Promotion of Nutritional Therapy, founder of the British Association of Nutritional Therapists, and author of *Principles of Nutritional Therapy* (Thorsons). She is also an adviser to the Institute for Complementary Medicine, BACUP, and *Here's Health* magazine.

Nutritional Health Bible

LINDA LAZARIDES

Thorsons
An Imprint of HarperCollins*Publishers*

Thorsons
An Imprint of HarperCollins*Publishers*
77–85 Fulham Palace Road,
Hammersmith, London W6 8JB
1160 Battery Street,
San Francisco, California 94111–1213

Published by Thorsons 1997
5 7 9 10 8 6 4

A catalogue record for this book
is available from the British Library

ISBN 0 7225 3424 8

Printed and bound in Great Britain by
Creative Print and Design (Wales), Ebbw Vale

Contents

Preface

I cannot claim the credit for what is in this book. I owe most of what I know to the research, writings and teachings of others, particularly those great champions of nutritional/environmental medicine Linus Pauling, Abram Hoffer, Carl Pfeiffer, Roger Williams, Jeffrey Bland, Melvyn Werbach, Theron Randolph, William Rea and Jean Monro. My patients have been my other great teachers. I would also like to thank Pharma Nord (UK) Ltd and Thorne Research Inc for the use of their databases in my research, ITServices for their excellent monthly research summaries in *Clinical Pearls News*, and HealthComm International Inc for *Functional Medicine Update*. Doctors will find both these publications especially helpful for keeping well informed in this field. I can also highly recommend Dr Melvyn Werbach's book *Nutritional Influences on Illness* (Third Line Press). For details of where to obtain these publications, *see Appendix V, Useful Addresses*.

Computer technology is allowing the huge number of nutritional medicine studies to be recognized as a coherent body of research which points with ever-increasing insistence towards the need for changes in our approach to chronic disease. I hope that this book will provide concise answers for the growing number of medical practitioners who are hungry for information.

The *Nutritional Health Bible* is for both the interested lay person and for students, doctors, dietitians and other health carers. It is a Learn as You Look reference: in defining most of the terms I have tried to enhance the reader's understanding of how each item relates to human health. In this sense I hope it is as complete a reference as possible, but if you the reader have any suggestions, please do let me know.

Linda Lazarides, April 1997

Foreword

Linda Lazarides is becoming a force to be reckoned with in the nutritional world – in the UK, in Europe, and now worldwide. With the publication of the *Nutritional Health Bible* she has shown that she has an encyclopaedic amount of data at her fingertips, and can collate and present that data in a reference work that will prove essential for anyone, anywhere, working in the field of nutrition. This is one of those books that we will all, eventually, have and use on CD-ROM, but until that time the text version is something that you will want to have on your bookshelves.

Consider this: you may be a doctor, a dietitian, an alternative therapist; a patient asks you about, for instance, Saw Palmetto, or Gerson Therapy, or alternatives to HRT – something about which you keep meaning to read up but have not yet. A quick look at this book will at least tell you what they are talking about. A later, more careful reading will enable you to put the whole thing into context, and rate its importance and usefulness. These days medicine is increasingly fragmented, with the different schools, orthodox, nutritional, alternative, all digging in behind their barricades. Indeed, as I write this a *Lancet* editorial arrives, declaring that 'A truce must be called' between conventional and unconventional cancer treatments. In this context, we have to remember that an expert opinion is still a personal one; objective truth seems further away every year. But Linda Lazarides doesn't put a foot wrong – her assessments of the many therapeutic options described here are always cautious and sound, and where there is a downside she is not afraid to describe it.

Consider also this: you may be a patient, or a concerned parent, or just interested in taking care of yourself. You have a problem, and perhaps your doctors aren't being a lot of help. Use this book to get an idea of what the nutritional options are, of how to start solving the problem, and of where to go for further help. Linda Lazarides won't give you any advice that isn't sound and well-founded, and she will help you to help yourself.

Dr Damien Downing, MBBS
Senior Editor, *Journal of Nutritional
and Environmental Medicine*
London, April 1997

A

Vitamin A (Retinol)

Vitamin (fat-soluble)
UK RNI 700 mcg (2300 iu)
US RDA 1000 mcg (3300 iu)

FUNCTIONS
Eyesight
Growth
Immune system
Mucous membranes
Normal development of tissues
Protein synthesis

GOOD FOOD SOURCES
Butter
Cheese
Fish liver oils
Liver
Margarine

Deficiency symptoms

- Acne
- Dandruff
- Dry eyes
- Dry scaly skin
- Frequent infections
- Frequent mouth ulcers
- Poor vision in dim light

Preventing deficiency

Preformed (ready-made) vitamin A is known as retinol, and can only be obtained from animal foods, where it is usually found in the fatty portion, as it is a fat-soluble vitamin. The bioavailability (*which see*) of vitamin A and other fat-soluble vitamins is improved by the consumption of fat or oil as well as protein in the same meal. The consumption of vitamins C and E in the same meal helps to protect vitamin A and therefore also enhances its bioavailability. The presence of a zinc deficiency on the other hand impairs the absorption and utilization of vitamin A. Food irradiation also reduces vitamin A bioavailability.

Vitamin A is said to be very quickly depleted by the presence of infections, and it may be wise to eat liver more frequently during these times.

Vegetarians have to rely on their body's ability to convert pro-vitamin A (beta-carotene, *which see*) found in many fruits and vegetables – to retinol. Most people probably have no problem with this conversion, with the exception of hypothyroid individuals – those whose thyroid gland is underfunctioning. Common symptoms of hypothyroidism are a tendency to put weight on too easily, and abnormal hair loss.

Comments

Animals store vitamin A in their liver, which is why liver is a good source of retinol – sometimes too good a source. Vitamin A supplements are used in modern intensive farming as a growth promoter, which can increase 20-fold the amount of vitamin A which naturally occurs in an animal's liver. This is why pregnant women are warned against consuming liver regularly, although the problem is less likely to occur with liver from organically-reared animals.

Supplementation

In research studies, Vitamin A supplements have been found to:

- Help cure acne
- Help cure psoriasis
- Help prevent the common cold
- Reduce the rate of complications from measles
- Improve eyesight
- Increase the healing rate of gastric ulcers

Preferred form and suggested intake
Recommended general health supplementation: 1 teaspoon cod liver oil or 1 capsule halibut liver oil daily.

For acne, 7,500 iu plus 15 mg zinc daily. For dry, scaly skin, 7,500 iu plus 15 mg zinc daily, plus 1–2 tablespoons of cold-pressed, good quality flax seed oil.

Cautions
It is easier to overdose on fat-soluble vitamins than others because they are stored in the body rather than excreted. While death is extremely rare, and single doses of several hundred thousand iu have been used in short trials without problems, headaches, nausea and loss of appetite may result from an excessive intake taken over a long period of time. This is toxic to the liver and can cause birth defects if consumed by pregnant women.

During pregnancy it is best to eat liver only from organically reared animals, and to take only minimal supplementation, as from a moderate multivitamin preparation,

or in the form of a little cod liver oil. Although vitamin A requirements are raised by pregnancy, and birth defects can be linked with vitamin A deficiency as well as vitamin A excess, your daily supplementation should not exceed a total of 7,500 iu while pregnant or if planning pregnancy.

Acetaldehyde

Acetaldehyde is a toxic substance produced in the body from alcohol and is one of the impurities found in cheap wine and 'moonshine' spirits. Its effects are often felt as a 'hangover'. Acetaldehyde is also found in cigarette smoke, and is produced by the yeast *Candida albicans*, which may account for much of the malaise experienced by those with a heavy overgrowth of this yeast in their intestines, since the acetaldehyde will be absorbed from their intestines into the bloodstream, to be circulated throughout the body.

Alcohols and aldehydes are formed as intermediary metabolites during the body's normal processes of detoxification. If the liver's detoxification pathways are impaired, aldehydes can, instead of being converted to the next intermediate product, build up to harmful levels and cause much damage since they are often more toxic than the original substances from which they are derived.

Acetaldehyde is said to destroy vitamins B_1, B_6 and C. Supplements of these nutrients, together with the amino acid cysteine, may help the liver to detoxify acetaldehyde.

Acetyl CoA
(also see Energy production)

Acetyl CoA is an intermediate product in the production of energy. It can be formed from pyruvate (which in turn is formed from glucose or glycerol), or from fats or some of the amino acids. It enters the Krebs cycle where its energy is released by oxidation.

Acetylcholine

Acetylcholine is a neurotransmitter – a chemical involved in the transmission of nerve impulses. It is made from a combination of acetyl with the nutrient choline, and is required for many functions, particularly memory and intestinal peristalsis.

Acetylcholinesterase (AChE), an enzyme which breaks down acetylcholine in junctions between nerve cells, is thought to maintain levels of acetylcholine within safe bounds. Organophosphate pesticides are known to inhibit this enzyme.

In Parkinson's disease, acetylcholine-containing nerve cells appear to be improperly controlled. Drugs which inhibit the action of acetylcholine can ease the symptoms of parkinsonism.

Neurochemical examinations of the brains of individuals dying with Alzheimer's disease show a significant reduction in acetylcholine and the enzymes associated with both its synthesis and destruction, in the parts of the brain most severely damaged by the disease.

Achlorhydria

Also known as hypochlorhydria, this describes a reduced ability to produce hydrochloric acid in the stomach. Since hydrochloric acid is a pre-requisite for protein digestion, and is also required to stimulate the next (pancreatic) stage of digestion, achlorhydria may result in significantly impaired digestion and absorption.

Dysbiosis and bacterial overgrowth of the stomach and small intestine may occur in achlorhydric individuals since hydrochloric acid normally destroys micro-organisms in the stomach.

Acid-alkaline balance

In healthy individuals the pH of the blood is maintained between 7.35 and 7.45. This balance is dependent on the excretion of carbonic acid (carbon dioxide in solution) through the lungs, and the excretion of an acid or alkaline urine by the kidneys.

Diet can contribute significantly to the body's acid-alkaline balance. Fruits and vegetables are metabolized to an alkaline ash and are known as alkaline-forming, whereas high-protein foods are metabolized to sulphuric acid and phosphoric acid and are therefore acid-forming.

Although fruits yield citric acid and malic acid, these acids are oxidized by the body as part of its energy-production process.

Alkaline-forming foods	Acid-forming foods
All fruits, most vegetables, honey, milk, wine and most nuts.	Most meats, poultry, fish and sea food, lentils, brazil nuts, peanuts, bread and cereals, chocolate, eggs and cheese.

Failure to maintain the acid-alkaline balance can result in acidosis or alkalosis.

Acidophilus (see Probiotics)

ACTH (Adrenocorticotropic hormone)

A hormone produced by the anterior pituitary gland, which stimulates the secretion of cortisol by the adrenal cortex.

Adenosylcobalamine
(see Vitamin B₁₂)

Adipose tissue

This is another term for body fat. The adipose tissue stores energy and provides cushioning for body organs as well as body insulation. 95 per cent of adipose tissue is white, but about five per cent is brown. Brown adipose tissue can oxidize glucose and fatty acids from food, releasing their energy as heat.

Adrenal glands

The adrenal glands rest like a cap on top of the kidneys. Each is a double gland consisting of the adrenal cortex and the adrenal medulla. The adrenal cortex produces so-called corticosteroid hormones, subdivided into:

- Mineralocorticoids (mainly aldosterone) which control sodium, potassium and water balance in the body),
- Glucocorticoids (mainly cortisol but also cortisone and corticosterone) which,

among many other actions, have important effects on glucose metabolism, reduce inflammation and help maintain normal blood pressure,
- Small amounts of androgens (sex hormones).

The production of glucocorticoids is increased during stress.

The adrenal medulla produces adrenaline (also known as epinephrine – the 'fight or flight' hormone) and noradrenaline, which acts as a neurotransmitter and, like adrenaline, can constrict blood vessels and raise blood pressure.

Some of the nutrients on which the adrenal glands are particularly dependent include vitamin C, pantothenic acid (vitamin B₅), the amino acid methionine, and zinc. High-dose vitamin B₅ supplementation results in an increase in the urinary excretion of 17,21 dihydroxy-20 ketosteroids – an unmistakable sign of a functional activation of the adrenal gland (*Fidanza A: Therapeutic action of pantothenic acid. Int J Vit Nutr Res, Suppl 24: In Vitamins in Medicine: Recent therapeutic aspects. A Hanck [ed], 1983*). The adrenal hormones (and other hormones) are made of cholesterol esters, hydroxyl groups and methyl groups. Methionine and choline are required in adequate amounts every day to supply methyl groups for hormone syn-thesis. Some nutritionists believe that methionine deficiency is relatively common. Methionine may be particularly low in vegetarian diets which rely mainly on pulses for protein.

Adrenaline
(see Catecholamines)

Aflatoxin (see Mycotoxins)

Agar

Also known as agar-agar, this is a seaweed extract used as a vegetarian substitute for gelatin.

Agnus castus

Herb

Agnus castus has been widely researched. It is best known as a female hormone balancer, especially helping to promote the production of progesterone by increasing luteinizing hormone and inhibiting the production of follicle-stimulating hormone by the pituitary. Its main indications are to treat frequent menstruation, premenstrual symptoms such as fluid retention and acne, and menopausal problems. In breast-feeding mothers, Agnus castus can help to stimulate milk production, although it takes a few weeks to take effect. This herb has a relaxing and calming quality.

Availability: From health food shops, herbalists and nutritional therapists.

Alanine

Amino acid

An amino acid formed from the conversion of pyruvate (a common compound formed during carbohydrate metabolism) or the breakdown of DNA or the dipeptides carnosine and anserine (this latter process requires a zinc-dependent enzyme), found in large amounts in chicken and turkey.

Alanine helps to prevent exercise-induced ketosis and may reduce the ketosis of diabetes. It can be converted quickly in the liver to usable glucose, thus acting as a major energy source, and by triggering the release of glucagon (*which see*) from the liver, it can stimulate an increase in blood sugar.

Alanine also acts as an inhibitory neurotransmitter and is important in the body's production of lymphocytes. According to environmental medicine expert Dr William Rea, it is frequently deficient in chemically sensitive individuals, resulting in a slow ability to conjugate toxins.

Availability: Not normally available as a food supplement.

Albumin

Albumin (or albumen) is synthesized in the liver and is a major protein of blood plasma. It is mainly responsible for maintaining osmotic pressure in blood vessels; a lack of albumin therefore explains fluid retention in protein deficiency states. Albumin also acts as a carrier for many substances in the blood.

Alcohol

Alcohol is formed by the fermentation of sugar. It is also known as ethanol or ethyl alcohol, and is readily absorbed from the stomach and intestines into the blood. The liver converts alcohol to acetaldehyde.

Alcohol consumption inhibits the enzyme delta-6-desaturase, which is required for the conversion of essential fatty acids into gamma-linolenic acid (GLA) and eicosapentaenoic acid (EPA). Cases of arthritis in heavy drinkers have responded to supplementation with GLA and EPA. Alcohol also interferes with the metabolism of folic acid and methionine. The risk of breast cancer increases in women who consume three or more drinks a day.

Alcohol consumption also depletes B vitamins, and probably also antioxidants, since these are required to quench the free radical activity stimulated by the liver's alcohol detoxification processes.

Alcoholic drinks may contain a number of contaminants such as benzopyrene and nitrosamines, which can promote cancers.

Alder buckthorn

Herb

A herb used as a bowel-stimulating laxative. It is considered to be less habit-forming and irritating than many other laxative herbs such as senna.

Availability: Available in the Arkopharma range of products, and from medical herbalists, but may be hard to find in health food shops.

Alfalfa
(also see Sprouted seeds)

Superfood

Alfalfa is also known as lucerne. It is a common forage plant fed to animals. Alfalfa products are available in the form of a tea, or as tablets or capsules of the dried plant. In Russia and China the leaves are served as a vegetable. Alfalfa seeds are often used for home sprouting, and produce highly nutritious fine, thread-like sprouts used in salads and as a sandwich filling. One tablespoon of alfalfa seeds can produce about 2 lb of sprouts.

Various health claims have been made for alfalfa products, particularly that they can help arthritis and prevent the absorption of cholesterol. However, there are many more effective natural products for these purposes. The best use for alfalfa is probably the consumption of sprouts for their phytoestrogen (plant oestrogen) content. Phytoestrogens are thought to have a balancing effect on female hormones: reducing an excess of oestrogen by competing for absorption sites in the body, and making up for a deficiency by providing substitutes with similar effects. Alfalfa sprouts are also rich in many nutrients.

The consumption of exceptionally large quantities of alfalfa seeds or sprouts on a regular basis is not advised since this has been associated with blood abnormalities and an aggravation of auto-immune diseases, particularly systemic lupus erythematosus. As with all foods, moderation is advised.

Availability: Widely available from health food shops.

Algae

Superfood

Algae are simple plants which grow in water. Some are cultivated and used as concentrated sources of nutrients and chlorophyll (*which see*). Many are rich in protein, beta-carotene and GLA. Some algae may contain vitamin B_{12} analogues, but these do not have true vitamin activity. Varieties of algae which are commonly available as food supplements include Spirulina, Chlorella, Blue-Green Algae and Pacific Algae. Spirulina is also promoted as a mild appetite suppressant.

Although sold for their nutrient-dense properties, the quantity of algae which an individual would need to consume daily to obtain significant amounts of nutrients from these sources would be a relatively expensive way of obtaining these nutrients. It is hard to tell whether the health benefits claimed for these products by some of their users would also have occurred with ordinary dietary supplements and/or by dietary improvement alone. Health benefits claimed by users include intestinal cleansing effects, greater overall energy and well-being, and increased mental acuity.

Quality control may be a problem for some algae grown outdoors in open lakes, since there are a number of potential sources of contamination. Users have occasionally reported problems like hair loss after beginning to consume some of these products. Deep-sea algae products (sometimes sold as 'Phyto-Plankton') are thought to be a less likely candidate for contamination and, being very rich in beta-carotene, are often used as an economical form of beta-carotene supplement.

Availability: From health food shops.

Alkaloids
(see Secondary plant metabolites)

Alkylglycerols

Alkylglycerols are oil-based chelating agents found in large amounts in shark liver oil, and also synthesized by the human body, where they are found in the bone marrow and in breast milk. They are capable of combining with toxic metals like mercury, and hastening their removal from tissues. Alkylglycerols differ from ordinary fats by linking their fatty acids to glycerol with ether bonds instead of ester bonds.

Research suggests that alkylglycerols may be protective of white blood cells, especially in situations such as radiotherapy for cancer.

Availability: Shark liver oil capsules often originate in Sweden and are available from health shops.

Allergy

Allergy can be loosely defined as an altered reaction to a normally harmless substance with which the body comes into contact. The strict definition of an allergy involves a rapid onset of symptoms which can be clearly linked with immune system responses, as in hay fever, coeliac disease, and asthma attacks which have been induced by contact with animal fur or house dust mites. Anaphylactic shock, where the blood pressure falls to life-threateningly low levels, is also a classical allergic reaction, and can cause deaths as a result of peanut allergy, for instance.

Another type of allergy is known as a 'food intolerance'. Reactions are often delayed, intermittent or chronic, and although they may involve the release of histamine by the mast cells of the immune system, they are not generally considered to be immune system mediated. Examples of these reactions include intermittent migraine, irritable bowel syndrome, joint pains, or chronic fatigue.

Foods which cause intolerance reactions may be rich in tyramine, which releases histamine from mast cells (e.g. chocolate, alcoholic beverages, mature cheese, salami, bean pods, bananas, yeast concentrates, soy sauce and stock cubes). Alternatively histamine may be released through effects which occur to cell membranes and prostaglandins as a result of the body's response to a problem food.

Food intolerances may be due to enzyme deficiencies, which may be inherited or induced by a toxic overload (*which see*) or by nutritional deficiencies or incomplete digestion. Any of us can react to any substance if the enzymes responsible for its metabolism are inefficient or absent. Symptoms are not related to the substance itself, but to our reaction to it. Thus one individual may develop migraine after eating bread; another may experience diarrhoea.

Adverse reactions to the consumption of high-protein foods may occur if the individual lacks the nutrients (such as magnesium) needed for the conversion of ammonia – a breakdown product of protein – to urea, which is excreted via the kidneys. The symptoms of ammonia overload may include fatigue, headache, lethargy, irritability and allergy-type reactions.

Aloe vera

Herb

Aloe vera refers to the gel in the centre of the leaf of Aloe vera plants. However, some preparations may be homogenized whole leaf extracts, which also contain aloes, the laxative substance found in the bitter, yellow juice which is also contained in the leaf.

Studies have found the gel to be effective against first- and second-degree burns, radiation burns, skin ulcers and peptic ulcers.

Availability: Widely available in health food shops and as an ingredient in skin care products.

Alpha-linolenic acid
(see Fats)

Aluminium

Toxic element

Although known for its light weight, aluminium is classed as a heavy metal because it may accumulate in the body. Aluminium is a neuro-toxin and can cause brain deterioration as well as depletion of phosphate and bone minerals. Aluminium can produce changes in brain structure similar to those seen in Alzheimer's disease. Sources of aluminium include cooking vessels, antacids, some baking powders and food additives, tea bags, dried milk, instant coffee, table salt and many anti-perspirants, as well as cereals and vegetables. Soya milk contains more aluminium than cow's milk but is unlikely to cause the consumer to exceed official safe intake levels. Babies, however, excrete aluminium poorly because their kidneys are not yet fully developed. Excessive levels of aluminium in the body can be detected by hair mineral analysis.

Aluminium is considered to be poorly absorbed from the intestinal tract (which has an alkaline environment) because it is insoluble at a pH of more than 5. Acid rain is causing aluminium to be dissolved out of soil and deposited in lakes.

Amazake

Amazake is a naturally sweet dessert or drink often consumed by macrobiotic enthusiasts, which has been made by traditionally culturing cooked whole cereal grains so that their starches turn into natural sugars.

Availability: Mainly from macrobiotic specialist suppliers.

Amino acids

Commonly referred to as 'the building blocks of protein', amino acids are needed to make almost all components of the body including enzymes, blood corpuscles, hormones, antibodies, hair, skin, bone and tissues.

Amino acids are generally linked together by peptide bonds, to form peptides. When 10 or more are linked, these are known as polypeptides. Very large polypeptides are known as proteins.

Amino acids are often classified according to whether they are 'essential' or 'non-essential'. This is a potentially misleading description since it is sometimes assumed to mean that most amino acids do not play an essential role in the body. In fact the term 'essential' does not refer to the role of the amino acids but to the body's ability to synthesize them. 'Essential' amino acids are those which the body is incapable of synthesizing and which must, therefore, be obtained from the diet. Although equally important, amino acids such as taurine, carnitine and tyrosine can, at least in healthy individuals, be synthesized from other amino acids and are therefore described as 'non-essential'.

Some authorities have made statements that amino acid supplementation is valueless because most people in the Western world already eat too much protein. However, this fails to take account of individual biochemistry and possible errors of metabolism. Some people may be less capable than others of synthesizing 'non-essential' amino acids and would therefore benefit from supplementation, especially if they do not regularly consume animal products in their diet.

Amino acids can be divided into a number of categories according to their structure and functions:

Amino acids with important metabolites: lysine, carnitine, histidine
Aromatic amino acids: phenylalanine, tyrosine and tryptophan
Branched chain amino acids: leucine, isoleucine, valine
Glutamate amino acids: glutamic acid, GABA, glutamine, proline, hydroxyproline, asparatic acid, asparagine
Sulphur amino acids: cysteine, glutathione, taurine, methionine, homocysteine
Threonine amino acids: threonine, glycine, serine, alanine
Urea cycle amino acids: arginine, citrulline, ornithine

Glucogenic amino acids are those which, after losing their amino group, give rise to metabolic intermediate substances which form glucose. These are: alanine, arginine, aspartic acid, cysteine, glutamic acid, glycine, histidine, hydroxyproline, methionine, proline, serine, threonine and valine.

Amino acids can occur in two isomer forms known as the 'D' and 'L' forms. This is why you will often see them described as L-tryptophan or L-tyrosine, for instance. The 'D' form of amino acids is not usually found in nature and, with the exception of D-phenylalanine, is not normally utilizable by the human body.

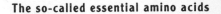

The so-called essential amino acids

Histidine
Isoleucine
Leucine
Lysine
Methionine
Phenylalanine
Threonine
Tryptophan
Valine

Ammonia

A toxic waste product of protein breakdown. Ammonia is converted to urea by the liver, and the urea is then excreted in the urine. If nutrients such as magnesium, needed for the conversion to urea, are deficient, and ammonia is not adequately broken down, one of its toxic effects is interference with the Krebs cycle of energy production (by depleting the supply of alpha-ketoglutarate). This can result in fatigue, headache, lethargy, irritability, and allergy-like reactions to high-protein foods.

Amylase (see Digestion)

Anaemia

A condition in which the oxygen-carrying capacity of the blood is reduced. It may be caused by a deficiency of one or more of the nutrients required for red blood cell formation, or by excessive bleeding or the abnormal destruction of red blood cells.

Symptoms of anaemia may include fatigue, breathlessness on exertion, dizziness and pallor.

Iron deficiency anaemia is the most common type of anaemia. Other nutritional anaemias include folic acid, vitamin B_2, vitamin B_6 (sometimes associated with taking the contraceptive pill), vitamin B_{12}, vitamins C and E, copper, zinc and protein; deficiencies of these nutrients result in inadequate red blood cell formation.

Macrocytic anaemia, characterized by reduced numbers of abnormally large, malformed red blood cells, is caused by vitamin B_{12} and folic acid deficiencies.

Pernicious anaemia, caused by a failure to absorb vitamin B_{12} (often because of a lack of intrinsic factor – *which see*) is a type of macrocytic anaemia.

Sickle cell anaemia is due to abnormal haemoglobin which results in distortion and fragility of red blood cells. Both sickle cell anaemia and thalassaemia (Mediterranean anaemia) may respond to high doses of vitamin E daily.

Androgens

Any steroid hormones, such as testosterone, which increase male characteristics. The androgens are not found exclusively in males but are also made by the female adrenal glands.

Angelica

Herb

A warming herb described as an aromatic digestive. It is used as an expectorant and against pleurisy and bronchitis, arthritic conditions and intestinal flatulence. Angelica is also widely used as a flavouring in foods.

Availability: As a medicinal herb, available mainly from medical herbalists.

Anorexia

Lack of appetite. This may be a symptom of zinc deficiency. Anorexia nervosa ('slimmers' disease') is a complex psychological condition characterized by a prolonged refusal to eat due to an abnormal fear of becoming fat and a distorted body image. Sufferers become severely emaciated. The condition is usually associated with emotional stress or conflict, and issues involving control.

Anthocyanosides
(see Antioxidants and Flavonoids)

Antigen

A substance, usually foreign to the body, which causes the immune system to form antibodies in response to it.

Antioxidants

Nutrients or enzymes which 'scavenge' free radicals by donating extra hydrogen electrons to them. This prevents the free radicals from taking hydrogen electrons from molecules in body tissues and damaging the tissues in the process. Vitamins A, C, E and beta-carotene are the best known antioxidant nutrients, although another carotene-like substance, lycopene (found in tomatoes), is now thought to be superior to beta-carotene in quenching singlet oxygen. Zinc and manganese are needed to form the antioxidant enzyme superoxide dismutase, which combats the superoxide radical; selenium is needed to form the antioxidant enzyme glutathione peroxidase, which combats hydrogen peroxide. The antioxidant enzyme catalase also combats hydrogen peroxide.

Many flavonoids (which see) also have antioxidant action. The herb Ginkgo biloba is a good source of antioxidant flavonoids known as proanthocyanidins. The skins of black cherries, blueberries and blackberries also contain proanthocyanidins. Extracts of bilberry (which see) contain flavonoids known as anthocyanosides, which have a very powerful antioxidant activity – some say even more so than vitamins C and E.

Other antioxidants include the flavonoid quercetin, the enzymes methionine reductase and catalase, a substance found in liver known as lipoic acid, and the vitamin-like substance coenzyme Q10.

Availability: Antioxidant supplements are now widely available in health food shops, pharmacies and through nutritional therapists.

Also see Free radicals

Arachidonic acid

A polyunsaturated fatty acid of the omega 6 series (*see Fatty acids*) which can be formed in the human body from dietary linoleic acid. It is a constituent of cell membranes and an immediate precursor to series 2 prostaglandins and leukotrienes, which are involved in many body functions such as blood vessel constriction, inflammation, pain and blood clotting.

Availability: Not available as a food supplement.

Arame

A type of seaweed ('sea vegetable') used in macrobiotic cookery.

Arginine

Amino acid

Arginine is one of the urea cycle Amino acids (*also see Amino acids*). It plays an important role in the conversion of ammonia from protein breakdown into urea, which can be excreted via the kidneys, and it stimulates the activity of the enzyme which starts off the process. Arginine is also a component of anti-diuretic hormone, a hormone which reduces the excretion of water by the kidneys.

Many people take arginine (together with another amino acid, ornithine) as a body-building supplement. There is some evidence that supplementation with these amino acids may stimulate the release of growth hormone, which is responsible for increasing muscle bulk, and also insulin. Arginine-rich foods include nuts, peanuts, seeds, chocolate and grains (cereals).

Vegetarian sources: Weight for weight, peanuts, tofu, pumpkin seeds, almonds, sunflower seeds and brazil nuts are as rich in arginine as animal proteins.

Availability of supplements: Arginine supplements are widely available in health shops.

Suggested dosage for body-building: 2 grams of arginine and 2 of ornithine on an empty stomach before retiring, and 2 grams on an empty stomach prior to vigorous exercise. 100 mcg of a chromium supplement may also be helpful. Arginine supplementation should be avoided in cases of schizophrenia and herpes virus.

Arsenic

Toxic element

Food and drink levels of arsenic are limited by law, due to its toxicity, although arsenic was once used as a treatment for syphilis. Symptoms of chronic arsenic poisoning include fluid retention in the face and eyelids, itching, sore mouth, loss of appetite, nausea and vomiting, loss of hair and fingernails.

Traces of arsenic are found in shellfish, and some meat may also contain arsenic if it was present in the animals' feed. Arsenic compounds are used as insecticides which can leach into the water table and thence into reservoirs, as well as remaining in trace amounts in food crops.

Excessive levels of arsenic in the human body can be tested for by hair mineral analysis.

Artemisia annua
(also see Dysbiosis)

Herb

This herb is described by Dr Leo Galland as highly effective against parasites, and particularly useful in chronic infections, since it is not toxic as are prescription drugs such as Flagyl.

Availability: This herb may not be easily available in shops, but is used by nutritional therapists and is available in their treatment programmes.

Artichoke

Herb

Extracts from the leaves of the globe artichoke have anti-toxic effects on the liver, similar to those of the herb extract silymarin (*which see*). They can also promote regeneration of the liver and increase the blood supply to that organ. Artichoke leaf extracts can reduce blood cholesterol by increasing the excretion of cholesterol, but also appear directly to inhibit the synthesis of cholesterol in the liver. The main use of artichoke leaf extract is against gall-bladder disease, reducing pain, nausea and digestive discomfort, and stimulating gall-bladder drainage.

Availability: It may be possible to purchase an artichoke syrup from some larger health food stores, otherwise you may need to consult a medical herbalist or nutritional therapist to obtain the leaf extract.

Asafoetida

Herb

Sometimes known as 'Devil's dung' because of its odour, this humble herb which is widely used in Indian cookery has been described by some medical herbalists as one of the most effective known agents against intestinal candidiasis (*which see*).

Availability: Widely available from Indian grocers.

Suggested intake for candidiasis: a quarter teaspoon before and after each meal, taken with ginger tea, or the equivalent in capsules.

Aspartame

A very widely used artificial sweetener (trade name *NutraSweet*) consisting of a synthetic dipeptide of aspartic acid and the methyl ester of phenylalanine. Much controversy surrounds this product, which has been blamed for a wide range of symptoms in heavy users of foods and drinks to which it has been added (*see table*). These symptoms have been passed off as 'unusual sensitivity' to aspartame, since studies carried out on monkeys have shown no ill-effects from the consumption of 3 grams of aspartame per kilo of body weight per day. However, food given to test animals is usually very nutrient-rich, not high in sugar, fat and a variety of artificial food

additives. It is possible that humans and animals who do not consume such diets rich in antioxidants which help the body to metabolize xenobiotics (foreign substances such as aspartame) may be more susceptible to developing problems.

In the digestive tract, aspartame is split into its two component amino acids and a methyl group. During metabolism, the methyl group is converted to the toxin methyl alcohol and then to another toxin, formaldehyde, which must be detoxified by the liver. Aspartame must not be used by individuals who have been diagnosed with the condition known as phenylketonuria, since they must ensure that their phenylalanine intake remains as low as possible.

The most common symptoms reported to the US Food and Drug Administration by aspartame users, which have resolved when aspartame use was ceased

---

Abdominal pain and cramps
Depression
Diarrhoea
Dizziness or poor balance
Eye problems
Fatigue and weakness
Headache (19 per cent of all complaints)
Memory loss
Mood changes
Numbness and tingling
Rash
Seizures and convulsions
Sleep problems
Urticaria
Vomiting and nausea

Aspartame (*NutraSweet*) is used commercially to sweeten yoghurt, diet drinks, fruit squashes and low-calorie desserts, and is also sold in tablets and granules for adding to food and drinks.

Aspartates

Some dietary supplements are made by combining minerals and trace elements with the amino acid aspartic acid (*which see*). They are then known as mineral aspartates, and effectively provide a double supplement of both mineral and amino acid. Potassium and magnesium, and possibly other mineral supplements appear to be more readily absorbed when taken as aspartates.

Aspartic acid

Amino acid

Known as a glutamate amino acid, aspartic acid is made from another amino acid, glutamic acid, by enzymes using vitamin B_6. It plays an important part in the urea cycle (the conversion of toxic ammonia from protein breakdown into urea which can be excreted by the kidneys), and in DNA metabolism. Aspartic acid is a major excitatory neurotransmitter (*which see*). Animal studies have found that both potassium and magnesium aspartate may be able to stimulate the proliferation and differentiation of the thymus gland, bone marrow and spleen tissue, as well as help the red blood cell-producing organs to regenerate after exposure to radiation.

With glutamine, aspartic acid forms asparagine, and with citrulline it forms arginosuccinate. It is involved in oxidative phosphorylation and energy production (*which see*).

Availability: Not easily available in its pure form. Best taken as mineral aspartates (e.g. magnesium aspartate).

Assimilation

The process by which digested foodstuffs which have been absorbed into the blood are taken up and used by cells and tissues.

Astragalus

Herb

A tonic herb, frequently used in Chinese herbal medicine.

Availability: Widely available from herb suppliers.

ATP (Adenosine triphosphate)

Sometimes known as the body's 'energy currency', ATP is the most important immediate source of energy for cell metabolism, and is the end product of glucose breakdown. It is used for all energy-dependent processes in the body.

B

Vitamin B₁ (Thiamine)

Vitamin (water-soluble)
UK RNI 1.0 mg
US RDA 1.5 mg

FUNCTIONS

Conversion of carbohydrate to energy
Energy production
Brain, heart, muscle and nerve function
Release of acetylcholine (*which see*) from nerve cells

GOOD FOOD SOURCES

Beans
Brown rice
Lentils
Pork
Whole grains

Deficiency symptoms

- Burning, tingling in toes and soles
- Depression
- Easy fatigue
- Insomnia
- Irritability
- Loss of appetite
- Muscle weakness
- Tender calves
- Low levels of several B vitamins have been found in psychiatric patients and in senile dementia

Preventing deficiency

Sugar metabolism requires vitamins B_1, B_2 and B_3, magnesium and chromium. A high sugar consumption uses up these nutrients without replacing them, because sugar does not contain any vitamins or other nutrients except calories. (Beware the advertisements about sugar giving you energy; energy is simply the scientific name for calories!) Alcoholism can also lead to B vitamin deficiency, and alcohol itself can impair the absorption of B vitamins from the intestines.

Many countries make the replacement of some of the lost B vitamins compulsory in products made from refined (white) flour, since the B vitamins are mostly found in the bran and germ of the flour, not in the white, starchy portion. Since white flour products are staple foods for many people, diets could otherwise become dangerously inadequate. Manufacturers may advertise this so-called fortification as 'added vitamins', giving rise to the mistaken impression that their products are nutritionally superior when this may be far from true.

To avoid thiamine and other B vitamin deficiencies, your diet should be low in sugar (for instance you could restrict your intake of sugary food or drink to just one small item a day), and you should use wholemeal bread, flour and cereals whenever possible, but not in raw form, since cooking is often needed to improve bioavailability (*which see*).

The bioavailability of vitamin B_1 is reduced in the presence of a folic acid deficiency and by the consumption of alcohol and so-called anti-thiamine factors found in fish, shellfish, blueberries, blackcurrants, brussels sprouts, red cabbage and beetroot, but only when these foods are eaten raw. Vitamin B_1 is one of the least stable of all the vitamins and huge losses occur during normal processing and cooking. The more finely ground a food (such as minced beef or pork) the greater the loss of vitamin B_1, which escapes via the juices. Vitamin B_1 is completely inactivated by the widely used preservative sulphur dioxide, and by sulphite solutions used, for instance, to keep chipped potatoes from turning brown. Uncooked freshwater fish and shellfish contain the enzyme thiaminase, which destroys 50 per cent of the vitamin B_1 found in the food. Tea also contains an anti-thiamine factor (ATF) which destroys vitamin B_1.

Comments

Doctors and other practitioners working in the field of nutritional medicine and therapy consider that an individual's requirements for B vitamins can be raised if he or she has gone without adequate amounts for any length of time. This may be why deficiency symptoms (*see above*) can exist even when the diet later becomes adequate by normal standards, and in these cases it may be necessary to take dietary supplements for a limited period of time to correct any damage to the B-vitamin dependent systems.

Supplementation

In research studies, vitamin B_1 supplements have been found to:

- Act as a painkiller in some cases of headache or joint pain
- Improve neurophysiological functions in epilepsy
- Improve trigeminal neuralgia
- Inhibit oxidation of the neurotransmitter dopamine
- Help optic neuritis
- Reduce sensory neuropathy in diabetics

Preferred form and suggested intake
B vitamins should not normally be taken singly, since they work together as a team and good nutrition is about avoiding imbalances. A B complex supplement providing 50 mg of each B vitamin is enough for most purposes. However, a practitioner or doctor of nutritional medicine or therapy may work for short periods with higher doses.

The co-enzyme form of vitamin B_1 is known as octothiamine, which is biologically more active than the more commonly available thiamine supplements as it is readily usable by the human body. Nutritional therapists sometimes use octothiamine for people with serious energy deficiency problems such as chronic fatigue syndrome.

Cautions
Vitamin B_1 is one of the safest known supplements. There is no known unsafe dosage. B complex supplements are also considered to be very safe.

Vitamin B₂ (Riboflavin)

Vitamin (water-soluble)
UK RNI 1.3 mg
US RDA 1.7 mg

FUNCTIONS

Activates vitamin B₆
Conversion of carbohydrate to energy
Conversion of tryptophan to vitamin B₃
Growth
Metabolism of fats, protein and carbohydrate

GOOD FOOD SOURCES

Dairy produce
Eggs
Liver
Meat
Soya flour
Whole grains

Deficiency symptoms

- Bloodshot, burning, 'gritty' eyes
- Cracks and sores in corners of mouth
- Dryness, cracking, peeling of lips
- Eyes sensitive to light
- Insomnia
- Sides of nose red, greasy and scaly
- Soreness and burning of lips and tongue
- Low levels of several B vitamins have been found in psychiatric patients and in senile dementia.

Preventing deficiency

See Vitamin B₁. The bioavailability (*which see*) of vitamin B₂ is reduced by the consumption of alcohol, and by high zinc levels, some antibiotics, and caffeine. Riboflavin in foods is destroyed by lengthy exposure to the light. Up to 14 per cent of vitamin B₂ is lost when milk is pasteurized, and a further 12–25 per cent when it is boiled.

Comments

See Vitamin B₁.

Supplementation

In research studies, vitamin B₂ supplements have been found to help against:

- Acne rosacea
- Carpal tunnel syndrome
- Cataracts
- Mitochondrial myopathies
- Some types of anaemia

Preferred form and suggested intake
See Vitamin B₁.

Cautions
See Vitamin B₁. There is no known unsafe dosage of vitamin B₂. Yellow colouration of urine after taking B complex supplements containing vitamin B₂ is harmless.

Vitamin B₃ (Niacin or nicotinic acid)

Vitamin (water-soluble)
UK RNI 18 mg
US RDA 19 mg

FUNCTIONS

Conversion of carbohydrate to energy
DNA synthesis
Health of skin, nerves, brain and digestive system
Synthesis of fatty acids and steroids

Beef liver

Chicken

Meat

Nuts

Peanuts

Salmon and other oily fish

Sunflower seeds

Whole grains

Deficiency symptoms

- Depression
- Dermatitis
- Fatigue
- Insomnia
- Irritability
- Loss of appetite
- Muscle weakness
- Red, swollen tongue
- Low levels of several B vitamins have been found in psychiatric patients and in senile dementia

Preventing deficiency

See Vitamin B₁. Alcohol severely inhibits vitamin B_3 bioavailability. In many grains (particularly wheat and corn), vitamin B_3 occurs in the form of a complex which cannot be digested or absorbed if the grain is unprocessed. Wheat requires baking with alkaline baking powder, and corn requires soaking in alkaline lime water before vitamin B_3 is released.

Comments

See Vitamin B₁. Some cases of severe vitamin B_3 deficiency are indistinguishable from schizophrenia, and Dr Abram Hoffer in Canada has pioneered the treatment of schizophrenia using vitamin B_3 megadoses,

with many successes. Experiences of World War II ex-POWs from Japanese camps suggest that the longer and more severe a B_3 deficiency, the higher the corrective dosages needed to restore normal function. Some schizophrenics may need more than 600 mg B_3 per day, but this should be under the care of a specialist practitioner.

Oestrogens reduce the rate of conversion of tryptophan to vitamin B_3, which means that when this vitamin is lacking, women in their child-bearing years are twice as likely as men to develop deficiency-related problems. Two enzymes required for the conversion are dependent on vitamins B_2 and B_6, so that deficiencies of either of these vitamins could also lead to vitamin B_3 deficiency.

Vitamin B_3 is also supplemented in large doses by many people for a cholesterol-lowering effect. However, this approach does not address the possible causes of the high cholesterol, and holistic practitioners generally prefer to investigate these first.

Supplementation

In research studies, vitamin B_3 supplements have been found to:

- Act as a mild anti-histamine
- Help relieve tinnitus
- Reduce cholesterol levels
- Reduce insulin requirements in some diabetics
- Reduce period (menstrual) pains
- Reduce the symptoms of schizophrenia when used in megadoses
- Reduce wheezing in asthmatics

Preferred form and suggested intake

See Vitamin B₁. Vitamin B_3 is available in two forms: the acid form (niacin, also known as nicotinic acid) and the amide form (niacinamide, also known as nicotinamide). The term niacin is often used as an umbrella for both forms. In most cases the preferred form for supplementation is the amide form. The acid form can produce an unpleasant 'flushing' effect as it causes the release of histamine.

Cautions
Doses of more than 500 mg vitamin B_3, especially in timed-release form, have been linked with a few cases of liver damage.

Vitamin B_5
(Pantothenic acid)

Vitamin (water-soluble)
UK estimated adequate intake: 7 mg
US estimated safe and adequate intake: 7 mg

FUNCTIONS
Conversion of carbohydrate to energy
Growth and development
Health of nervous system
Production of anti-stress hormones

GOOD FOOD SOURCES
Eggs
Liver
Meat
Nuts
Whole grains
Yeast

Deficiency symptoms

- Burning feet
- Depression
- Fatigue
- Loss of appetite
- Poor muscle co-ordination
- Weakness
- 'Wind pains' in intestines

Low levels of several B vitamins have been found in psychiatric patients and in senile dementia.

Preventing deficiency

See Vitamin B_1. The vitamin B_5 content of foods is considerably reduced by storage and freezing. Green beans lose more than 50 per cent of their B_5 after 12 months' storage while frozen. Canned vegetables lose up to 85 per cent of their vitamin B_5 if stored for lengthy periods.

Comments

Vitamin B_5 is known as the 'anti-stress' vitamin because such large quantities of it are found in the adrenal glands where the anti-stress hormones are made.

Supplementation

In research studies, vitamin B_5 supplements have been found to:

- Alleviate allergic reactions
- Help in stress situations
- Help rheumatoid arthritis
- Treat some cases of anaemia

Preferred form and suggested intake
See Vitamin B_1. Vitamin B_5 is normally available as calcium pantothenate. 100– 500 mg per day of vitamin B_5 are often taken in addition to a B complex product by individuals with allergies, rheumatoid arthritis and other health problems associated with adrenal stress. The co-enzyme form of vitamin B_5 is known as pantethine, which is biologically more active than the more commonly available pantothenate supplements as it is readily usable by the human

body. Nutritional therapists sometimes use pantethine for people with serious energy deficiency problems such as chronic fatigue syndrome.

Cautions

Vitamin B₅ is one of the safest known vitamins, and does not appear to be toxic at any dose.

Vitamin B₆
(Pyridoxine or Pyridoxal)

Vitamin (water-soluble)
UK RNI 1.5 mg
US RDA 2.2 mg

FUNCTIONS

Blood and haemoglobin formation

Calcium and magnesium metabolism

Conversion of glycogen to glucose

Conversion of tryptophan to vitamin B₃ or serotonin

Energy production

Histamine metabolism

Magnesium metabolism

Protein, carbohydrate and fat metabolism

Selenium metabolism and transportation

Synthesis of prostaglandins from essential fatty acids

Zinc absorption

GOOD FOOD SOURCES

Avocados

Bananas

Fish

Meat

Nuts

Seeds

Whole grains

Deficiency symptoms

- Anaemia
- Convulsions (in infants)
- Inability to remember dreams
- Insomnia
- Irritability
- Kidney stones
- Morning sickness of pregnancy
- Nervousness
- Premenstrual syndrome
- Red, scaly patches at sides of nose and corners of mouth
- Skin rashes, especially on the forehead

Vitamin B₆ and vitamin B₂ deficiency symptoms are very similar.

Low levels of several B vitamins have been found in psychiatric patients and in senile dementia.

Preventing deficiency

See Vitamin B₁. The bioavailability of vitamin B₆ is reduced by alcohol, by consumption of the B₆ antagonists linseeds and mushrooms, and, in milk, by sterilization. B₆ bioavailability in peanut butter, soya products and cereals processed with dry heat is low. The contraceptive pill and hormone replacement therapy may greatly increase a woman's requirements for vitamin B₆, although some scientists dispute this. 75–90 per cent of vitamin B₆ is lost when flour is refined, and 37–56 per cent is lost from vegetables by the freezing process.

Vitamin B₆ deficiency is probably more common than is generally realized: in one study which measured the B₆ status of 35 pre-school children, 17 per cent of the children had B₆ intakes less than two thirds of the RDA. Of these children, 9 per cent had inadequate vitamin B₆ levels in their blood plasma. (*Fries M E et al.: Vitamin B₆ status of a group of preschool children. Am J Clin Nutr 34(12):2706-10, 1981.*)

Comments

One type of schizophrenia, known as pyrroluric schizophrenia, is caused by an abnormally high requirement for both vitamin B$_6$ and zinc.

An example of how a vitamin deficiency can lead to widespread problems which may not be recognized as deficiency-related is the role of B$_6$ in the breakdown of beta-alanine. Beta-alanine is a nonprotein amino acid obtained from dietary sources and formed by intestinal bacteria. In healthy individuals it is found at very low levels in the urine. If the body fails to metabolize it, and it therefore reaches high levels in the urine, the conservation of other amino acids, particularly taurine, by the kidneys, can become impaired. The result of this is abnormally high losses of taurine through the urine, and the potential development of a taurine deficiency. Since taurine is needed for the detoxification of pollutants and other foreign substances, this could have serious consequences. According to environmental medicine expert Dr William Rea, beta-alanine levels are often high in the chemically sensitive, and some cases are associated with a severe exacerbation of their symptoms, which may turn into 'total allergy syndrome'.

Supplementation

In research studies, vitamin B$_6$ supplements have been found to:

- Effectively treat childhood autism
- Help asthma
- Help carpal tunnel syndrome
- Help morning sickness of pregnancy
- Help Parkinson's disease
- Help premenstrual acne
- Help premenstrual syndrome
- Improve insulin resistance (which is associated with maturity-onset diabetes)
- Promote the conversion of toxic homocysteine to cystathione, thus helping to prevent heart disease
- Reduce fluid retention
- Reduce sensitivity to monosodium glutamate
- Reduce urinary oxalate, thus helping to prevent kidney stones
- Together with a reduction in beta-alanine-yielding foods, treat some cases of Tourette syndrome and hyperactivity disorder
- Treat premenstrual acne
- Treat some types of anaemia, including sickle cell anaemia

Preferred form and suggested intake

See Vitamin B$_1$. The preferred form of B$_6$ supplementation is pyridoxal-5-phosphate, which is the active (or co-enzyme) form of the vitamin. 100–200 mg a day of P-5-P can, if needed, be safely added to a daily B complex supplement.

Cautions

The cheapest and most widely available form of vitamin B$_6$ supplement is pyridoxine, which, if taken in large amounts (more than 200 mg per day) over a long period of time, without magnesium and the other B complex vitamins, can in some cases cause numbness and tingling in hands and feet (peripheral neuropathy). This is thought to be because pyridoxine requires adequate amounts of other B vitamins and magnesium in order to be converted to its active form pyridoxal-5-phosphate, and if these are not available, pyridoxine can build up to undesirable levels. The effects of pyridoxine excess are completely reversible when the supplements are discontinued.

Vitamin B$_{12}$ (Cobalamin)

Vitamin (water-soluble)
UK RNI 1.5 mcg
US RDA 3 mcg

FUNCTIONS

Detoxifies cyanide (found in tobacco smoke and some foods)

DNA synthesis

Growth and development

Healthy nerves

GOOD FOOD SOURCES

Cheese

Eggs

Fish

Liver

Meat

Yoghurt

Found only in animal foods, although some vegan products are fortified with extra B$_{12}$ by the manufacturers.

Deficiency symptoms

- Agitation
- Anaemia
- Disorientation and confusion
- Fatigue
- Hallucinations
- Increased risk of heart disease (by promoting raised homocysteine levels)
- Loss of sensation in feet and legs
- Nerve and spinal cord degeneration (with unsteadiness and mental deterioration)
- Sore, smooth tongue

Low levels of several B vitamins have been found in psychiatric patients and (for B$_{12}$ in particular) in senile dementia.

Preventing deficiency

Although vitamin B$_{12}$ is only found in animal foods, vegans (who do not eat any animal foods) survive because our requirements for this vitamin are very small. Yeast extracts used as food flavourings are often fortified with vitamin B$_{12}$, and vegans should ensure that they consume such foods regularly, or some other product with a guaranteed vitamin B$_{12}$ content, such as a B$_{12}$ supplement. Algae and seaweeds are sometimes promoted as plant sources of this vitamin, but it is now known that they contain only vitamin B$_{12}$ *analogues* – substances which are quite similar to vitamin B$_{12}$ but may actually block the bioavailability of the real vitamin.

Between 16 and 75 per cent of vitamin B$_{12}$ in a meal is absorbed. The more B$_{12}$ is ingested, the lower the percentage of absorption. The bioavailability of vitamin B$_{12}$ is reduced by a lack of intrinsic factor (*see below*), by parasitic infections and by bacterial overgrowth of the small intestine. Chronic diarrhoea, tapeworm and other intestinal disorders can also inhibit B$_{12}$ absorption.

Comments

Vitamin B$_{12}$ contains the trace element cobalt, and provides its only known function in the human body.

Pernicious anaemia, which is the vitamin B$_{12}$ deficiency disease, is not usually caused by a poor intake of this vitamin, but by a lack of 'intrinsic factor', a substance found in the stomach which combines with vitamin B$_{12}$ and allows it to be absorbed by the lower part of the small intestine. Elderly people are particularly susceptible to a lack of intrinsic factor. Without it, only about 1 per cent of dietary vitamin B$_{12}$ can be absorbed. Intestinal parasites can also cause vitamin B$_{12}$ malabsorption.

Vitamin B_{12} deficiency is common even in the presence of normal blood levels, particularly in the elderly. In a study carried out on 548 surviving members of the original Framingham study, serum B_{12} and folate levels were compared with levels of metabolites (biochemical markers) which are raised if the nutrients are not available in sufficient quantities to enable them to be broken down. The rate of B_{12} deficiency was found to be 12 per cent. (*Lindenbaum J et al.: Prevalence of cobalamin deficiency in the Framingham elderly population. Am J Clin Nutr 60(1):2-11, 1994.*)

Supplementation

In research studies, vitamin B_{12} supplements (administered by injection) have been found to help:

* Chronic pain
* Fatigue
* Mental confusion
* Multiple sclerosis
* Numbness of the extremities
* Some cases of mental illness
* Some cases of tinnitus

Preferred form and suggested intake

Vitamin B_{12} is best taken by injection (administered by a doctor) when there is an absorption problem. Other forms of supplementation are vitamin B_{12} tablets or capsules, or B complex supplements (typically providing up to 100 mcg each), and vitamin B_{12} nasal gel. There is some evidence that the nasal gel is better absorbed than oral supplements.

Cautions

No cautions are required with vitamin B_{12} supplementation as there is no known unsafe dose.

Vitamin B_{15} (Pangamic acid)

Vitamin-like substance

Although commonly called vitamin B_{15}, pangamic acid is not in fact a vitamin. It was first isolated from apricot kernels by Drs Ernst Krebs (father and son), and is said to stimulate the carriage of oxygen from lungs to blood and from blood to organs and tissues. Russian studies claim that B_{15} supplements can lower the body's oxygen needs, thus helping athletes by transporting oxygen to their muscles more efficiently.

There appears to be some difficulty in obtaining a natural source of B_{15}, and some doubt about whether pangamic acid is in fact the active ingredient in the products sold as vitamin B_{15}, which are manufactured under a Russian patent. Dr Eric Braverman's excellent book *The Healing Nutrients Within* claims that B_{15}'s active effects are due to its content of dimethylglycine (DMG), an intermediate product made from choline, found in very small amounts in the human body, and eventually converted to the amino acid glycine. On the basis of his research with DMG, Dr Braverman believes that many of the effects of B_{15} are in fact attributable to glycine, and also to choline, the breakdown of which is slowed down by DMG.

Availability: Available from specialist suppliers.

Barberry

Herb

Also known as *Berberis vulgaris*, barberry bark contains an alkaloid known as berberine, which is found helpful as a wash for hypersensitive eyes, inflamed lids and chronic or allergic conjunctivitis. This herb also has an anti-bacterial effect which, when it is taken orally, makes it useful against dysbiosis (*which see*). It also stimulates bile flow and eases liver congestion. It is frequently used to combat an inflamed gall-bladder as well as intestinal inflammation, which is often associated with dysbiosis.

Availability: Mostly from herbalists or nutritional therapists.

Basal Metabolic Rate (BMR)

This is the energy required when the body is completely at rest, for the functioning of the internal organs and to maintain body temperature. The BMR is calculated as energy expenditure per metre of body surface area. It is high in growing children and in people who live in cold climates.

Bayberry

Herb

A warming, astringent herb, often used against inflammatory conditions of the intestines, and regarded as a digestive tonic.

Availability: Mostly from herbalists or nutritional therapists.

Bearberry (see Uva-ursi)

Bee pollen

Superfood

The microscopic male seed in flowering plants. It is gathered by bees as they collect nectar for honey. Bee pollen contains all the water-soluble vitamins and is a good source of carotene and vitamin E, as well as minerals, trace elements, rutin (a flavonoid) and hormonal substances. Enthusiasts claim that it rejuvenates the skin and controls hay fever, and it is used by athletes to increase strength and endurance.

Availability: From health food shops.

Beetroot juice

With a long tradition of use as a liver cleanser in naturopathic regimes, beetroot juice stimulates the emptying of the gall-bladder, into which liver toxins are drained before elimination via the gall-bladder, intestines and stools.

Benzopyrenes

Carcinogenic polycyclic hydrocarbons formed by the browning of fat and protein-containing foods during their preparation. In char-grilling, some of the fat which drips on hot coals is converted into smoke containing benzopyrenes, which rises and forms deposits containing these carcinogens on the food. It is thought that garlic contains natural chemicals which can detoxify benzopyrenes.

Benzoates

Anti-microbial and flavouring agents used as food additives. Benzoates cause enlarged kidneys and liver in rat studies.

Berberis (see Barberry)

Beri-beri (see Nutritional deficiencies)

Beta-carotene (see Carotenoids)

Betaine

Found mainly in beetroot, betaine is an intermediate in the conversion of choline to glycine. It can help to break down fats, thus preventing some types of fatty liver.

Betaine hydrochloride

A dietary supplement used to provide hydrochloric acid as an aid to digestion. *Caution*: betaine hydrochloride should always be taken during or just after a meal, on a full stomach, dissolved in water. It should not be used by individuals with an over-acid stomach or with peptic ulcers. *Availability*: From health food shops and nutritional therapists.

Bicarbonate

Sodium or potassium bicarbonate (a quarter teaspoon dissolved in water) can be used to help neutralize an over-acid condition of the body. Some people find that it also helps to 'switch off' allergic symptoms after the accidental consumption of an allergy-causing food.

Bifidobacteria (see Probiotics)

Bilberry

Superfood

Bilberries – European cousins of the American blueberry – yield large quantities of red juice which contains a blue pigment. According to German doctor and herbalist Rudolf Fritz Weiss, this pigment is a wonderful gut healer which enters into the intestinal wall and forms a firmly adhering deep purple protective layer which shields against all mechanical irritation and reduces inflammatory secretions. The blue pigment also has an affinity for bacterial cells and damages the bacteria as it enters them. This effect is probably not enough to kill the bacteria, says Weiss, but their growth will be inhibited, and strained bilberry juice or tea made from steeping dried bilberries in hot water can be most effective against some forms of bacteria-induced diarrhoea.

The blue pigment of the bilberry is identified as an anthocyanoside-type flavonoid (*which see*). It also has many other health benefits. During World War II, pilots for the British Royal Air Force noticed that they had better night vision if they ate bilberry jam before night flying. Now Italian scientists have demonstrated that anthocyanosides increase the production of enzymes in the retina of the eye, which are responsible for energy production. Studies have confirmed that bilberry extract speeds light/dark adaptation, which frequently diminishes as we age.

Bilberry extract also increases the blood flow to the retina. This is thought to be due to its properties as an antioxidant, improving the flexibility of cell membranes and capillaries, so that red blood cells can carry nutrients and oxygen more easily to the eyes. Bilberry extract may even reduce the pressure inside the eye. This may be found useful in preventing the blindness-causing disease glaucoma, and, in combination with vitamin E, the extracts have been found 97 per cent effective against cataract formation. Short-sightedness too was improved by bilberry extract in one study. By strengthening capillaries, bilberries can reduce a tendency to bruise easily and they improve the circulation generally.

Availability: May be more easily available frozen than fresh. Dried bilberry extract is available in capsules through nutritional therapists.

Bile

A bitter, greenish-yellow fluid secreted by the liver and stored in the gall-bladder, from which it is released into the small intestine, enabling waste products and cholesterol from the liver to be excreted from the body. Bile also plays a role in the digestive process by mixing with food after it emerges from the stomach, emulsifying fats and neutralizing acidity.

Bioavailability

Refers to the body's ability to absorb and use a particular nutrient. Much may depend on the form in which the nutrient is supplied. For instance, magnesium oxide and calcium carbonate supplements, though commonly sold in pharmacies, dissolve poorly in stomach acid. If a substance cannot dissolve, it is not very bioavailable, as it cannot get into the bloodstream. Some dietary supplements are coated with shellac, which prevents them from disintegrating. This, and packing powdered products too tightly together when tableting them, causes 'bed pan bullets' – products which emerge unchanged in the stools.

Supplements of inorganic minerals in the form of sulphates, chlorides, oxides and carbonates (called inorganic because they do not normally occur naturally in the plant or animal kingdom) tend to be less bioavailable than organic mineral compounds like gluconates, citrates, lactates and picolinates, which do. These compounds can be ingested in food or can be formed in the human body by the process of chelation (*which see*) and are highly bioavailable.

For the bioavailability of nutrients in foods, see the individual nutrients.

Bioflavonoids (see Flavonoids)

Biotin

Member of the B complex of vitamins (water-soluble)
UK safe adequate intake 10–200 mcg
US safe adequate intake 100–200 mcg

Deficiency symptoms

- Anorexia
- Depression
- Dermatitis
- Hair loss
- Loss of sebaceous glands
- Nausea
- Smooth, pale tongue
- Severe cradle cap in babies can be due to biotin deficiency

Preventing deficiency

See Vitamin B₁. Biotin is manufactured by the bacteria in our intestines, therefore long-term use of antibiotics could result in deficiency. The white part of raw eggs contains a substance called avidin, which binds biotin and makes it unavailable to the human body. The regular consumption of raw egg white should therefore be avoided.

Comments

See Vitamin B₁. Biotin deficiency in vitro is associated with the conversion of Candida albicans to the more pathogenic fungal form. Biotin may work synergistically with insulin and help to lower blood sugar levels.

Supplementation

In research studies, biotin supplements have been found to:

- Help some cases of hair loss and scalp disease
- Help some cases of seborrhoeic dermatitis and other skin complaints
- Reduce blood sugar in some insulin-dependent diabetics
- Reduce diabetic peripheral neuropathy

Preferred form and suggested intake
See Vitamin B₁. Biotin supplements of up to 1,000 mcg may be used by nutritional therapists as an aid against candidiasis.

Cautions
See Vitamin B₁. There is no known unsafe dose of biotin.

Biotransformation (see Detoxification)

Bismuth

A mineral which has a variety of medical uses, including as an antacid to treat indigestion, and as a protective agent and astringent for mucous membranes and raw surfaces in people who have had part of their intestinal tract removed by surgery. Bismuth inhibits the growth of Helicobacter pylori, a stomach acid-resistant microorganism recently found to be associated with peptic ulcer disease.

Normally prescribed by doctors, bismuth treatment should be limited to a maximum of six to eight weeks with an eight-week interval before a further course of treatment since long-term use of bismuth may cause damage to the nervous system.

Bladderwrack

Herb

A form of seaweed used (like kelp) for its high iodine content. May be beneficial in hypothyroidism.
Availability: Mainly through medical herbalists.

Blood

A fluid consisting of plasma, red cells, white cells and platelets, which carries nutrients and oxygen to the tissues and transports waste materials to the kidneys, lungs, liver and skin for excretion. Blood cells are formed in the bone marrow.

Blood sugar

Blood sugar, or, more correctly, blood glucose, simply means glucose which is found in the blood. The glucose is normally obtained from carbohydrate in food and absorbed from the intestinal tract into the bloodstream. Blood glucose rises after a carbohydrate meal and falls during fasting. The body attempts to maintain blood glucose levels between strict limits during fasting conditions because the brain relies on glucose as fuel, and a lack of blood glucose could lead to unconsciousness.

A battery of hormones is responsible for this regulation.

Insulin is released from the beta cells of the pancreas in response to a rise in blood glucose, and helps the glucose to diffuse into muscle and fat (adipose) cells. It also promotes the storage of glucose as glycogen (stored sugar) in the liver and muscle cells, and enhances the uptake of glucose by fat and liver cells for conversion into fat. *Effect*: to lower blood sugar.

Glucagon is released from the alpha cells of the pancreas in response to low blood glucose levels, and has exactly the opposite effect. It causes a rise in blood glucose by converting glycogen back into glucose and promoting the conversion of amino acids and glycerol (from fat) into glucose, and stimulates the release of insulin from the pancreas. *Effect*: to raise blood sugar.

Cortisol and **corticosterone** (also known as 'glucocorticoids') are produced by the adrenal cortex in response to low blood glucose levels, and, like glucagon, they reduce the utilization of glucose by the tissues. They also increase the rate at which amino acids are converted into glucose. *Effect*: to raise blood glucose.

Thyroxine is produced by the thyroid gland in response to severely decreased blood glucose levels. Like glucagon, it promotes both the conversion of glycogen back into glucose, and the conversion of amino acids and glycerol into glucose. Thyroxine also increases the absorption of another sugar, hexose, from the intestines. *Effect*: to raise blood sugar.

Growth hormone, released by the anterior pituitary gland, also reduces the cellular uptake of glucose. *Effect*: to raise blood sugar.

Adrenaline (known in the United States as epinephrine) is produced by the adrenal medulla gland in response to anger or fear, and, like glucagon, favours the breakdown of glycogen to yield glucose. It also decreases the release of insulin from the pancreas. *Effect*: to raise blood sugar specifically in order to provide extra energy for dealing with stressful situations.

Also see Energy production, Glycaemic index, Hyperglycaemia and *Hypoglycaemia*

Blood-brain barrier

To protect itself from undesirable substances in the blood, the brain has a complex set of mechanisms which control both the types of substances which enter the brain's extracellular fluid (fluid surrounding the cells) and the rate at which they enter, thus precisely regulating this fluid's chemical composition and minimizing the ability of harmful substances to reach brain tissues.

Water, carbon dioxide and oxygen readily cross the blood-brain barrier. Ketone bodies, amino acids and fatty acids cross more slowly, and other substances like proteins and hormones are highly restricted. Some areas of the brain lack a blood-brain barrier.

Blue-green algae (see Algae)

Boldo

A herb used as a gall-bladder stimulant and mild diuretic.

Availability: From health food shops.

Borage oil

Borage oil, being a rich source of GLA (*which see*), is often sold as a GLA supplement.

Boron

Trace element
UK RNI None
US RDA None

FUNCTIONS

May be involved in bone mineralization
May help to reduce calcium loss from urine in post-menopausal women

GOOD FOOD SOURCES

Apples
Pears
Prunes
Pulses
Raisins
Tomatoes

Deficiency symptoms

Not known, but may include osteoporosis and menopausal symptoms.

Preventing deficiency

Consumption of good food sources and vegetables generally.

Comments

It is not yet considered proven that boron is an essential nutrient for man. However there is some evidence that boron is protective of bone minerals, and countries with the highest boron intake due to high soil levels (Israel and parts of some other countries) have the lowest incidence of arthritis.

Supplementation

In research studies, boron supplements have been found to:

• Increase concentrations of circulating oestrogen and testosterone in post-menopausal women
• Reduce calcium excretion through the urine in post-menopausal women
• There are also claims that boron supplementation can reduce symptoms of arthritis

Preferred form and suggested intake

For most purposes it is best taken as part of a multi-nutrient formula. Also available as a separate supplement. No more than 3 mg supplementation per day is required under normal circumstances, but individuals with arthritis may wish to start at 6–9 mg daily for a few weeks before dropping to 3 mg per day.

Cautions

Not enough is known about boron to give guidance, but there are no reports of toxicity from supplementation.

Availability: From health food shops and nutritional therapists.

Boswellic acid

An antioxidant extract from the resin known as frankincense which is produced by plants of the Boswellia species.

Availability: Mainly through medical herbalists or nutritional therapists.

Branched-chain amino acids (also see Amino acids)

These are the three amino acids leucine, isoleucine and valine, comprising about 40 per cent of the total minimum daily requirement for essential amino acids. They are particularly involved in energy and muscle metabolism, and can be used directly as an energy source by muscles. They are also anabolic, promoting protein synthesis.

Branched-chain amino acids (BCAAs) are particularly depleted by stress, and studies have suggested that starvation, injury, surgery or infection raise requirements for BCAAs more than other amino acids. They may be elevated in diabetics since low insulin levels reduce the uptake of BCAA by muscle. BCAAs compete with each other and with tyrosine, phenylalanine, tryptophan and methionine for transport to the brain. BCAAs can act as neurotransmitters (*which see*) and are constituents of neuropeptides which have neurotransmitter functions.

BCAAs stimulate protein synthesis, inhibit protein breakdown, and can substitute for glucose, providing an alternative energy source for the body. Because of their ability to maintain blood sugar levels, some doctors believe that BCAAs may be a more ideal energy source than glucose in intravenous feeding solutions, particularly as they decrease the rate of breakdown and utilization of other amino acids. Nitrogen retention in critically ill patients seems to be proportional to the amount of BCAAs, and BCAA supplements seem to be able to correct most hypercatabolic states.

Cases of unexplained anorexia may respond to BCAA supplements.

Brassicas

This is a sub-species of the plant family known as the Cruciferae (cruciferous vegetables).

Broccoli
(see Cruciferous vegetables)

Bromelain

A dietary supplement extracted from pineapples, used as an aid to protein digestion. It may be combined with papain, a similar enzyme extracted from papaya fruit. Bromelain can also be used in cookery as a meat tenderizer.

Cautions
Take after a meal on a full stomach.
Availability: Widely available in health food shops.

Brown fat
(see Adipose tissue)

Buckwheat

Buckwheat is not a variety of wheat and is not related to wheat. It is the seed of a herbaceous plant related to dock and rhubarb, and is a rich source of the flavonoid rutin. A Russian porridge-like cooked cereal called kasha is made from roasted buckwheat. Buckwheat is free of gluten, and can be cooked like rice. It is also ground into flour.

Bulghar wheat

Wheat grains which have been cracked between rollers and then hulled, steamed and roasted. Bulghar wheat swells when water is added and can be combined with chopped raw vegetables and salad dressing to make a cold dish which is high in complex carbohydrates.

Bulimia nervosa

An eating disorder involving compulsive binge eating, usually in secret, often accompanied by self-induced vomiting and laxative abuse to control weight. As with anorexia nervosa, there is a morbid fear of becoming fat.

Butyric acid

A short-chain fatty acid found in butter, which gives butter its characteristic smell and taste. It is also formed during the colonic fermentation of dietary fibre and is an important energy source for the colonic mucosa (mucous membrane), accounting for the major part of its energy needs even in the presence of glucose. This makes it an important nutrient for growth and repair and nutritional therapists may accordingly administer it in supplement form for this purpose. Individuals who have been on a diet low in fibre may develop deficiencies of this nutrient.
Availability: From nutritional therapists.

C

Vitamin C (ascorbic acid)

Vitamin (water-soluble)
UK RNI 40 mg
US RDA 60 mg

FUNCTIONS

Aids the absorption of iron from vegetables

Antioxidant

Collagen formation (maintains healthy connective tissue and bone)

Immune system

Stress hormone production

Tyrosine production

Wound healing

GOOD FOOD SOURCES

Broccoli

Brussels sprouts

Cabbage

Fresh fruit, especially citrus

Green peppers

Kiwi fruit

Raw leafy vegetables

Tomatoes

Deficiency signs and symptoms

- Bleeding gums or loose teeth
- Easy bruising
- Fatigue
- Frequent infections (e.g. colds, flu, thrush)
- Fragile blood vessels

A chronic shortage of vitamin C, even if mild, can promote a wide range of illnesses and diseases since vitamin C is a vital nutrient for the immune system.

Preventing deficiency

Fresh fruit and vegetables must be consumed regularly, preferably at the rate of five portions daily, to prevent vitamin C deficiency. Vitamin C is rapidly lost from vegetables when they are boiled, since it leaches out into the cooking water. Steaming, or cooking vegetables quickly, as in stir-frying, minimizes losses. Since the cooking water retains the lost vitamin C, this should also be used (e.g. made into soup or stock). The longer fruit and vegetables are stored before consumption, the more vitamin C is lost, for instance 30 per cent of vitamin C in potatoes is lost after 1–3 months' storage. Vitamin C is also lost when the surface of fruit and vegetables is exposed to the air. To minimize this, do not chop them until just before consumption. By the same principle, vitamin C losses are also high from fruit juices. Losses of up to 100 per cent can occur once the container has been opened, shaken, and kept for a week in the refrigerator. Baking soda destroys vitamin C.

Vitamin C in the body is depleted by alcohol consumption, smoking, surgery, trauma, stress, exposure to pollutants, the use of certain medications such as aspirin-based painkillers, antacids and the contraceptive pill, and by infectious illness. Most researchers now recommend a minimum intake of 200 mg vitamin C daily for smokers and those exposed to tobacco smoke.

Comments

Humans are virtually the only mammals who cannot make their own vitamin C from glucose in their liver. This is because we are lacking the final enzyme which other mammals have. Other mammals can make the equivalent of 13 grams a day of vitamin C within their own bodies – more if under stress. This amount would be impossible to obtain from the diet. The roles of vitamin C in the body, its ready depletion by exposure to pollutants, smoking and stress, and the enhanced immunity afforded by a raised vitamin C intake have led many individuals to take a daily vitamin C supplement.

The view that, because the body excretes supplemented vitamin C, supplementation cannot make any difference to health is now considered outdated. Considerable research now supports the case for maintaining a high tissue saturation level of vitamin C in a variety of situations.

A severe deficiency of vitamin C (blood levels below 0.7 mg/100 ml) results in highly raised blood histamine levels. Vitamin C supplementation to 11 selected volunteers resulted in a reduction of the blood histamine level in every instance (*Clemetson CA: Histamine and ascorbic acid in human blood. J Nutr 110(4):662-8, 1980*).

Supplementation

In research studies, vitamin C supplements have been found to:

- Act as a mild anti-histamine
- Control and cure the common cold
- Cure some cases of cancer
- Cure some cases of the blood disease idiopathic thrombocytopenic purpura
- Enhance the number, size and motility of white blood cells
- Enhance wound healing
- Help asthma
- Help with the clearance of toxic chemicals from the body
- Improve blood sugar control in diabetics
- Improve manic depression
- Inhibit the formation of adrenochrome, which is found at raised levels in schizophrenia
- Lower blood cholesterol
- Protect the eye lens against oxidative damage
- Reverse pre-cancerous conditions
- With vitamin E, slow the progression of Parkinson's disease

Preferred form and suggested intake

Recommended preventive health level: 1 gram daily.

Common cold: At the first sign, take 1 level teaspoon (3 grams) of vitamin C powder dissolved in lukewarm water. Repeat every two hours between meals until symptoms subside. (*See Appendix IV for full instructions.*)

For immune enhancement, cancers, or high cholesterol (especially with high lipoprotein A or high apolipoprotein A2 levels): 1 level teaspoon of vitamin C powder dissolved in lukewarm water 2–3 times daily between meals (see cautions below). For Aids and severe viral infections, this amount can be increased to bowel tolerance (see cautions below). Like all water-soluble vitamins, vitamin C is best taken at several intervals daily rather than in one single dose.

The preferred form of supplementation is magnesium ascorbate capsules (for smaller doses) and powder or crystals for a larger daily intake. This is a buffered, non-acidic form which also provides magnesium – a nutrient which is often in short supply in the diet. The magnesium content also helps to prevent vitamin C from combining with minerals and removing them from the intestinal contents.

Cautions

- Do not take more than 1 gram a day of vitamin C if using the contraceptive pill, since vitamin C competes with oestrogen for excretion mechanisms.
- When supplementing large amounts of vitamin C, and especially if you are using the acidic form (ascorbic acid), take it away from meals to prevent interference with the absorption of other nutrients. The use of powdered or crystalline vitamin C dissolved in plenty of water is less irritating to the digestive system than large numbers of tablets or capsules.
- Body levels of copper and other trace elements should be monitored if very large doses of vitamin C are taken on a long-term basis.
- Excess amounts of vitamin C may cause bowel discomfort and loose motions. If this occurs, reduce your intake. This effect is lessened by taking vitamin C powder or crystals dissolved in warm (not hot) water rather than cold.
- The theory that vitamin C supplements may cause kidney stones has been disproven. Researchers have found that the high oxalate levels found in test subjects' urine were due to the analysis method used, not to the vitamin C. (*Wandzilak et al.: Effect of high dose vitamin C on urinary oxalate levels. J Urol 151:834-7, 1994.*) However, the subjects in this trial were normal individuals. There is some evidence that those who already have a tendency to form oxalate kidney stones should exercise caution with vitamin C supplements.

- Vitamin C supplements do not cause 'rebound scurvy'. Scurvy is a life-threatening disease caused by long-term severe vitamin C deprivation.
- Speculation that vitamin C supplements could cause the excessive absorption of iron has also been disproved by a review of the scientific literature. (*Bendich A et al.: Ascorbic acid safety: analysis of factors affecting iron absorption. Toxicol Lett 51(2):189-201, 1990.*)

Cabbage
(see Cruciferous vegetables)

Cadmium

Toxic element

One of the group of so-called heavy metals, cadmium accumulates in the body, especially in the liver and kidneys, as excretion is very slow. A high level of accumulation can eventually result in kidney damage. Other effects of cadmium excess can include anaemia (probably because cadmium competes with copper and iron, needed for blood formation), high blood pressure (probably due to kidney damage), and itai-itai disease (*which see*) in Japan.

Cadmium is a pollutant which is present in the air around industrial smelting and plating plants, and can be inhaled through the lungs. It is also present in galvanized water pipes, which may contaminate drinking water that passes through the pipes. Tobacco smoke contains cadmium (and lead) and may cause smokers to inhale up to 5 mcg of cadmium per day. Silver (amalgam) tooth fillings may also contain cadmium.

Some foods are contaminated with small amounts of cadmium: oysters, liver and kidneys, and crops which have been grown on soil contaminated with cadmium or dressed with cadmium-containing fertilizer.

Caffeine (see Methylxanthines)

Calcitonin

A hormone secreted by the thyroid gland in response to high blood calcium levels. Its action is to reduce blood calcium by increasing the deposition of calcium in bone.

Calcitriol

The active, hormonal form of vitamin D which promotes the absorption of calcium.

Calcium

Mineral
UK RNI 700 mg
US RDA 800 mg

FUNCTIONS
Acetylcholine synthesis
Action of many hormones
Activation of saliva and many enzymes
Blood clotting
Blood pressure regulation
Conversion of glycogen to glucose
Muscle contractions
Nerve impulses (release of neurotransmitters)

Structure of cells
Structure of bones and teeth
Vitamin B_{12} absorption

GOOD FOOD SOURCES
Broccoli
Cheese (especially hard cheeses)
Canned fish (if bones are consumed)
Cow's milk
Leafy green vegetables
Nuts
Pulses
Root vegetables
Yoghurt

Deficiency symptoms

- Convulsions and seizures
- Some cases of gum disease
- Loss of muscle tone
- Muscle cramps
- Osteoporosis (brittle bone disease)
- Rickets or osteomalacia (bone softening)

Preventing deficiency

The bioavailability (*which see*) of calcium is reduced by deficiencies of vitamin D and stomach acid, by high levels of dietary fibre, phytic acid (found in raw whole grains), oxalic acid (found in spinach) or saturated fat, and by a high protein or phosphorus intake, which causes increased losses of calcium in the urine. Sodium and caffeine also cause increased urinary losses of calcium. Very low-fat diets or fat malabsorption may impair calcium absorption. Stress can significantly increase calcium excretion.

60 per cent of calcium is lost when flour is refined. Although by law many countries require white flour to be fortified with calcium to compensate for this, the form of

calcium which is used (chalk) is considered to have low bioavailability.

A 1985 research study points out that the conditions which produce calcium deficiency may also lead to a shift of calcium from bone to soft tissue. This may promote not only osteoporosis but also arteriosclerosis and high blood pressure, due to increased levels of calcium in the blood vessel walls. Motor neurone disease and senile dementia could result from the calcium being deposited in the central nervous system. Another effect of calcium deficiency may be a shift of calcium from outside the cells (normal) to inside the cells (abnormal), which would encourage the development of diabetes and immune deficiency. (*Fujita T: Aging and calcium as an environmental factor. J Nutr Sci Vitaminol 31(Suppl):S15-19, 1985.*)

Comments

Many people believe that the regular consumption of dairy produce (milk, cheese, yoghurt, etc.) is essential to prevent calcium deficiency. This is in fact only true for individuals who eat a diet which would otherwise be very poor in calcium. The consumption of a good wholefood diet rich in vegetables and nuts ensures not only a high calcium but also a high magnesium intake. On the other hand, dairy products are a poor source of magnesium, and individuals who rely on dairy produce for their nutrient intake can end up with a relative magnesium insufficiency. Calcium deficiency sometimes does not respond to supplementation unless any concurrent magnesium deficiency is also treated. High dietary levels of calcium and potassium can help to prevent some of the harmful effects of excess sodium consumption.

Supplementation

In research studies, calcium supplements have been found to:

- Help prevent and treat some cases of muscle cramps (*also see Magnesium*)
- Help prevent and treat some cases of osteoporosis
- Help remove lead, mercury, aluminium and cadmium from the body
- Reduce allergic symptoms
- Reduce some cases of high blood pressure (*also see Magnesium*)
- Together with vitamin D, help treat migraine
- Together with vitamin D, help treat some cases of hearing loss
- Treat period pains
- Treat premenstrual emotional symptoms and fluid retention

Preferred form and suggested intake

Calcium carbonate supplements (usually sold in pharmacies and sometimes described as dolomite) are in fact identical to chalk or limestone. They are insoluble in water and cannot be absorbed by individuals who have reduced levels of stomach acid. Calcium citrate is an economical form of calcium which is well absorbed. It is usually also advisable to take magnesium when supplementing calcium, and many combination products are available. Those with the highest ratio of magnesium to calcium are preferable.

Cautions

A high calcium intake in conjunction with a low magnesium intake may lead to magnesium deficiency problems such as premenstrual syndrome and over-excitable nerve impulses.

Calorie

A unit of energy considered to be the amount of heat needed to raise the temperature of 1 gram of water by 1 degree Celsius. In nutrition what is described as a calorie is in fact a kilocalorie (or 1,000 calories).

1 gram of carbohydrate yields 4 kcal
1 gram of protein yields 4 kcal
1 gram of fat yields 9 kcal
1 gram of alcohol yields 7 kcal

Candida albicans (also see Dysbiosis)

A yeast which can colonize the mouth, vagina or intestinal tract, and may be able to migrate to other parts and organs of the body. When it forms an overgrowth in the mouth or vagina it is known as thrush, and is visible as a creamy white deposit or discharge which in the vagina can cause intense itching. An overgrowth of *Candida albicans* in the intestinal tract is known as candidiasis, and is particularly encouraged by the use of antibiotics. This is because Candida is normally kept under control by so-called 'friendly' bacteria in the intestines. Antibiotics destroy these friendly bacteria, allowing Candida to proliferate out of control. Systemic candidiasis, where Candida colonizes many parts of the body, can also occur, usually in individuals with a severe, life-threatening depletion of the immune system as in terminal cancer or Aids.

Intestinal candidiasis is capable of causing much ill-health, including symptoms such as bloating, fatigue, digestive disturbances, headaches and malaise. The yeast's waste products, which are absorbed into the bloodstream and include the highly poisonous acetaldehyde, are responsible for some of the symptoms. Damage and irritation caused by the growth of Candida on the intestinal wall are responsible for others. In some circles candidiasis has become something of a bandwagon, blamed for all occurrences of these symptoms when no other cause is found by standard medical tests. In fact all the symptoms of candidiasis are non-specific and can also be caused by food allergy, other micro-organisms, digestive enzyme dysfunction, or by some other source of toxins.

Candida is often linked with food and inhalant allergies, which it promotes in two ways. First, because Candida is a yeast, a Candida overgrowth can cause an individual to become sensitized not only to Candida but also to other yeasts. The presence of Candida in the intestines then causes chronic allergic reactions like bloating and inflammation, diarrhoea and skin rashes. The consumption of yeast in the diet, from bread, wine, beer, stock cubes and yeast extract, can aggravate these symptoms or cause additional allergic reactions. Nutritional deficiencies can develop in time as the absorptive surface of the intestine becomes coated with Candida overgrowth.

Many microbiologists have pointed out that under the right conditions, the Candida yeast can change into a so-called mycelial form, developing a fungus-like structure which is capable of burrowing roots into the intestinal walls. The damage which this can cause to the intestines promotes further malfunction, and in particular a condition known as 'leaky gut syndrome' (*which see*). A leaky or over-permeable intestine can result in undigested food particles coming more easily into contact with the bloodstream, and thus further inflammation. Toxins are also more easily absorbed into the blood from a leaky, over-permeable gut, resulting in increased stress on the liver, which is already overburdened with Candida toxins. As liver detoxifying enzymes become overloaded, sensitivity to odours, environmental factors and natural chemicals in many foods can develop, producing varied symptoms and often a severely debilitating fatigue.

It is difficult to diagnose intestinal candidiasis, since it is normal for most individuals to have some of this yeast harmlessly resident in their digestive tract. Some specialist centres now provide tests based on stool cultures, available through nutritional therapists. Such tests should always be used if there is no significant history of antibiotic or contraceptive pill use, and no history of vaginal or oral thrush.

Candidiasis
(see Candida albicans)

Caprylic acid

Fatty acid

A fatty acid found mainly in coconuts, which has anti-fungal properties and is often used in natural anti-candidiasis regimes.

Availability: Usually as calcium/magnesium caprylate, from health food shops and nutritional therapists.

Capsicum

Herb

Also known as chilli, red pepper and cayenne pepper, capsicum is widely used as a spice for its hot, pungent flavour which is mainly due to the alkaloid capsaicin. Capsicum can stimulate the production of adrenal cortex hormones. It is described by herbalists as a strong circulatory stimulant which stimulates gastric secretions, counteracts irritation and also acts as a carminative (counteracts flatulence).

Caraway

Herb

Caraway seeds contain the active ingredients carvol and limonene and are used in medical herbalism as a powerful carminative – to counteract flatulence. For this reason caraway seeds are often added to dishes like cabbage which are liable to produce gas.

Carbohydrates
(also see Energy production)

The collective name given to starches, glycogen, sugars and dietary fibres which can be converted to glucose and used as fuel for energy. They are classified as monosaccharides and disaccharides (simple carbohydrates or sugars), polysaccharides (starches, glycogen and fibre), and oligosaccharides (carbohydrates which fall somewhere in between sugars and starches, or are formed during the digestion of polysaccharides).

Chemically speaking, carbohydrates consist of various combinations of carbon, hydrogen and oxygen, and are classified into three main groups, according to their complexity. Least complex are the monosaccharides and disaccharides (also known as the sugars), and most complex are the polysaccharides (also known as starch or complex carbohydrate).

Carbohydrates come from plants, which store them as their chief source of energy.

Monosaccharides	Main food sources	Broken down to
Glucose	Fruits, honey, corn syrup	
Fructose	Fruits, honey	
Galactose	Does not occur in free form in food	
Sorbitol	Fruits, vegetables, dietetic products	
Disaccharides		
Sucrose	Cane and beet sugars, maple syrup	Glucose and fructose
Lactose	Milk and milk products	Glucose and galactose
Maltose	Malt products	Glucose and glucose

Water, minerals and nitrogen in the soil are taken up by the plant's roots and sent to the leaves. With the aid of chlorophyll, these nutrients combine with carbon dioxide and sun energy to form sugars via photosynthesis.

The most common of all the sugars is sucrose, or ordinary table sugar. Like lactose and maltose, sucrose is a disaccharide, which simply means a combination of two simple sugars, or monosaccharides. Some common sugars and their sources are shown in the box above.

Disaccharides are broken down into their component monosaccharides by the processes of digestion. As we can see, all disaccharides have a glucose component. A daily supply of glucose is needed for all the body's metabolic functions.

The end product of starch digestion is also mainly glucose. Starches may be fully or partially digestible, or completely indigestible, depending on the type. They are found in grains, roots, vegetables and pulses, encased within plant cells. Cooking softens and ruptures the plant cell to make the starch available for enzymes to work on in our intestines.

Once sugars and starches have been broken down into monosaccharides by the digestive processes, the monosaccharides enter the bloodstream and travel to the liver, where those that are not already glucose are converted into glucose and released into the circulation. Within 30 minutes to one hour after a meal, the blood glucose peaks.

High blood glucose (blood sugar) levels stimulate the production of the hormone insulin by the pancreas. Insulin encourages the uptake of glucose from the blood into the body's muscle and fat cells, where it goes through successive chemical changes. Energy is released when the end products of glucose are combined with oxygen.

Cardamom

Herb

A herb widely used in Indian cookery. It also has a valuable use in medical herbalism as a warming digestive stimulant for congestive digestion with symptoms such as abdominal distension, nausea and lack of appetite.

Carminative

A substance – often herbal – which prevents and removes the accumulation of gases in the stomach and intestines, thus counteracting flatulence.

Carnitine

Amino acid

The most important function of carnitine is thought to be its role in regulating fat metabolism – carrying fat across a membrane to the energy-burning mitochondria of each cell. The more carnitine is available, the faster fat is transported, and the more fat is used for energy. This is a particularly vital function in the heart muscle.

Carnitine also helps the body to break down branched-chain amino acids into fuel for the muscles when necessary, and it controls ketone levels in the blood. Ketones are the result of the incomplete oxidation of fats in energy production. They are high in diabetics (whose hearts often metabolize carnitine abnormally) and they also rise in high-protein or high-fat diets and tend to acidify the blood.

In a double-blind study which administered 2 grams of carnitine or a placebo to 10 volunteers 1 hour before they began working on an exercise cycle, it was found that at the maximum exercise intensity, treatment with L-carnitine significantly increased the maximum oxygen uptake and power output. Oxygen uptake, carbon dioxide production, pulmonary ventilation and plasma lactate were reduced. The researchers concluded that carnitine supplementation results in a more efficient performance at maximum exercise intensity. (*Vecchiet L et al.: Influence of L-carnitine administration on maximal physical exercise. Eur J Appl Physiol 61(5-6):486-90, 1990.*)

Availability: From health food shops.

Carotenes
(see Carotenoids)

Carotenoids

Carotenoids are plant pigments which give yellow, orange and red fruits and vegetables their colour. Over 600 carotenoids have now been identified, and about 60 of these are found in food. Some carotenoids are emerging as powerful antioxidants with even greater ability to quench reactive oxygen species or free radicals (*which see*) – particularly singlet oxygen – than the more 'established' antioxidants. (*Di Mascio P et al.: Lycopene as the most efficient biological carotenoid singlet oxygen quencher. Arch Biochem Biophys 274(2):532-8, 1989.*) Evidence is also building that the most effective protection from free radicals may come from a combination of antioxidants rather than from large amounts of single nutrients. Certain carotenoids can also activate the expression of genes which encode the message for production of a protein required for communication between cells. Great interest is being shown in lycopene, which is thought to be even more effective than beta-carotene at quenching free radicals and preventing cancer. In addition, lycopene may be able to slow down the growth rate of cancer cells by inhibiting an insulin-like growth factor which they produce. Lutein and zeaxanthin can help to reduce the risk of macular degeneration, a leading cause of blindness.

Beta-carotene is the best known of the carotenoids, and, like another 60 or so, can be converted by the human body into vitamin A.

Some carotenoids and their best sources
Alpha carotene: carrots, red and yellow peppers, pumpkin
Beta-carotene: carrots, apricots, canteloupe, parsley, spinach, kale, sweet potatoes
Cryptoxanthin: tangerines, oranges, papaya

Lutein: kale, spinach, lettuce, parsley, broccoli
Lycopene: tomatoes, pink grapefruit, guava, watermelon
Zeaxanthin: spinach, chicory leaf, okra, corn.

It is best to obtain carotenoids from food, but to augment a food intake, mixed carotenoid supplements are now available in health food shops.

Cascara

Herb

Also known as cascara sagrada, this herb is used as a laxative to treat constipation. It has been described as one of the most gentle but effective stimulating laxatives available, able to produce a bowel movement without undue griping, especially if combined with fennel, chamomile and other carminatives.

In the Chinese classification system, cascara is a 'cold bitter' which means that it is best applied in conditions of excessive vitality and avoided in any conditions involving coldness, such as depressed circulation or low metabolic rate, frequent urination or chronic respiratory congestion.

Availability: Widely available from health food shops, pharmacies and herbalists.

Casein

A protein derived from milk.

Catalase (see Antioxidants)

Catecholamines

Stimulating compounds made from the amino acid dopa, which is in turn derived from tyrosine. The catecholamines form part of a larger family of substances known as monoamines (*which see*). The best known catecholamines found in the human body are adrenaline (known in the United States as epinephrine) and noradrenaline, both produced by the adrenal medulla in response to stress. Dopamine, found mainly in the brain, is also an important catecholamine. Catecholamines may also be formed when the amino acid tyrosine is taken up by the terminals of nerve cells. The enzymes present in these terminals determine which catecholamine will be formed.

The main functions of these compounds include the peripheral excitation or inhibition of certain muscles, cardiac excitation, metabolic actions, endocrine actions, and central nervous system actions. Catecholamines bind to receptors in nerve terminals, and their effects depend on the receptors.

Adrenaline and noradrenaline

Also known as the 'fight or flight' hormone, adrenaline prepares the body for dealing with stress situations. Like noradrenaline, when it combines with alpha receptors on the muscles of blood vessel walls, it causes them to contract. However, the small arteries which supply skeletal muscle also have beta receptors, and when adrenaline combines with these, there is an opposite, relaxing effect. The net result is that more blood is made available to the skeletal muscles, which are then able to respond to extra physical demands such as running, self-defence or competitive sports. Both adrenaline and noradrenaline also increase the force of contraction of the heart muscle and raise blood pressure, and adrenaline speeds up the heart rate.

Low blood sugar stimulates the release of adrenaline for the metabolic tasks of inhibiting insulin secretion, stimulating glucagon secretion, stimulating the breakdown of glycogen (stored carbohydrate), mobilizing fat stores, and promoting the conversion of amino acids, lactate and glycerol into glucose. The effect of these actions is to raise the blood sugar (*which see*). Other effects of adrenaline include an increase of 30 per cent or more in the body's heat production, and a raised metabolic rate.

The catecholamines are thought to be involved in the mechanisms of clinical depression and mania. Individuals with depression excrete reduced amounts of catecholamines and other monoamines in their urine. Individuals with mania, on the other hand, excrete increased amounts. Monoamine oxidase inhibitors, which are drugs used to treat depression, work by inhibiting an enzyme which breaks down catecholamines, thus allowing higher concentrations of them to circulate in the body. The drug lithium, which is used to treat mania, is thought to work by reducing the release of noradrenaline from nerve terminals and enhancing its uptake.

Dopamine

Dopamine is primarily known for its role as a neurotransmitter, and as a precursor of adrenaline and noradrenaline. Virtually all drugs which improve or worsen the mental illness schizophrenia have some effect on levels of dopamine in the body. In particular the antipsychotic drugs work by blocking dopamine receptors. Dopamine is also involved in Parkinson's disease, where the dopamine-releasing nerve cells in the substantia nigra, a portion of the brain, start to degenerate, thus reducing the availability of dopamine to other cells in the brain. (This explains why dopamine-inhibiting drugs given to schizophrenics can cause a parkinsonian-like syndrome known as tardive dyskinesia.)

Another important effect of dopamine is its ability to inhibit the secretion of prolactin, in which role it is known as prolactin release-inhibiting hormone, or PIH.

Celery

Herb

Both celery seeds and the juice of celery stalks are used as a herb to promote alkalinization and as a mild diuretic. These effects may act together to reduce the inflammation of arthritis, and celery seed extract is commonly used by natural medicine practitioners in arthritis treatment. The juice of celery stalks is a rich source of organic sodium which is said to help counteract some of the harmful effects of inorganic sodium chloride.

Cell membrane

The outer membrane of the cell, which controls the entry of nutrients into the cell and the release of wastes. Also known as the plasma membrane, it consists of a thin layer of phospholipid and cholesterol molecules in which proteins are embedded. A variety of binding sites are located on the outer surface of the cell membrane, for the attachment of hormones and other chemical messengers. The cell membrane can therefore receive chemical signals which regulate the cell's activity. Chemical reactions can also take place on the inner or outer surface of the cell membrane. Other roles include cell-to-cell recognition and communication. Fatty acids are converted to prostaglandins (*which see*) in the cell membrane.

Free radical (*which see*) damage to the cell membrane reduces the membrane's ability to transport nutrients, oxygen and water into the cell and to regulate the excretion of waste matter from the cell. Free radical damage can also cause cell membranes to rupture.

Celloid minerals

Supplements prepared from the inorganic minerals originally identified by Dr Wilhelm Schüssler in Germany in 1873, using a process developed by Dr Maurice Blackmore of Australia in 1938. The minerals are:

Calcium fluoride
Calcium phosphate
Calcium sulphate
Iron phosphate
Magnesium phosphate
Potassium chloride
Potassium phosphate
Potassium sulphate
Silicon dioxide
Sodium chloride
Sodium phosphate
Sodium sulphate

Whereas Schüssler's tissue salts (*which see*) are sold in homoeopathic potencies, Blackmore's celloids are sold in small physiological doses. However, the prescribing indications used by celloid mineral practitioners often have more in common with homoeopathy than with nutritional therapy.

Cellulase

An enzyme capable of breaking down cellulose (*which see*). Does not occur naturally in the human digestive tract, but may be found in digestive enzyme supplements.

Cellulose

An important dietary fibre which is a constituent of plant cell walls. It is not digestible by the enzymes of humans or animals, only by bacteria in the rumen of some animals.

Cereals

Also known as grains, cereals are the seeds of domesticated grasses, including wheat, rice, millet, oats, maize, barley and rye. Wheat, oats, rye, maize and barley contain gluten; rice and millet do not. Unrefined cereals are a good source of B vitamins. Except for maize (which is short of the amino acid tryptophan), cereals are usually short of the amino acid lysine and do not therefore constitute complete proteins.

Chamomile

Herb

A herb which, when made into tea, can be used medicinally and as a recreational drink to aid sleep and relaxation. As a medicine it is used to reduce inflammation in the digestive system, relieve digestive spasms (often quite rapidly) and counteract flatulence.

Availability: Chamomile tea is widely available in health food shops and supermarkets.

Char-grilling (char-broiling)

Cooking food over hot coals (as with barbecuing) or with the heating element below the food. Some of the fat which drips on to the coals is not completely combusted and forms a smoke containing carcinogenic benzopyrene which rises and is deposited on the food.

Charring of the exterior of fat- or protein-rich food during grilling results in the formation of some mutagenic and possibly carcinogenic substances. Several scientific studies have found a greatly increased risk of cancer associated with the frequent consumption of charred or fried foods.

Charcoal

Charcoal can attach itself to almost anything it comes into contact with, and if ingested can therefore help to prevent toxins from being absorbed from the stomach and intestines, and carry them out of the body. It can also help to absorb gas in the intestinal tract. Charcoal tablets are available from health shops and pharmacies as a dietary supplement for these purposes.

Chelates
(also see Bioavailability)

Minerals released from food by gastric acid in the stomach combine with dietary proteins, amino acids and acids such as ascorbic acid, citric acid, gluconic acid and lactic acid during the digestive process to form compounds called 'chelates' which can easily cross the intestinal wall into the bloodstream. Examples of such chelates are zinc picolinate, zinc monomethionine, ferrous aspartate, calcium lactate or proteinate and magnesium citrate or gluconate. Mineral supplements bound with protein or amino acids are sold as chelated minerals, and are thought to be highly bioavailable because they imitate the body's own processes. These are not to be confused with some cheaply made products which may also be sold as chelates, but in which there has been no proper binding process. When buying chelates, select those which the manufacturer guarantees to be properly chelated.

Chelation
(also see Bioavailability)

The process whereby an inorganic mineral is converted to an organically bound compound known as a chelate.

Chlorella
(see Algae)

Chloride

Minerals can combine with the element chlorine to form chlorides, compounds such as sodium and potassium chloride.

Chlorophyll

A green pigment found in all green plants which enables them to synthesize carbohydrates from carbon dioxide and water, using the sun's energy. It is often described as the 'haemoglobin' of the plant world. Chlorophyll is used as a natural green colouring, and is also taken as a dietary supplement for its ability to combine with gut toxins and remove them from the body. It is sometimes used as a breath deodorant.

Cholecystokinin

A hormone secreted by the upper part of the small intestine, which stimulates gallbladder contraction and the release of digestive enzymes and hormones from the pancreas.

Cholesterol

Uses and sources

Cholesterol is a fatty substance found in animal tissues and in eggs. It is a vital component of cell membranes, and especially of the myelin sheath which insulates nerves, and is used to make bile acids which play a part in fat digestion. It is also required for the production of steroid hormones and vitamin D. Very little of our blood cholesterol is obtained from dietary sources, the majority is synthesized by the liver. Elevated blood cholesterol levels are not therefore necessarily linked with a high cholesterol consumption, but they do tend to be associated with a diet high in saturated fat. This tendency depends to some extent on the types of saturated fat consumed. The formation of different prostaglandins and leukotrienes (*which see*), which have different regulatory effects on metabolism and physiological function, probably plays a part in this.

Excretion

Cholesterol once made cannot be broken down by the body except into bile acids. It can only be excreted via the stools, in the form of bile acids (which are released into the gut during the process of digestion) and cholesterol molecules. When adequate dietary fibre, especially pectins and other soluble fibre, is consumed in the diet, it binds bile acids and carries them out of the body via the stools. The reduced transit time of the gut contents, which is promoted by a high-fibre diet, also helps to enhance the excretion of bile acids. If bile acids are not removed from the gut, they are reabsorbed and eventually re-converted to cholesterol. Low-fibre diets therefore encourage this reabsorption.

Forms of cholesterol

Like all fats, cholesterol is not soluble in water and therefore has to be transported in the blood in the form of fat/protein complexes known as lipoproteins. This gives rise to several common forms of blood cholesterol:

- VLDL (very low density lipoproteins). These transport triglycerides and cholesterol out of the liver and deposit them in peripheral tissues and arteries. VLDLs eventually become LDLs.

- LDL (low density lipoproteins, or 'bad cholesterol'). These contain predominantly cholesterol, which they deposit in the peripheral tissues and arteries and in the liver.
- HDL (high density lipoproteins or 'good cholesterol'). These consist of mainly phospholipids and 35–40 per cent cholesterol. The phospholipid picks up cholesterol from the peripheral tissues and arteries and deposits it in the liver.

It is thought that LDL cholesterol may have to be oxidized before it can form harmful atherogenic deposits in the arteries, which is the reason why a high intake of antioxidant nutrients such as vitamins A, C, E, selenium and beta-carotene is thought to be valuable in preventing heart disease.

Methods of reducing blood cholesterol levels

Increasing fibre intake
Increasing the rate of loss of bile acids and cholesterol through the stools by increasing fibre intake can reduce blood cholesterol levels by 10–25 per cent. Pectin, found mainly in fruit, is the most effective type of fibre for this purpose. Bran and cellulose are not so effective. Fibre also enhances the production of propionic acid by intestinal bacteria. Once absorbed into the blood, propionic acid may inhibit the synthesis of cholesterol by the liver.

Increasing consumption of plant foods
- Substances known as sterols, found in beans and in many vegetable and seed oils, inhibit the absorption (or reabsorption) of cholesterol.

- Vitamin E-like substances known as tocotrienols (*which see*), also found in many plants, particularly palm oil and barley oil, also help to inhibit enzymes involved in cholesterol synthesis, resulting in a lowering of cholesterol. It is thought that the often-observed cholesterol-lowering effect of palm oil and cocoa butter – which are, paradoxically, saturated fats – may be due to their tocotrienol or plant sterol content.

Correcting nutritional deficiencies
- Copper-, vanadium- or chromium-deficient diets or a diet with a high ratio of zinc to copper, can result in hypertriglyceridaemia and high blood cholesterol.
- Inuit Eskimos are well known for being free of heart disease, and consume a great deal of oily fish. It is now known that the synthesis of VLDLs (cholesterol-depositing lipoproteins which eventually form LDL, or 'bad cholesterol') is reduced by EPA, a substance found in the oils from these fish. Fish oils may also depress the synthesis of cholesterol by the liver.

Dietary supplementation
- Large doses of supplementary vitamin C can reduce blood cholesterol levels, possibly by stimulating the conversion of cholesterol to bile acids.
- Niacin supplementation (3,000–9,000 mg per day) may be prescribed by doctors to reduce serum cholesterol through a reduction in synthesis of VLDL. Niacin is also thought to enhance HDL ('good cholesterol') synthesis. However, most holistic practitioners believe that because of the association of such large doses of niacin with possible liver damage, other nutritional avenues should be explored first.

Cholestyramine

Anti-cholesterol drug which works by binding bile acids. Can cause depletion of folic acid.

Choline

Vitamin-like substance

FUNCTIONS
Component of all lipoproteins
Lipotropic (helps to remove fat from the liver)
Structural role in cell membranes
Synthesis of the neurotransmitter acetylcholine

GOOD FOOD SOURCES
Egg yolk
Grains
Heart
Lecithin
Liver
Nuts
Pulses

Deficiency symptoms

- Fatty liver and liver impairment
- Possible memory or thought impairment
- Retarded growth

Preventing deficiency

Choline is relatively low in fruits and vegetables, so those most at risk of choline deficiency (and other deficiencies) are those on long-term 'fad' diets such as fruit-only regimes. Choline may also be deficient if liver function is impaired, since a limited amount of choline can be synthesized in the liver, using the amino acid methionine. As with all other nutrients, a wide variety of foods, preferably for the most part unrefined, is the best health protection.

It would be difficult to develop a choline deficiency without also developing a number of other deficiencies.

Supplementation

In research studies, choline supplements have been found to:

- Foster healing of fatty liver changes in ex-alcoholics
- Reduce the cholesterol content of bile and increase bile phospholipids
- Reduce the tremors of tardive dyskinesia, a Parkinson's disease-like syndrome caused by major tranquillizer drugs used in schizophrenia

Preferred form and suggested intake
The preferred form of choline supplementation is phosphatidyl choline, also known as lecithin. It can be bought in granules and sprinkled on food or in hot drinks. The usual dosage is 1–2 tablespoons per day.

Cautions
Some forms of choline used in medical practice can give the body a fishy odour. Phosphatidyl choline (lecithin) does not, and there is no known unsafe dosage of this form of choline.

Chondroitin sulphate

A long-chain mucopolysaccharide (*which see*) found in connective tissue, which assists bonding between protein filaments. It may be commercially extracted from cartilage and used as a dietary supplement to help problems such as arthritis.

Availability: May be available only through specialist suppliers.

Chromium

Trace element
UK minimum suggested intake 25 mcg
US safe adequate intake range 50–200 mcg

FUNCTIONS

As part of Glucose Tolerance Factor (*see below*), promotes good blood sugar balance and enhances the effectiveness of insulin.

GOOD FOOD SOURCES

Liver
Mushrooms
Whole grains
Yeast

Deficiency symptoms

- Adult-onset diabetes
- Atherosclerosis
- Elevated blood cholesterol, blood sugar and triglycerides
- Muscle weakness
- Reactive hypoglycaemia (with symptoms such as fatigue, dizziness and mood swings)

Preventing deficiency

Sugar metabolism requires chromium, B vitamins and magnesium. A high sugar consumption uses up these nutrients without replacing them, because sugar does not contain any vitamins or other nutrients except calories. (Beware the advertisements about sugar giving you energy; energy is simply the scientific name for calories!) Chromium is also lost in the urine whenever sugar is consumed.

Many countries make the replacement of some of the lost B vitamins compulsory in products made from refined (white) flour, since the B vitamins are, like chromium, mostly found in the bran and germ of the flour, not in the white, starchy portion. Unfortunately chromium is not replaced in this way although 98 per cent of the chromium in wheat is lost when flour is refined.

To avoid a chromium deficiency, your diet should be low in sugar (for instance you could restrict your intake of sugary food or drink to just one small item a day), and you should use wholemeal bread, flour and cereals whenever possible.

Dietary chromium in the US and other developed countries is roughly half of the minimum suggested intake of 50 micrograms. This marginal intake may lead to health problems. Supplementation with chromium has demonstrated many health benefits but it will only benefit those people whose signs and symptoms are due to chromium deficiency (*Anderson RA: Essentiality of chromium in humans. Sci Total Environ 86(1-2)75-81, 1989*).

Comments

GTF (Glucose Tolerance Factor), which is a water-soluble component of liver, blood plasma and brewer's yeast, and is the form in which chromium exerts its blood sugar controlling activity, has never been chemically identified, but is thought to consist of a combination of chromium with the B vitamin nicotinic acid and three amino acids: glycine, glutamic acid and cysteine. However, artificial complexes made with these ingredients do not result in the same degree of biological activity as found in the material produced by living cells.

Chromium supplements are popular as weight-loss aids in some circles. The correction of chromium deficiency with dietary supplements may help to stabilize blood sugar. This may in turn assist appetite control since low blood sugar leads to feelings of hunger.

Small amounts of chromium may leach from stainless steel cookware if it comes into contact with acidic food.

Research paper

Wallach S: Clinical and biochemical aspects of chromium deficiency. J Amer Coll Nutr 4:107-120, 1985.

Supplementation

In research studies, chromium supplements have been found to:

- Increase the density of insulin receptors (thus assisting the function of insulin)
- Reduce high blood cholesterol levels
- Reduce symptoms of hypoglycaemia, especially when used together with magnesium

Preferred form and suggested intake

Chromium supplements are only available as trivalent chromium (chromium III). Hexavalent chromium (chromium VI) is the form used for metal-plating and other industrial uses, and is highly toxic. There is some dispute about which chromium supplements have the highest 'GTF activity' (are most effective in assisting blood sugar control). Chromium polynicotinate is considered by many experts to be the best form, and chromium yeast (where yeast is grown in a chromium-rich environment and absorbs much chromium as it grows) also has high GTF activity. A daily dosage of 100–200 mcg is adequate for most purposes.

Cautions

No symptoms of excess intake have been reported. Chromium is generally very poorly absorbed. However there may be some doubt about the safety of chromium orotate. One little-known side-effect of chromium supplementation for some individuals is an increased tendency to experience bad dreams.

Cider vinegar

Used as a condiment, and also medicinally, against arthritis and as an appetite suppressant to promote weight loss.

Cinnamon

Herb

Widely used in cookery, cinnamon also has antispasmodic and anti-microbial properties. It is a warming digestive and circulatory stimulant and helps to counteract flatulence and diarrhoea. It is capable of suppressing the growth of numerous micro-organisms, including *Escherichia coli*, *Staphylococcus aureus* and *Candida albicans*, and some parasitic worms.

Citrates

Many dietary supplements are manufactured by complexing minerals with citric acid, forming weak chelates (*which see*) known as citrates. For the most part highly bioavailable, these supplements include magnesium citrate, calcium citrate and zinc citrate.

Citrulline

Amino acid

An amino acid which takes part in the urea cycle (*see Amino acids*) and is converted to arginine. Onions and garlic are good sources of citrulline. This amino acid is not normally available as a dietary supplement.

Cleansing diets
(see Therapeutic diets)

Clinical ecology
(see Environmental medicine)

Cobalt (also see Vitamin B$_{12}$)

Trace element

Cobalt is a constituent of vitamin B$_{12}$ and has no other known function in the body.

Cod liver oil

Superfood

Cod liver oil contains sufficient amounts of vitamins A and D to act as a good source of supplementation for these nutrients. However a survey by the international environmental organization Greenpeace has found significant levels of pesticide residue in many brands of cod liver oil. Consumers should seek a brand whose producers guarantee good quality control. Cod liver oil is not a good source of EPA (eicosapentaenoic acid) or DHA (docosahexaenoic acid) (*which see*). The consumption of oily fish or fish oil (oil extracted from the flesh of oily fish, not the liver) is required to obtain these nutrients.

Coenzyme Q10
(also see Energy production)

Vitamin-like substance

FUNCTIONS
Antioxidant nutrient
Transfer of oxygen and energy between components of the cells
Transfer of oxygen and energy between the blood and tissues

GOOD FOOD SOURCES
Beef
Chicken
Mackerel
Nuts
Sardines
Soya oil
Whole grains

Deficiency symptoms

- Chronic fatigue
- Gum disease and deterioration
- Heart failure and other heart problems
- Infections
- Some mental problems
- Reduced muscular strength and endurance

Preventing deficiency

Coenzyme Q10 does not need to be ingested from food, since the body is capable of making it. However the synthesis of coenzyme Q10 is dependent on vitamin E, so you should ensure that your daily diet contains vitamin E-rich foods such as whole grains and nuts.

Comments

Coenzyme Q10 is a fat-soluble nutrient with a structure similar to those of vitamins E and K. Its functions overlap to some extent with these vitamins.

Supplementation

In research studies, coenzyme Q10 supplements have been found to:

- Bring clinical improvements in Aids
- Cure some cases of breast cancer
- Improve glucose tolerance in diabetics
- Improve congestive heart failure
- Improve heart function (including angina and irregular heart rhythms)
- Reduce high blood pressure

Preferred form and suggested intake

Although it may be difficult to obtain, an emulsified form of coenzyme Q10 is said to be more bioavailable than the usual non-emulsified forms, since emulsified nutrients and fats are taken up by the lymphatic system rather than the bloodstream, thus temporarily bypassing the liver. Supplementation with 30–90 mg CoQ10 (in divided doses) daily is adequate for most purposes, but studies using the nutrient against breast cancer have obtained their best results by gradually increasing the dosage to about 400 mg daily.

Cautions

There is no known unsafe dose of CoQ10 but it is probably wise not to exceed 400 mg daily since we do not yet know enough about possible effects at higher doses.

Availability: Coenzyme Q10 is a very expensive product. Widely available in health food shops and through nutritional therapists.

Coffee

Coffee contains methylxanthines (*which see*) such as caffeine, which act as central nervous system stimulants.

The over-consumption of coffee may produce any of the following effects:

- Addiction (even from the consumption of as little as one cup a day)
- Anxiety and nervousness
- Birth defects (if consumed by expectant mothers)
- Exacerbation of psychiatric symptoms
- Fibrocystic breast disease or breast lumps
- Increased insulin production, resulting in symptoms of hypoglycaemia
- Palpitations
- Raised blood cholesterol levels (only if coffee is boiled)
- Rapid heartbeat
- Temporarily raised blood pressure

Reports of a link between coffee consumption and pancreatic cancer have not been confirmed, but research does suggest that the consumption of more than five cups of coffee a day raises the risk of heart disease. Instant coffee contains more caffeine than the drink made from ground coffee. Coffee is a rich source of vitamin B_3 (in its nicotinic acid form).

Collagen

The main protein which forms the skin, joints, bones, teeth, muscles and many other tissues throughout the body. The body's production of collagen is dependent on vitamin C.

Colloidal minerals

Colloidal minerals are described as the smallest particles which minerals can be divided into while still keeping individual characteristics. They remain in solution in water rather than going into suspension, because of their negative charge and size/weight ratio. It is claimed that these characteristics, together with the large surface area which results from their small size, gives them special qualities of absorption and assimilation. Colloidal mineral supplements may be manufactured from humic shale – a type of rock consisting of prehistoric plant life. The mineral content is therefore in organic, colloidal form.

Availability: Not easily available. May be sold under different names or through specialist suppliers.

Colon

The large intestine. Absorbs water from digested food and contains many bacteria.

Colostrum

Human breast milk is known as colostrum in the first two weeks of production. It is a yellowish transparent fluid containing more protein, sodium, potassium and chloride and less fat and carbohydrate than mature milk.

Coltsfoot

Herb

An old-established cough remedy and member of the daisy family, coltsfoot tea taken daily on waking has been found effective for the symptomatic relief of chronic emphysema and silicosis.

Availability: Widely available in health food shops.

Comfrey

Herb

A plant which may be eaten as a vegetable (like spinach) or used medicinally. Comfrey is found to be particularly effective against osteoarthritis and other conditions involving chronic pain. It is a tissue-builder, and its beneficial effect on wound and bone healing is legendary. It is also an important herb for the digestive system, helping to soothe and heal inflamed tissues and ulceration.

Worries about small amounts of toxic ingredients in comfrey known as pyrrolizidine alkaloids have led to the banning of tablets and capsules made from comfrey root in some countries. This is because three cases of a rare form of liver disease have been found among comfrey users worldwide, and these cases have been attributed to pyrrolizidine alkaloids. However, a survey of 600 comfrey users in the UK, including individuals who had consumed comfrey products for up to 40 years, found no reports of liver damage or any other symptoms which could be attributed to comfrey. It has been suggested that the three cases of liver damage may have been due to accidental contamination of comfrey products rather than to any inherent toxicity of comfrey itself at normal levels of intake.

Contraceptive pill

The Pill can cause metabolic changes which affect the status of many nutrients. It raises blood levels of vitamin A, impairs tryptophan metabolism and increases the body's requirements for vitamin B_6, vitamin B_{12}, folic acid, vitamin C, vitamin E, manganese and zinc.

High supplementary doses of vitamin C (more than 1 gram per day) are best avoided when taking oral contraceptives as they can increase their bioavailability.

Control group

In a scientific study, the control group (sometimes known simply as the 'controls') is a group selected for comparison purposes, often matched as closely as possible to the experimental group. For instance the experimental group may all have the same illness and receive the same medication, while the control group also has this illness, but receives a placebo (dummy) medicine. This allows the effectiveness of the medicine to be evaluated. Likewise an experimental group may have an illness whereas the controls do not. This setup is common in studies which measure differences in nutritional status between sick and healthy individuals.

Copper

Trace element
UK RNI 1.2 mg
US safe adequate intake 2–3 mg

FUNCTIONS
Assists iron absorption and transport
Connective tissue and blood vessel maintenance
Cholesterol regulation
Energy production
Haemoglobin
Inactivation of histamine
Maintenance of myelin sheath around nerve fibres
Needed to make ceruloplasmin
Needed to make antioxidant enzyme SOD
Needed to make cytochrome oxidase (detoxifying) enzymes
Pigments in skin and hair
Production of adrenal hormones

GOOD FOOD SOURCES
Avocado pears
Liver
Molasses
Nuts
Olives
Pulses
Shellfish
Whole grains

Deficiency symptoms

- Anaemia (resulting in fatigue)
- Depigmentation of skin
- Haemorrhaging of blood vessels
- Hypothermia
- Kinky hair

Preventing deficiency

As for most nutrients, a diet high in whole grains and other wholefoods is protective against deficiencies. Large doses of vitamin C or zinc taken daily on a long-term basis may result in depletion of copper levels, therefore it would be prudent to include a daily copper supplement (which should not be taken at the same time) to prevent this. Many multimineral or multi-nutrient supplements exclude copper because of theories that many individuals are already consuming excessive amounts of copper from non-dietary sources. If copper intake is in fact too low rather than too high, such supplements may aggravate a copper deficiency by providing large amounts of nutrients (such as zinc) which compete with copper for absorption.

Comments

Copper is not just obtained from the diet. Copper pipes carrying household water supplies, copper cookware, processed food, pesticide and fungicide residues in food, and copper containers can add significant amounts of copper to our dietary intake. Use of the contraceptive pill can result in elevated blood copper levels.

Environmental medicine specialists find that patients suffering from chemical sensitivities may need supplementary copper to help in their detoxification process.

Supplementation

In research studies, copper supplements have been found to:

- Help anaemia
- Help rheumatism (copper bracelet)
- Help rheumatoid arthritis
- Inhibit chemical carcinogenesis (in animal studies)

Preferred form and suggested intake

Copper supplements are generally provided as chelates. Take 1–2 mg daily, preferably not at the same time as zinc.

Cautions

Copper bracelets are thought to result in copper uptake (in unknown quantities) through the skin. If found helpful this route of supplementation can be continued, although it might be advisable to monitor blood copper levels from time to time. An excess intake of copper can result in symptoms like depression, irritability, joint or muscle pain, nervousness or abnormal mental states.

Cori cycle (also see Energy production)

Also known as the lactic acid cycle, this describes the process whereby glucose is recycled when there is insufficient oxygen for normal glucose metabolism via the Krebs cycle. In the Cori cycle, blood glucose is converted to lactic acid, which is then converted back to glucose or glycogen.

Corticosteroids

Hormones produced by the adrenal glands (*which see*).

Cortisone

One of the glucocorticoid hormones made by the adrenal glands (*which see*).

Cranberry

Herb

Cranberry juice (which should be undiluted and unsweetened or used in the form of a commercially prepared extract) is capable of helping to prevent bacteria from adhering to the walls of the bladder and genitourinary tract, thus preventing cystitis.

Cruciferous vegetables

Vegetables belonging to the plant family known as the *Cruciferae*. See *Food families* for a list of the members of this family. Cruciferous vegetables contain natural chemicals which reduce cancer risks, for instance sulphoraphane in broccoli.

Cyclic AMP
(adenosine monophosphate)

A substance involved in the hormonal control of metabolism.

Cyclooxygenase
(see Prostaglandins)

Cysteine

Amino acid

Cysteine belongs to the sulphur group of amino acids. It is obtained from dietary sources and can also be synthesized from methionine. Cysteine contributes to the structure of proteins, in the form of cystine. (Cystine is created when two molecules of cysteine bond together; the two amino acids can for most purpose be considered as the same). It also plays a role in energy metabolism and can be converted to glucose if necessary. Cysteine supply may be a limiting factor for white blood cell (lymphocyte) function. Research has shown that cysteine supply is impaired in a number of conditions associated with immunodeficiency, including Aids.

In the liver, cysteine is used to form the amino acid glutathione (*which see*) which helps to detoxify potentially harmful substances and free radicals. It is also a precursor of the detoxifying amino acid taurine.

A cysteine deficiency can result in allergic-like chemical sensitivities and in abnormal glucose metabolism, since cysteine is involved in glucose metabolism and holds the insulin molecule together.

Do not supplement cysteine or glutathione in insulin-dependent diabetes because cysteine acts as a coenzyme for insulin degeneration.

Vegetarian sources: Weight for weight, soya protein concentrates, almonds, sesame seeds and walnuts are as rich in cysteine as animal proteins.

Availability of supplements: N-acetyl cysteine (*which see*) is becoming the preferred form of cysteine supplementation, and is available in health food shops or through practitioners. As a detoxification aid, the suggested dose is about 1 gram per day.

Cystine (see Cysteine)

Cytochrome P450 oxidase
(see Detoxification)

D

Vitamin D (Calciferol)

Vitamin (fat-soluble)
UK RNI None
US RDA 5 mcg (200 iu)

FUNCTIONS

Absorption of magnesium, iron, calcium, zinc
and other minerals
Bone health
Calcium metabolism
Kidney metabolism
Cell differentiation

GOOD FOOD SOURCES

Butter
Cod liver oil
Halibut liver oil
Herrings
Kippers
Mackerel
Salmon
Sardines
Tuna

Deficiency symptoms

- Osteoporosis or osteomalacia in adults: loss of bone minerals with bone pain and tenderness, brittle bones, weakness of some muscles (e.g. in climbing stairs), waddling gait, deafness.
- Rickets in children: softening and deformity of the bones, bowed legs, knee pains and poor growth.

Preventing deficiency

Vitamin D can be produced in the body from the action of sunlight on the skin, therefore when exposure to the sun is sufficient, dietary sources of vitamin D are not required. Most individuals obtain dietary vitamin D from dairy produce and eggs, or from margarine (to which vitamin D is artificially added by law in many countries). Vegans living in cold climates should take particular care not to become deficient in vitamin D and it may be best to err on the side of caution and take vitamin D supplements during the winter months. This especially applies to dark-skinned people, who have a reduced ability to produce vitamin D from sunlight. Uncovering the skin when outdoors allows the body to absorb more sunlight to make vitamin D. So-called 'heavy' metals (*which see*) can block the synthesis of active vitamin D by the kidneys.

Non-vegetarians who avoid dairy produce should instead regularly eat oily fish such as herrings, mackerel and salmon.

The bioavailability (*which see*) of vitamin D decreases in the elderly. Malabsorption of dietary fats can result in vitamin D deficiency. Vitamin D absorption is enhanced by the consumption of fat or oil along with the vitamin.

Comments

Vitamin D_3 (cholecalciferol) is the natural form of vitamin D, found in food and is produced in the body. Vitamin D_2 (ergocalciferol), which is often used in supplementation products, is artificially produced.

Supplementation

In research studies, vitamin D supplements have been found to:

- Clear psoriasis (D_3 form only, when applied to the skin and taken orally)
- Improve bone density in osteoporosis
- Improve calcium absorption in the elderly
- Inhibit the growth of some tumours
- Reverse some cases of hearing loss
- Together with calcium, help treat migraine

Preferred form and suggested Intake
For most purposes, natural cod liver oil 1 teaspoon daily (which provides 360 iu or 9 mcg of vitamin D) is sufficient and popular. However, some cod liver oil products were found in a recent survey to be contaminated with pesticides. Products consumed should have a manufacturer's quality control guarantee of low pesticide levels.

Cautions
Although the body is unlikely to make excessive vitamin D from exposure to sunlight, orally ingested vitamin D can build up to toxic levels if heavily over-supplemented. Toxic effects can include high blood pressure, irregular heartbeat, nausea and vomiting, seizures, hardening of the arteries and kidney damage.

Dandelion

Herb

Dandelion is one of the oldest medicinal herbs. Both root and leaf can be used, or the juice extracted from the fresh plant. The root acts as a gentle liver cleansing tonic, promoting bile flow. It may be purchased as 'dandelion coffee', either in instant granules or as dried root pieces. The leaves are more often used as a diuretic, and are eaten fresh in salad or dried and made into a tea.

Because of its liver-draining effects, helping to clear toxins from the body, dandelion is useful in chronic rheumatic or arthritic conditions.

In the Chinese classification system, dandelion is a 'cold bitter' which means that it is best applied in conditions of excessive vitality and avoided in any conditions involving coldness, such as depressed circulation or low metabolic rate, frequent urination or chronic respiratory congestion.

Deoxyribonucleic acid (see DNA)

Detoxification

One of the body's most vital functions is to convert metabolic products and toxins into soluble, safe substances which can then be eliminated via the urine or via the gall-bladder into the intestines. The liver plays an all-important role in this process, which is known as detoxification or *biotransformation*.

Recent research has shown that many patients with chronic fatigue syndrome or ME have a disordered liver biotransformation ability. We simply don't know what other diseases and health disorders may be promoted by a toxic overload resulting from such dysfunction, but progress is beginning to be made in looking at specific detoxification pathways and relating underfunctioning of these to the development of diseases like parkinsonism, motor neurone disease (also known as ALS) and Alzheimer's disease.

A number of biochemical pathways are involved in liver biotransformation. These are normally grouped into oxidation, reduction or hydrolysis reactions (Phase I) and conjugation reactions (Phase II).

Phase I detoxification

Phase I reactions, which are catalysed by a group of liver microsomal enzymes known as cytochrome P450 oxidases, introduce oxygen into the structure of toxins or metabolites. Typically the toxins are converted to alcohols and aldehydes by this process, then into acids, which are water-soluble and can be excreted via the urine.

The intermediate substances created during Phase I detoxification, which include reactive oxygen species (free radicals), can be extremely toxic – far more so than the original toxins. Their harmful effects are primarily controlled by antioxidant nutrients and enzymes, therefore a plentiful supply of these substances is essential. Apart from free radicals, other intermediate metabolites include epoxides, chloral hydrate (which is identical to the knock-out drug often known as the 'Mickey Finn') and endogenous benzodiazepines – substances similar to Valium and other tranquillizers and sleeping pills. This makes it easier to understand how chronic fatigue can develop when a toxic overload is present.

The more P450 enzymes have to be induced, the more toxic intermediates will be present in the human body. These enzymes are induced by caffeine, alcohol, dioxin and other pollutants, exhaust fumes, high-protein diets, oranges and tangerines, organophosphorus pesticides, paint fumes, steroid hormones, and a variety of drugs including paracetamol (acetaminophen), diazepam tranquillizers and sleeping pills, the contraceptive pill and cortisone. Substances which can inhibit P450 enzymes include carbon tetrachloride, carbon monoxide, barbiturates, quercetin and naringenin (found in grapefruit). The oxidation reaction can also be blocked by an excess of toxic chemicals, a lack of enzymes, lack of nutrients and/or loss of oxygen. Such blocking results in a build-up of more toxic substances such as formaldehyde and other aldehydes in the target tissue. This can in turn lead to a spreading phenomenon, with increasing sensitivity to more chemicals such as ketones and alcohols, and eventually even to natural chemicals occurring in foods, pollen and mould. A build-up of aldehydes can in severe cases lead to tissue crosslinking, causing vasculitis with possible seizures and brain damage.

Intestinal overgrowth with *Candida albicans*, as well as the peroxidation of polyunsaturated fats, are known sources of aldehydes. The fatigue, foggy thinking and 'brain fag' linked with candidiasis may be due to an overloading of the detoxification system with aldehydes, which can even lead to a reverse reaction of aldehyde to alcohol. Extreme intolerance to alcohol consumption may occur in these individuals, as it does in those diagnosed with ME or chronic fatigue syndrome.

Although most aldehydes in the body are thought to occur as intermediate metabolites, external sources include exposure to formaldehyde gas (which is given off by new carpets, curtains and other furnishings) and breakdown products of ethylene glycol and methanol.

Cytochrome P450 and other oxidizing enzymes also oxidize amines such as phenylethylamine found in chocolate, tyramine found in cheese, and catecholamines (*which see*) (adrenaline, noradrenaline and dopamine). These are oxidized into aldehydes by mitochondrial monoamine oxidase (MAO). If this enzyme is blocked, for instance by MAO inhibitor drugs used to treat depression, tyramine, for instance, cannot be metabolized and hypertension can develop as a chemical sensitivity reaction.

Phase II detoxification (conjugation)

There are five main conjugation categories, including acetylation, acylation (peptide conjugation with amino acids), sulphur conjugations, methylations and conjugation with glucuronic acid. Some substances enter Phase II detoxification directly, others come via Phase I pathways. Conjugation involves the combining of a metabolite or toxin with another substance which adds a polar hydrophilic molecule to it, converting lipophilic substances to water-soluble forms for excretion and elimination. Individual xenobiotics and metabolites usually follow a specific path, so whereas caffeine is metabolized by P450 enzymes, aspirin-based medications are conjugated with glycine, and paracetamol with sulphate.

Acetylation
Acetylation requires pantothenic acid to function. It is the chief degradation pathway for compounds containing aromatic amines such as histamine, serotonin, PABA, P-amino salicylic acid, aniline and procaine amide. It is also a pathway for sulphur amides, aliphatic amines and complex hydrazines.

A proportion of the general population – perhaps up to 50 per cent – are slow acetylators. This rises to as high a level as 80 per cent among the chemically sensitive population. Their N-acetyltransferase activity is thought to be reduced, and this prolongs the action of drugs and other toxic chemicals, thus enhancing their toxicity.

Acylation
Acylation uses acyl CO-A with the amino acids glycine, glutamine and taurine. Conjugation of bile acids in the liver with glycine or taurine is essential for the efficient removal of these potentially toxic compounds. Disturbed acylation by pollutant overload decreases proper levels of bile in the gastrointestinal tract, resulting in poor assimilation of lipids and fat-soluble vitamins, and disturbed cholesterol metabolism.

Toluene, the most popular industrial organic solvent, is converted by the liver into benzoate, which, like aspirin and other salicylates, must then be detoxified by conjugation with the amino acid glycine (glycination). Large doses of glycine and N-glycylglycine are used in treating aspirin overdose. Benzoate is present in many food substances and is widely used as a food preservative.

Glycine is a commonly available amino acid, but the capacity to synthesize taurine may be limited by low activity of the enzyme cysteine-sulfinic acid decarboxylase. Damage can occur to this enzyme directly by pollutants, or by overload/overuse resulting in depletion.

Both taurine- and glycine-dependent reactions require an alkaline pH: 7.8 to 8.0. Environmental medicine specialists may alkalinize over-acidic patients by administering sodium and potassium bicarbonate in order to facilitate these reactions.

Glutathione conjugation, using the amino acid glutathione in its reduced form, is used for the transformation of xenobiotics such as aromatic disulphides, naphthalene, anthracene, phenanthacin compounds, aliphatic disulphides and the regeneration of endogenous thiols from disulphides. There is a cycle of replenishment for glutathione, allowing it to be reformed after conversion to glutathione reductase. Heavy metals can inhibit this cycle, thus preventing replenishment.

Sulphate conjugation (sulphation)

Neurotransmitters, steroid hormones, certain drugs and many xenobiotic and phenolic compounds such as oestrone, aliphatic alcohols, aryl amines and alicyclic hydroxysteroids employ sulphation as their primary route of detoxification. Steventon at Birmingham University (UK) has found that many sufferers from parkinsonism, motor neurone disease and Alzheimer's disease as well as environmental illness, tend to have a reduced ability to produce sulphate from the amino acid cysteine in their body, and instead accumulate cysteine. Sulphate may be ingested from food, but is also produced by the action of the enzyme cysteine dioxygenase on cysteine. This process is known as sulphoxidation. The body's ability to conjugate toxins with sulphate is 'rate limited' by the amount of sulphate present; if there is inadequate sulphate, toxins and metabolites can accumulate, perhaps building up to levels which cause degeneration of nervous tissue after several decades. Steventon's findings are a matter for serious concern. How many individuals are given the opportunity to find out whether they are poor sulphoxidizers and to reduce their chances of developing the above mentioned diseases by improving their sulphoxidation ability?

Large doses of N-acetyl-cysteine (NAC) are a standard treatment for paracetamol overdose.

Methylation

According to environmental medicine specialist William Rae, the process most often disturbed in the chemically sensitive involves methylation reactions catalysed by S-adenosyl-L-methionine-dependent enzymes. Methionine is the chief methyl donor to detoxify amines, phenols, thiols, noradrenaline, adrenaline, dopamine, melatonin, L-dopa, histamine, serotonin, pyridine, sulphites and hypochlorites into compounds excreted through the lungs. Methionine is needed to detoxify the hypochlorite reaction. The activity of the methyltransferase enzyme is dependent on magnesium, and, due to the frequency of magnesium deficiency, supplementation with this nutrient will often stabilize chemically sensitive patients.

Glucuronidation

Glucuronic acid is a metabolite of glucose. It can conjugate with chemical and bacterial toxins such as alcohols, phenols, enols, carboxylic acid, amines, hydroxyamines, carbamides, sulphonamides and thiols, as well as some normal metabolites in a process known as glucuronidation. For most individuals glucuronidation is a supplementary detoxification pathway. It is a secondary, slower process than sulphation or glycination, but is important if the latter pathways are diminished or saturated. Obese people seem to have an enhanced capacity to detoxify molecules that can use the glucuronidation pathway. However, damage to the capacity for oxidative phosphorylation, which takes place in the mitochondria, is likely to diminish the capacity for glucuronide conjugation.

If the liver's detoxification pathways are excessively stimulated and overly utilized, they eventually become depleted or begin to respond poorly – being suppressed by toxic chemicals. Once breakdown of the main pathways occurs as a result of pollutant overload, toxins are shunted to lesser pathways, eventually overloading them, and disturbing orderly nutrient metabolism.

Chemical sensitivity may then occur, followed by nutrient depletion and finally fixed-name disease.

Interesting facts

- Dr William Rae of the Environmental Health Centre in Dallas says that the most severely ill chemically-sensitive patients not only have abnormally low antipollutant enzymes in addition to toxic suppression and nutrient depletion, but in some instances antibodies are produced against cytochrome P450 and these may inhibit or decrease its effectiveness.
- Environmental medicine specialists have found that almost 35 per cent of chemically sensitive patients are deficient in intracellular sulphur. Not only can this hinder the detoxification of some sulphur-containing and other toxic chemicals, it can enhance the harmful effects of exposure to cyanide from foods such as cassava and almonds as well as from tobacco products. The hereditary disease known as Leber's optic atrophy involves a genetic defect in the ability to detoxify cyanide, and leads to sudden, permanent blindness on first exposure to cyanide in small amounts such as those ingested from smoking cigarettes.
- Many practitioner multimineral supplements in the UK omit iron and copper due to theories that individuals may already be overloaded with these nutrients. However, if no overload is present, an unbalanced supplement may promote depletion of the minerals. The Environmental Health Centre in Dallas finds that intravenous infusions to replenish iron stores brings dramatic improvements for the chemically sensitive patient as part of their detoxification process. Copper is also found to help catalyse the cytochrome systems. (*NB*: self-supplementation with iron and copper should be cautious, to avoid iron and copper overload conditions).
- Although the liver microsomal system is the primary site for oxidation of xenobiotics, the cytochrome P450 system is found in other tissues that are exposed to environmental compounds like the skin, lungs, gastrointestinal tract, kidneys, placenta, corpus luteum, lymphocytes, monocytes, pulmonary alveolar macrophages, adrenals, testes and brain, in both the mitochondria and in the nuclear membrane.
- Always rinse your washing-up carefully. Pollutants in the form of solvents and detergents can damage and penetrate the cell membrane and damage the contents of the cell.
- Vitamin B_3 has been shown to accelerate the clearance of aldehydes in some chemically sensitive patients.
- Molybdenum, although an essential element, competes with sulphate in its activation step to the important enzyme PAPS and can thus lower sulphate levels and impair sulphation ability. Environmental medicine experts warn that molybdenum supplementation may be contraindicated in individuals with poor sulphation ability.
- The substance naringenin, found in grapefruit, can significantly inhibit Phase I detoxification, as can grapefruit itself. This may prove clinically useful in some situations where Phase I activity is too high (as shown in liver function tests available from nutritional therapists).
- Persons who have been exposed to toxic chemicals, drugs and other xenobiotics (foreign substances), have increased requirements for some vitamins. Functional nutritional assays for vitamins B_1, B_2, B_3, B_6, B_{12} and folate, and

serum levels of vitamins A, D, C and beta-carotene were performed in a random sample of 333 environmentally-sensitive patients prior to treatment. 57.8 per cent were found to be deficient in B_6, 37.7 per cent in vitamin D, 34.9 per cent in B_2, 32.2 per cent in folate, 27.7 per cent in vitamin C, 21.4 per cent in niacin, 14.9 per cent in B_{12}, 5.6 per cent in vitamin A and 4.6 per cent in beta-carotene. (*Ross GH et al.: Evidence for vitamin deficiencies in environmentally-sensitive patients. Clinical Ecology 6(2):60-6, 1989.*)

Foods to aid detoxification

- Beetroot: helps with liver drainage
- Broccoli, cauliflower and other cruciferous vegetables: these aid cytochrome P450 activity
- Protein
- Radish, watercress: rich in sulphur

Supplements to aid liver detoxification

- B complex vitamins
- Digestive enzymes: may be necessary to ensure that protein is adequately digested and glycine is readily available
- Essential fatty acids
- N-acetyl cysteine (NAC)
- Reduced glutathione
- Selenium, zinc, magnesium and manganese; possibly iron and copper if used with caution
- Taurine (a useful combination product is magnesium taurate)
- Vitamins C and E and beta-carotene

Liver herbs to aid detoxification (traditionally known as 'blood-cleansing' herbs)

- Dandelion root: cholagogue (stimulates liver secretions and bile flow)
- Globe artichoke leaf: promotes regeneration of the liver and promotes blood flow in that organ
- Silymarin (*which see*): according to recent research, this herbal extract stabilizes the membranes of liver cells, preventing the entry of virus toxins and other toxic compounds including drugs. Promotes regeneration of the liver.
- Turmeric: a cholagogue like dandelion, but may irritate the gastric mucosa. Its advantages are its cheapness and ability to be used in cookery.

These herbs are best combined with wild yam, which helps to prevent liver spasms caused by gall-bladder stimulating herbs. (*Also see Secondary plant metabolites.*)

Dextrose (see Sugars)

DGLA Dihomo-gamma linolenic acid (see Fats)

DHA Docosahexaenoic acid (see Fats)

DHEA (dehydroepiandrosterone)

A hormone secreted by the adrenal glands, and sold as an anti-ageing supplement, mainly in the US. By the age of 40 DHEA production drops to half the level produced at the age of 20. Benefits claimed for DHEA include effects against adult-onset diabetes, atherosclerosis, Parkinson's and Alzheimer's diseases and auto-immune diseases such as multiple sclerosis and lupus.

DHEA should not be used by those at risk of prostate enlargement as it may cause increased dihydrotestosterone levels, which would exacerbate the problem.

Availability: In US health food shops and through practitioners. In the UK, DHEA is classed as a licensable medicine.

Dietary fibre

That portion of our diet which is not broken down by our digestive enzymes and does not therefore serve as a (direct) source of nutrients. Also known as non-starch

Types of fibre			
Cellulose	Insoluble	Less digestible by bacteria. Adsorbs bile acids and cholesterol.	Found in plant cell walls (eg leafy vegetables, peas, beans, wheat bran).
Gums	Soluble	Can be digested by bacteria. Adsorb bile acids and cholesterol. Retard the rate of absorption of simple sugars from the small intestine.	Found in seeds and plant secretions. May be used as food additives.
Hemicellulose	Insoluble	Less digestible by bacteria. Adsorbs bile acids and cholesterol.	Found in plant cell walls.
Inulin	Soluble		Can be digested by bacteria. Found in Jerusalem artichokes.
Lignins	Insoluble	Less digestible by bacteria. Adsorb bile acids and cholesterol.	Found in bran.
Mannosans, raffinose, stachyose, verbacose	Soluble	Can be digested by bacteria.	Found in pulses.
Mucilages	Soluble	Can be digested by bacteria.	Found in seeds (e.g. psyllium) and seaweeds.
Pectins	Soluble	Can be digested by bacteria. Adsorb bile acids and cholesterol. Retard the rate of absorption of simple sugars from the small intestine.	Found in fruit and vegetables, especially apples and the white part of citrus fruit.

polysaccharides. Fibre is not, as is often thought, calorie-free; bacteria digest soluble fibre to form short-chain fatty acids, principally acetate, propionate and butyrate, which are used as energy sources for the intestinal lining (mucosa) and can also be absorbed into the bloodstream.

Dietary fibre holds water and thus softens the stools and adds bulk, assisting stool propulsion (peristalsis) and evacuation. Diets low in fibre promote constipation.

To prevent a deficiency of dietary fibre, a variety of whole grains, nuts, pulses, root vegetables and fruit should be consumed daily.

Dietary Reference Values

Three sets of figures used to assess the adequacy of diets for populations. The first set of figures is the *Reference Nutrient Intake* (RNI) which represents the amount of a nutrient that is deemed by a country's government to be sufficient to meet the needs of practically all healthy people – even those with higher than normal needs. In the UK it is roughly equivalent to the old Recommended Daily Amount (RDA) which was formerly the only set of figures used.

The *Estimated Average Requirement* (EAR) represents the amount of a nutrient that is deemed sufficient to meet the needs of the average individual. Dietitians are taught that if a group of people are consuming these levels of nutrients, they are unlikely to develop nutritional deficiencies. According to a spokesperson for the British Dietetic Association, meals in institutions will, generally speaking, be considered adequate if they achieve vitamin and mineral levels between the RNI and the EAR.

Finally, the Lower Reference Nutrient Intake (LRNI) represents an amount of a nutrient that is virtually certain to be inadequate. (The average intake of the trace

element selenium in the UK falls well below this figure).

See Appendix III for UK and US Dietary Reference Values for different nutrients.

Dietary supplements

Preparations of vitamins, minerals, amino acids, essential fatty acids, enzymes, fibre and other factors which fulfil a useful or necessary physiological function and are found in food or synthesized within the body from food. These preparations may be chemically synthesized or natural extracts. Dietary supplements can also be concentrated plant- or animal-source preparations such as fish oils, yeast, probiotics, algae and plant or herb extracts, used to supplement the diet with the nutrients they contain, or for their health-giving properties.

Digestion

The process whereby food is broken down by digestive juices to enable nutrients to be absorbed into the blood and lymphatic system and used for energy, growth and repair.

The digestive process begins in the mouth, with chewing of the food and mixing with saliva, which contains the enzyme salivary amylase that begins the breakdown of starch. Once the food is swallowed and reaches the stomach, it is mixed with acid and pepsin, which begins the breakdown of protein in the food.

When food leaves the stomach it is in the form of a thick creamy liquid called chyme, and is very acidic. As chyme leaves the stomach and enters the duodenum (the first part of the small intestine) its acidity stimulates the liver and pancreas to release bicarbonate, which changes the pH of the chyme, making it alkaline. This alkalinity is necessary for the next stage of digestion, using enzymes secreted mainly by the pancreas but also by the small intestine itself. The pancreas contributes lipase for fat (lipid) digestion, amylase for starch digestion, and protease for protein digestion. Bile released by the gall-bladder emulsifies fat particles, enabling pancreatic enzymes to work on them more easily.

Once digested, the nutrients from the food, including vitamins and minerals, are absorbed into the cells which line the small intestine. Finger-like projections called

---

Substances which aid digestion

Produced by	Name	Action
The saliva glands in the mouth	Salivary amylase, also known as ptyalin	Begins to break down starch
The stomach	Gastrin (gastric juice)	Hormone stimulating the production of gastric juice
	Hydrochloric acid	Kills microbes, solubilizes protein
	Pepsin	Enzyme which begins protein breakdown
The liver and gall bladder	Bicarbonate	Neutralizes acid coming from the stomach
	Bile salts	Emulsify fats
The pancreas	Aminopeptidase and carboxypeptidase	Enzymes required for the final stages of protein digestion
	Amylase	Carbohydrate digesting enzyme
	Bicarbonate	Neutralizes acid coming from the stomach
	Lipase	Fat digesting enzyme
	Proteases (trypsin and chymotrypsin)	Protein digesting enzymes
Small intestine	Carboxypeptidase	Enzyme required for final stages of protein digestion
	Cholecystokinin	Hormone stimulating the gall-bladder to release bile
	Disaccharidases (sucrase, lactase, maltase)	Enzymes needed to split disaccharides to simple sugars (see Carbohydrate)
	Gastric-inhibitory peptide	Hormone slowing the production of gastric juices and gastrointestinal motility
	Secretin	Hormone stimulating the production of pancreative juice

'villi' increase the surface area of the small intestine approximately to the size of a tennis court, thus optimizing absorption. Fatty substances pass into the lymphatic system, only entering the bloodstream after they have travelled up to the large veins in the neck. Other substances are absorbed into the blood and carried straight to the liver for processing, after which nutrients are distributed and taken up (assimilated) by the cells of the body's various tissues.

Dimethylglycine (DMG)
(see Vitamin B₁₅)

Disaccharides
(see Carbohydrates)

Diuretic

A substance that increases the flow of urine.

DLPA (DL-phenylalanine)
(see Phenylalanine)

DMG
(see Vitamin B₁₅)

DNA (see Nucleic acids)

Dolomite

Mineral

A rock similar to limestone (chalk) but containing more magnesium. Dolomite consists of calcium magnesium carbonate. Often sold as a dietary supplement, but poorly absorbed by those with reduced stomach acidity or when taken on an empty stomach. The manufacturer's quality control should guarantee that the product is not contaminated with lead.

Dong quai

Herb

Also known as dang gui, the Latin name for this herb is *Angelica sinensis*. Dong quai is a Chinese herb, known as one of the great nourishing blood tonics and often used to help regulate the menstrual cycle, ease period pain or improve weakness after childbirth.
  Availability: From health food shops.

Dopamine (see Catecholamines)

Double-blind clinical trials

In single-blind clinical trials, the researcher knows whether the patient has been given the active treatment or the placebo (dummy) treatment but the patient does not. In double-blind trials neither the patient nor the researcher knows.

Dysbiosis

A state of imbalance of the intestinal flora (bacteria and other micro-organisms), which may lead to excessive bacterial fermentation in the gut and 'autointoxication' from endotoxins (toxins produced by undesirable bacteria within the body). In the 1980s an increasing number of reports began to be published about injury to intestinal cells by intestinal bacterial toxins. Bacterial growth appears to destroy enzymes (such as the disaccharidases which are needed to digest sugars) on the intestinal cell surface, thus preventing carbohydrate digestion and absorption, and making carbohydrates available for bacterial fermentation. Excess mucus may then be triggered as the intestine attempts to flush out the microbial toxins and acidic by-products, and the partially digested, unabsorbed carbohydrates. The result may be chronic diarrhoea or 'mucus colitis'.

Dysbiosis is promoted by the consumption of antibiotics, which destroy 'friendly' (useful) bacteria such as lactobacilli and bifidobacteria much more readily than undesirable putrefactive varieties such as *E coli* and Clostridium. A reduced ability to produce gastric acid may also lead to an overgrowth of bacteria in the small intestine. Such an overgrowth may promote nutrient malabsorption, particularly that of vitamin B_{12}.

One particularly common form of dysbiosis is known as candidiasis, where the intestinal tract becomes colonized by the yeast *Candida albicans* (*which see*).

Natural medicine practitioners treat dysbiosis and conditions promoted by autointoxication, by using herbal anti-microbials, gut healing products, and probiotics (*which see*) together with an appropriate dietary programme.

E

Vitamin E (Tocopherol)

Vitamin (fat-soluble)
UK RNI None
US RDA 10 mg (15 iu)

FUNCTIONS

Antioxidant, especially combating peroxidation
of unsaturated fats in cell membranes
Development and maintenance of nerve and
muscle function
Fertility
Immunity
Preventing photooxidative damage to eye lens
Prostaglandin modulation
Red cell membrane stability
Reduces oxygen needs of muscles
Spares vitamin A

GOOD FOOD SOURCES

Almonds
Butter
Leafy green vegetables
Oats
Peanuts
Soya oil
Sunflower oil and seeds
Wheat germ and wheat germ oil
Whole grains

Deficiency signs and symptoms

- Age spots (accumulation of lipofuscin)
- Cataracts
- Damage to cell membranes
- Increased red cell fragility and haemorrhaging
- Infertility
- Muscle weakness
- Neuromuscular damage
- Possibly auto-immune diseases (*see Section II Lupus erythematosus*)

Preventing deficiency

Many countries make the replacement of some of the lost B vitamins compulsory in products made from refined (white) flour, since the B vitamins are, like vitamin E, mostly found in the germ of the flour, not in the white, starchy portion. Unfortunately vitamin E is not replaced in this way although 92 per cent of vitamin E in wheat is lost when flour is refined, and most of the rest is destroyed by bleaching.

Cooking food in fats destroys 70 to 90 per cent of the fats' vitamin E content, especially when the fats are old or rancid. Boiling destroys about one third of the vitamin E in carrots, cabbages and brussels sprouts. The storage of foods, even when frozen, can result in heavy vitamin E losses, e.g. frozen French fries can lose up to 74 per cent after two months' storage. Two thirds of the vitamin E can be lost during the production of commercial vegetable oils. Fat malabsorption causes deficiency.

Vitamin E needs are related to the intake of polyunsaturated fats because vitamin E is used up in the process of preventing their oxidation. The bioavailability (*which see*) of vitamin E is decreased by an excessive intake of polyunsaturated fats.

Vitamin C and the amino acid glutathione have a sparing effect on vitamin E.

Smoking can lead to a vitamin E deficiency (*Pacht ER et al.: Deficiency of vitamin E in the alveolar fluid of cigarette smokers. Influence on alveolar macrophage cytotoxicity. J Clin Invest 77(3):789-96, 1986*). Levels of vitamin E are also significantly lower in users of the contraceptive pill (*Tangney CC et al.: Vitamin E status of young women on combined-type oral contraceptives. Contraception 17(6):499-512, 1978.*)

Comments

Vitamin E is one of a group of nutrients known as tocopherols. The tocopherol with the greatest vitamin E activity is thought to be alpha-tocopherol, but as yet we know very little about the roles of the other tocopherols in health, and it cannot be assumed that they are without value. Tocopherols are found in conjunction with plant oils, especially those with polyunsaturated oils, and are concentrated in the germ.

Severe vitamin E deficiency has marked similarities to two diseases: muscular dystrophy and myasthenia gravis, which both involve increasing muscle weakness and dysfunction. Other symptoms of these diseases which also occur in vitamin E deficiency include lipofuscin deposits (*which see*), low plasma vitamin E concentrations, creatinuria, and increased plasma creatine phosphokinase activity (all indicative of muscle cell damage). The same symptomatology is also seen in conditions where there is intestinal malabsorption of fat: cystic fibrosis of the pancreas, biliary atresia or cirrhosis, sprue and chronic pancreatitis.

Supplementation

In research studies, vitamin E supplements have been found to:

- Delay the progress of Parkinson's disease
- Enhance a variety of immune system responses
- Halve the risk of heart attack in those with heart disease
- Heal some cases of gangrene
- Help heal sunburn when applied directly to the skin
- Help reduce tardive dyskinesia (jerky movements) in patients taking anti-schizophrenic drugs
- Improve epileptic seizure control
- Improve macular degeneration of the eyes
- Improve mobility and reduce pain in osteoarthritis
- Improve premenstrual syndrome
- Improve systemic lupus erythematosus
- Increase levels of HDL ('good') cholesterol
- Inhibit platelet adhesiveness (blood stickiness)
- Prevent cataracts
- Reduce capillary fragility and hyperpermeability
- Reduce some complications of diabetes and enhance insulin action
- Reduce liver damage from carbon tetrachloride
- Reduce pain from shingles as well as other types of chronic pain
- Reduce scars when applied directly to the skin
- Reduce the harmful effects of inhaling ozone, nitrogen oxides and other constituents of smog or cigarette smoke
- Reduce the incidence of mammary tumours in experimental animals
- Reduce the number of irreversibly sickled cells in sickle cell anaemia
- Suppress the formation of faecal mutagens

- Treat cystic breast disease and mammary dysplasia
- Treat intermittent claudication (painful condition of the legs in cardiovascular disease)
- Treat menopausal symptoms
- Treat some types of neuropathy
- With selenium, improve muscular dystrophy
- With vitamin A, improve some cases of hearing loss

Preferred form and suggested intake

Although vitamin E is available as mixed tocopherols, most supplements consist only of alpha tocopherol, which has the highest vitamin E activity. For preventive health purposes 100–200 iu a day is probably more than adequate. For longstanding symptoms thought to be related to vitamin E deficiency, up to 1,000 iu can be taken safely by most individuals.

Cautions

Do not take vitamin E supplements without a doctor's advice if you are taking anti-coagulant drugs, since vitamin E can itself act as an anti-coagulant (and is probably a much safer anti-coagulant than the pharmaceutical variety). Large amounts of vitamin E can interfere with vitamin K activity.

In some individuals with high blood pressure, beginning vitamin E supplementation may result in a temporary rise in blood pressure. Caution should be applied and blood pressure monitored while vitamin E levels are raised gradually.

Echinacea

Herb

Also known as purple coneflower, echinacea is a well-documented immune system stimulant which activates T and B lymphocytes. It also has marked anti-viral properties. Echinacea enhances resistance, stimulates the lymphatic system, and is often used against colds and flu. It is best taken in small, frequent doses. If used on a long-term basis, take echinacea for only six days a week, or three weeks out of four, since it is more effective if not taken continuously. *Availability*: Health food shops.

EDTA (edetic acid)

This is a substance which forms complexes with lead and other heavy metals and can therefore be used as a chelating agent to combine with and remove these substances from soft tissues in the body.

Availability: From specialist chelation clinics.

Eicosanoids
(see Prostaglandins)

Eicosapentaenoic acid (EPA)
(also see Fats)

The active ingredient in fish oil supplements. EPA can be produced from the essential fatty acid alpha linolenic acid in the body, and is then used to form series 3 prostaglandins and leukotrienes. It also forms a structural part of cell membranes.

Oily fish provide a rich source of ready-formed EPA.

Fish oil supplements have become popular with individuals seeking to prevent and treat heart disease. Studies have shown that populations (mainly Eskimos) who consume particularly large amounts of EPA suffer very low rates of heart disease despite their high-fat, high-cholesterol diet. It is now thought that this is due to EPA's ability to reduce platelet adhesiveness (thus reducing the blood's tendency to clot), very low density lipoprotein (VLDL) levels, plasma triglycerides, and the synthesis of cholesterol by the liver.

Availability: Health food shops and pharmacies.

Elderberry

Herb

Elderberries are not often sold as a herbal product, but can be picked in the wild in Europe (in the autumn) and are often made into wine. They have limited use as a herb, and can cause nausea if consumed in large quantities. They also have a mildly laxative action. Elderberry juice or purée consumed regularly is considered to be a good remedy for chronic rheumatism, neuralgia and sciatica.

Electrolytes

Electrically charged elements or compounds found in blood plasma and fluids occurring inside and between cells.

Positively charged electrolytes are known as anions and negatively charged electrolytes are known as cations. The correct quantities and proportions of the main electrolytes are critical for normal metabolism and function, for maintaining the body's acid/alkaline balance and the water balance inside and outside cells, transmission of nerve impulses and the contraction and relaxation of muscles. Potassium can be seriously depleted by diuretics, certain other drugs, or by the over-consumption of liquorice. Sodium can be depleted by very low-sodium diets used against high blood pressure, and by profuse sweating. Severe diarrhoea can cause depletion of all electrolytes *(see table below)*.

Endocrine system

The network of glands which secrete hormones directly into the bloodstream, affecting the function of specific target organs. Endocrine glands include the thyroid and parathyroid, the pituitary, pancreas, adrenal glands, gonads (sex glands) and pineal gland. (*See Hormones*)

Electrolytes

Anions	Mainly found	Cations	Mainly found
Chloride (Cl-)	Outside cells	Sodium (Na+)	Outside cells
Bicarbonate (HCO3-)	Outside cells	Calcium (Ca++)	Outside cells
Phosphate (PO4=)	Inside cells	Potassium (K+)	Inside cells
Sulphate (SO4=)	Inside cells	Magnesium (Mg++)	Inside cells

Endotoxins

Poisons produced within bacterial cells. Endotoxins can be absorbed from the gut into the bloodstream, adding to the body's overall toxic load. If the individual's gut is chronically overloaded with unfavourable bacteria at the expense of the so-called 'friendly' bacteria (mainly Lactobacilli and Bifidobacteria), endotoxin levels can represent a significant challenge to the liver's detoxification capacity. Endotoxins produced by an acute infection from pathogenic (disease-producing) bacteria such as Salmonella can be life-threatening.

Energy production (also see Carbohydrates and Blood sugar)

The raw material of energy is glucose, which can be obtained by eating sugars and starches in the diet, or from stored sugar (glycogen). The liver can convert glycerol (from fat), and some of the amino acids into glucose.

Glycolysis is the first pathway involved in converting glucose into energy, and, like all the energy-producing reactions, takes place in a part of the cell known as the mitochondrion. Unlike the Krebs cycle and oxidative phosphorylation, glycolysis requires no oxygen, and can even produce a little energy itself (two molecules of the 'energy currency' known as ATP – adenosine triphosphate – for every one molecule of glucose). So as well as starting off the rest of the process, glycolysis is important when the oxygen supply to the body is inadequate – as for instance under intense exercising conditions when exertion exceeds the capacity of the heart and lungs to clear carbon dioxide from the muscles.

In glycolysis a phosphate molecule is attached to glucose, producing glucose-6-phosphate. A series of chemical reactions then takes place, resulting in the production of pyruvate. If enough oxygen is present, pyruvate can then form acetyl CoA (*which see*), which then enters the next pathway, known as the Krebs cycle, citric acid cycle or tricarboxylic acid (TCA) cycle. If oxygen is in short supply, pyruvate is instead converted to lactic acid, which accumulates until oxygen becomes available and can then be converted back to pyruvate or can enter the Cori cycle (*which see*) to be converted back to glucose. Lactic acid accumulation in the muscles causes the burning pain normally associated with over-exertion. Glycolysis is dependent on vitamin B_3, which it uses in its coenzyme form known as NAD.

The Krebs cycle consists of a complex series of chemical reactions which use oxygen, the vitamin B_5-dependent CoA, and vitamins B_1, B_2 and B_3 (in their coenzyme forms TPP, FAD and NAD) to gradually convert acetyl CoA to carbon dioxide and water, releasing electrons in the process.

The final pathway in energy production is known as oxidative phosphorylation, using the 'electron transport chain'. This chain is a series of proteins mounted in sequence on a membrane inside the mitochondria. These proteins receive the electrons released by the Krebs cycle, and pass them to one another, releasing a little energy at each step of this process. Some of the energy is released as heat, and some as ATP molecules. When all the energy has been released, the remaining hydrogen atoms are combined with oxygen to form water.

One of the molecules involved in oxidative phosphorylation is coenzyme Q10 (*which see*), often taken as a dietary supplement to assist energy production.

If glucose is not available for use as fuel, the body can use fatty acids to form acetyl CoA. Some amino acids can form pyruvate or acetyl CoA, or can even enter the Krebs cycle directly.

Environmental medicine

A branch of medicine concerned with maladaptive or allergic reactions to food, air and water. Formerly known as *clinical ecology*. As environmental medicine expert Dr Richard Mackarness said:

> As pollution of our environment grows, so more and more of us are becoming ill in mysterious ways attributable to an inability to adapt and stay healthy in our increasingly contaminated chemical environment.
>
> (*Chemical Victims*, Pan Books, 1980)

Practitioners of environmental medicine use nutritional detoxification techniques to improve the individual's ability to adapt to their environment, thus resulting in relief from many chronic conditions. Conditions which may respond to these techniques include Gulf War syndrome, chronic fatigue syndrome, multiple allergy syndrome, chemical sensitivity, failure of children to thrive, and fixed-name diseases such as migraine, epilepsy, rheumatoid arthritis, hypothyroidism, asthma and eczema.

Enzymes

Proteins produced by living cells which enable metabolic reactions to take place. The best known enzymes are the digestive enzymes which break down food, allowing it to be absorbed by the body. Practically every chemical reaction which takes place in the body requires an enzyme. Names of enzymes are recognizable by ending in '-ase', such as protease, lipase, sucrase, desaturase, synthetase, kinase, oxidase.

The substance which an enzyme works on is known as a *substrate*, and the substance produced by the action of the enzyme is known as a *product*. Enzymes do not themselves undergo any net chemical change during the reaction, rather they *catalyse* (facilitate) reactions.

EPA
(see Eicosapentaenoic acid)

Epinephrine
(see Catecholamines)

Epsom salts

Magnesium sulphate crystals, often sold as a laxative. The laxative effect is produced when enough crystals are dissolved in water to form a strong solution which prevents the normal absorption of water from the intestine. The bowel is stimulated by the increased fluid content, and opens within a few hours.

Erucic acid (also see Fats)

A fatty acid found in large amounts in rape and mustard seed oils, and widely (but mistakenly) thought to be toxic. As reported by nutritionist and oil expert Udo Erasmus PhD, the rat studies which showed fatty degeneration of heart, kidneys and glands after the consumption of erucic acid, were interpreted to mean that erucic acid is also toxic to humans. What was not considered was that sunflower seed oil, which contains no erucic acid, has the same effect on rats, because rats metabolize fats and oils poorly.

Meanwhile a whole industry has grown up around the production of 'low erucic acid' rape seed oil.

Erucic acid has been used to treat a fatal degenerative disease known as adreno-leukodystrophy (ALD) and is sometimes known as 'Lorenzo's oil', after the boy who inspired the development of the treatment.

Essential amino acids (see Amino acids)

Essential oils

Volatile oils which can be distilled or extracted from plants and used for medicinal or cosmetic purposes or as aromatherapy oils. Examples are garlic oil, rosemary oil, peppermint oil and bergamot oil (the latter used to flavour Earl Grey tea).

Essiac

A Native American herbal treatment for cancer discovered by a Canadian nurse René Caisse. (The letters Essiac are her surname spelled backwards). In 1938, after much public lobbying, Essiac came very close to being legalized by the Ontario government as a remedy for terminal cancer patients. Its ingredients are turkey rhubarb (*Rheum palmatum*), burdock root (*Arctium lappa*), the inner bark of slippery elm (*Ulmus fulva*), and sheep sorrel (*Rumex acetosella*). Campaigners who benefited from the treatment believe that organized medicine was responsible for marginalizing it.

Availability: Better known in the US than in the UK. Not widely available but may be made at home by combining the above herbs, or obtained from specialist practitioners and clinics.

Esters

Compounds formed between acids and alcohols.

Estrogen (see Oestrogen)

Ethanolamine phosphate (EAP)

A substance found within the body which can be used as a natural chelator to assist the absorption of minerals from food. (*Also see Chelates*.)

Evening primrose oil (Also see Fats)

The oil of seeds from the evening primrose plant, which yields about 8 to 10 per cent of its fatty acids as gamma linolenic acid (GLA). Evening primrose oil is also rich in linoleic acid.

Excipients

Also known as 'fillers and binders', excipients are additives used in tablet- and capsule-making, which help to bind the active ingredients together, to act as carrier substances, or to 'fill out' a capsule.

F

Fats (also see Adipose tissue)

Also known as lipids, fats are components of the diet and the human or animal body which are insoluble in water but soluble in organic solvents. Fats may be solid or liquid, in which case they are known as oils. Butter, lard, meat fat, oils and margarine are the foods with the highest fat content.

Other high-fat foods

Biscuits	Deep-fried foods
Buttercream	Fatty meats (e.g.
Cakes	burgers, streaky
Cheese (especially	bacon, salami,
cream cheese and	sausages)
processed cheese)	French fries
Cheesecake	(especially if thinly
Chocolate	cut)
Cookies	Fried bread
Creamy desserts	Fritters
Creamy dips (e.g.	Full fat milk and
taramasalata)	yoghurt
Creamy sauces (e.g.	Icecream
mayonnaise,	Pastry
Hollandaise)	Pâté
Crispy snacks	Pork Pies
Croissants	Potato crisps
Dairy cream	

The fat content of food plays a large part in its palatability. For instance the taste of meat comes from the flavour of its fat. Fat makes ice cream creamy and pastry crumbly or flaky. Without fat, cakes become rubbery and milk watery. Many people eat a high-fat diet (the average in the Western diet is around 40 per cent of the total calorie intake) without realizing this, owing to large quantities of fats being hidden in processed foods such as biscuits and burgers. The law in most countries compounds the problem; for instance in the UK meat may legally be described as 'lean' even if it is one-third fat.

Chemistry

Dietary fats and oils are composed of units called triglycerides which in turn consist of carbon, hydrogen and oxygen formed into chains of fatty acids attached to a 'backbone' of glycerol. Fatty acids are classed as 'essential' or 'non-essential', depending on whether the body is capable of synthesizing them or not. Those which it cannot make and must obtain from the diet are known as essential fatty acids (EFAs). A deficiency of EFAs can have a widespread impact on health.

Fatty acids are classified according to four characteristics:

- Whether or not they are essential
- The length of the chain
- Whether they are saturated or unsaturated
- The position of the first double bond (a double bond occurs in an unsaturated fatty acid molecule at points where there is no hydrogen atom for a carbon atom to bond with)

Linoleic acid, which is an essential fatty acid, is described as an 'omega 6' fatty acid because the first double bond appears after the 6th carbon atom. The other essential fatty acid is known as alpha linolenic acid. It is described as an 'omega 3' fatty acid because the first double bond appears after the third carbon atom.

GOOD FOOD SOURCES OF LINOLEIC ACID

Corn oil

Fresh nuts and seeds

Groundnut oil

Safflower oil

Sunflower seed oil

GOOD FOOD SOURCES OF ALPHA LINOLENIC ACID

Linseed (flax seed) oil

Soybean oil

Vegetable leaves

Walnuts

Saturated fats have no double bonds – all the carbon atoms in their fatty acid molecules are attached to a hydrogen atom.

Monounsaturated fatty acids, such as oleic acid, found in olive oil, have one double bond – one carbon atom is not attached to a hydrogen atom. Polyunsaturated fatty acids have two or more double bonds. The more unsaturated a fat, the more it tends to be liquid at room temperature. However, unsaturated fats can be turned into saturated fats by artificially adding hydrogen atoms to which the carbon atoms can attach. This is how oils can be turned into margarine.

FUNCTIONS

After a meal, emulsified fat droplets are absorbed from the gut into the lymphatic system and then drain into the bloodstream at the thoracic duct in the neck. Within hours, the triglycerides are broken down into fatty acids and glycerol and then removed from the blood and into the adipose (fat) cells where they are reconstituted into triglycerides and stored for use as a future source of energy. This is the ultimate function of dietary saturated fat.

The essential fatty acids, which are polyunsaturated, have many other functions:

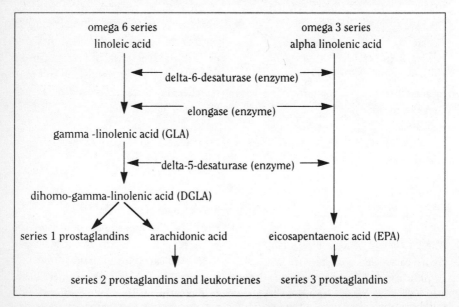

How EFA's are metabolized (broken down) to prostaglandins

- Components of plasma and mitochondrial lipoproteins
- Controlling cholesterol levels
- Fat transport and metabolism
- Precursors of prostaglandins and leukotrienes (*which see*)

Prostaglandins are hormone-like substances which control many essential functions in the body in relation to disorders such as high blood pressure, arthritis, menstrual pain, allergies, asthma, eczema, migraine and fertility.

The diagram on page 76 shows how the EFAs are metabolized (broken down) to prostaglandins.

As the fatty acids are metabolized, their chains become longer and more unsaturated. Each step in metabolism depends on an enzyme, the name of which is shown in the figure, and always ends in '-ase'. If these enzymes are in short supply, the production of prostaglandins may be impaired. Factors which we know interfere with the optimum function of delta-6-desaturase (D-6-D) are:

- A high intake or blood level of cholesterol
- A high intake of saturated fats and 'trans' fats (see below)
- High adrenaline levels
- A high alcohol consumption
- Diabetes
- Atopy (an inherited susceptibility to allergic diseases)
- Deficiencies of magnesium, vitamin B$_6$, biotin or zinc

Some health problems which make us suspect a deficiency of EFAs, or a lack of efficiency in converting them to prostaglandins are:

- Dry eye syndrome
- Eczema, psoriasis or dry skin
- Inflammatory disorders of all types
- Premenstrual syndrome (especially breast pain)
- Tendency to clot formation in blood

Supplements prescribed to correct these deficiencies may be more effective if they bypass a defective D-6-D enzyme. This is why GLA and EPA supplements are sometimes given instead of their precursors, and studies have shown them to be often effective in the clearance of the above conditions. GLA is the active ingredient in evening primrose oil, borage oil and blackcurrant seed oil, and EPA is obtained from fish oils. Other possible signs of essential fatty acid deficiency are split fingernails, a history of ear problems or hyperactivity in children, and extreme thirst (where no other cause can be found).

Essential fatty acids have been found helpful in the treatment of schizophrenia (see Section II).

Cis and Trans

Essential fatty acids have an active form (known as 'cis') and an inactive form (known as 'trans') depending on the arrangement of their atoms. Only the cis form can be turned into prostaglandins.

Plant oils contain large amounts of cis fatty acids. But commercial processing of oils to improve stability and odour, and the partial hydrogenation of oils to form margarines or 'vegetable fat', converts a large proportion of cis fatty acids into the inactive trans form. So it is possible to develop an essential fatty acid deficiency even if we appear to eat adequate amounts of oils.

Though not thought to be actively toxic, the primary adverse effect of trans fatty acids is to inhibit the metabolism of EFAs by competing with them for the important liver enzyme delta-6-desaturase.

This increases EFA requirements, affects EFA utilization, impairs prostaglandin production, and aggravates the symptoms of EFA deficiency. Trans fatty acids are also incorporated differently into cell membranes, triglycerides and phospholipids within the body, and there is evidence that a high consumption of partially hydrogenated vegetable fats (which are high in trans fatty acids), is associated with a greater risk of heart disease.

Fatty acids (see Fats)

Feingold diet
(see Therapeutic diets)

Fennel seeds

Herb

Fennel seeds are consumed in the form of tea as a digestive aid since they have a carminative action, helping to counteract flatulence. Fennel tea may also be given to children with dyspepsia and diarrhoea since it helps to relieve intestinal spasms. It is said to have a mild expectorant effect and, if applied as a loose compress to the eyes, to help relieve inflammatory eye conditions such as blepharitis and conjunctivitis.

Availability: Widely available from health food shops in tea bags.

Fenugreek

Herb

Fenugreek seeds are rich in mucilage and are made into a tea and consumed as a cough remedy in Mediterranean countries. In Germany they are sometimes used externally to soften abscesses and boils. In Chinese medicine, fenugreek is used as a yang tonic to support the energies of the kidneys, heart and spleen, and help conditions such as poor circulation, listlessness and frequent urination. In clinical trials fenugreek ingested orally has demonstrated an insulin-like effect in the treatment of maturity-onset diabetes.

Ground fenugreek seeds are widely used in Indian cookery.

Availability: Supermarkets, delicatessens and Asian grocers.

Feverfew

Herb

Feverfew has a vasodilatory (warming) effect, and this may explain why a proportion of migraine sufferers who consume it regularly experience a reduction in the number of migraine attacks suffered. However, not all migraine attacks are associated with the vasoconstriction (tightening of the blood vessels) which this herb helps to combat.

Availability: Usually as capsules, from health food shops.

Few Foods Diet
(see Therapeutic diets)

Fibre (see Dietary fibre)

Fish oils

Superfood

Fish oils contain the active ingredients EPA and DHA (*which see*). The oils are extracted from the flesh of oily fish such as herrings, mackerel and salmon. These oils are not the same as fish liver oils, which are taken for their vitamin A and D content and are not significant sources of EPA and DHA.

Flavones

Yellow pigments found in plants. Flavones belong to the group of compounds known as flavonoids (*which see*).

Flavonoids
(also see Bilberries)

Also known as bioflavonoids, flavonoids are colourful antioxidants found in plants. They are responsible for the colours of fruits (e.g. the red or blue of grape and berry skins) and vegetables. Twelve basic classes (chemical types) of flavonoids have been recognized: flavones, isoflavones, flavans, flavanones, flavanols, flavanolols, anthocyanidins, catechins (including proanthocyanidins), leukoanthocyanidins, chalcones, dihydrochalcones, and aurones. Anthocyanidins and closely related flavonoids such as proanthocyanidins may collectively be referred to as anthocyanosides.

Apart from their antioxidant activity, flavonoids are known for their ability to strengthen capillary walls, thus assisting circulation and helping to prevent and treat bruising, varicose veins, bleeding gums and nosebleeds. They may also be useful in the treatment of heavy menstrual bleeding, where no apparent cause for this is found on medical investigation. A third beneficial effect of some flavonoids such as quercetin, rutin, curcumin, silymarin and green tea polyphenols is their reputed anti-inflammatory effect, which may be related to their ability to inhibit the enzymes cyclo-oxygenase and lipoxygenase, which can act on arachidonic acid in cell membranes to form potent inflammatory substances known as prostaglandins (*which see*), some of which promote swellings and possibly symptoms such as headaches, rashes and joint pains.

Lemons (outer skin and white pith), and the central white core of citrus fruit generally, are a particularly rich source of flavonoids. The white pith of green peppers is also rich in flavonoids, as is the skin of colourful berries and grapes. Some herbs (such as *Ginkgo biloba*) are taken partly for the action of their flavonoids.

The names of some of the flavonoids

Anthocyanidins: Blue pigments (which may appear red under some conditions) found in the skins of some berries, especially bilberries. Beneficial effects on eyesight and circulation, and some antibacterial action.

Hesperidin: Found in citrus peel. Improves abnormal capillary fragility.

Myricetin: One of the beneficial antioxidants found in *Ginkgo biloba*. Helps to prevent free radical damage to nerve cells.

Nobiletin: Found in citrus fruits. Has anti-inflammatory action and assists detoxification.

Proanthocyanidins: (also known as pycno-genols) Related to tannins, these are poly-phenolic flavonoids found in pine bark, tea, peanut skins, cranberries and grape seeds and skins. Their antioxidant potency (particularly the varieties found in grape seeds) is reputedly 20 times greater than that of vitamin E.

Quercetin: (which see) Found in apple peel, onions, tea, *Ginkgo biloba* and cabbage. Helps to prevent cataract formation. May help allergy-related problems such as hay fever, asthma and eczema. Promotes the more efficient cross-linking of collagen. Quercetin is structurally related to the anti-allergic drug disodium chromoglycate.

Rutin: Found in buckwheat. Helps in the treatment of high blood pressure, bruising and haemorrhages under the skin, including redness due to radiation.

Flax seed
(also see Fatty acids)

Also known as linseeds, these seeds come from the flax plant, which is also the source of linen fibre. Both the seeds and their oil are used for their health benefits.

Flax seeds are rich in mucilaginous fibre and are often consumed as a gentle, bulking laxative. They may be ground and stirred into water, or chewed and swallowed, but must be consumed with a large quantity of fluid to allow them to swell. If not taken with sufficient fluid they will absorb water from the digestive system instead, which could result in constipation. The usual dose is one tablespoon in the morning and evening with a large glass of water. Their nutritious oils cannot be digested and absorbed by the body unless the seeds are crushed or ground before consumption.

A tea made by infusing linseeds in hot water for a few minutes and then adding

honey and lemon juice, may help to soothe coughs and sore throats.

Cold-pressed flax oil is a particularly rich source of alpha-linolenic acid (see Fats), which is frequently deficient in individuals with skin ailments, menstrual problems and prostate enlargement.

Flax seed oil should not be exposed to light during storage, and should be kept refrigerated until use.

Availability: The seeds are readily available in health food shops. Since flax seed oil easily degrades, it is sometimes best obtained by mail order from a supplier who stores it in light-resistant containers and guarantees to keep it frozen until the time of despatch.

Fluoride

Trace element

Fluoride is normally present in the human body in amounts similar to those of iron. Most fluoride is found in bone, where it combines with calcium or hydroxyapatite to form fluorapatite, helping to strengthen bones and teeth. It is known that a high fluoride intake by children results in a lower incidence of dental decay (caries). Many studies have also shown that a higher fluoride intake corresponds to greater bone density. Most foods contain small quantities of fluoride. Particularly rich sources are seafood and black tea.

Unlike most trace elements, there is a very small margin between beneficial and toxic levels of fluoride intake. Children who regularly consume a little too much fluoride may develop permanently mottled teeth. Chronic exposure to excessive fluoride may result in osteoporosis, calcification of the tendons and ligaments, and the growth of bone spurs, probably through the overstimulation of the parathyroid glands. Fluoride is also an inhibitor of the enzymes enolase, involved in glycolysis (see Energy production) and adenylcyclase, which stimulates the production of cyclic AMP. It may therefore have potentially adverse effects on energy production and its consumption should be particularly discouraged in those with chronic fatigue syndrome.

Many health campaigners oppose the addition of fluoride to public water supplies, on grounds that potential long-term adverse health effects of this compulsory mass medication are unknown.

Folate (see Folic acid)

Folic acid (Folate or folacin)

Vitamin (water-soluble)
UK RNI 200 mcg
US RDA 200 mcg

FUNCTIONS
Blood formation
Protein, RNA and DNA synthesis
Synthesis of purines and pyrimidines
Synthesis of the amino acids glycine and methionine

GOOD FOOD SOURCES
Leafy green vegetables, especially raw spinach
Liver
Freshly squeezed orange juice
Soya flour
Whole grains
Yeast extract

Deficiency signs and symptoms

- Anaemia
- Anorexia
- Apathy
- Birth defects in children
- Breathlessness
- Constipation and digestive disturbances
- Fatigue
- Growth impairment
- Habitual miscarriage
- Increased risk of cancer
- Increased risk of heart disease (by causing raised homocysteine levels)
- Insomnia
- Memory impairment
- Mental confusion
- Paranoid delusions
- Reduced immunity
- Sore tongue
- Weakness
- Low levels of several B vitamins have been found in psychiatric patients and in senile dementia

Preventing deficiency

Folic acid is one of the vitamins most easily destroyed by heat, therefore vegetables should be cooked for as short a time as possible. Whole grains rather than their refined counterparts should be eaten as regularly as possible. The cumulative losses of folic acid which occur during food processing often amount to 65 per cent, leaving many foods with only one third of their original folic acid content. Prolonged boiling alone can cause losses of up to 50 per cent. Like vitamin B_2, folic acid is sensitive to light. The bioavailability (*which see*) of folic acid is reduced by alcohol intake, the contraceptive pill, anti-epileptic drugs, aspirin, cimetidine (Zantac), antacids, zinc deficiency, vitamin B_{12} deficiency, and the ageing process. Folic acid deficiency is relatively common in malnourished hospitalized patients. Certain tissues can be more folate-deficient than others: for instance precancerous changes can occur in the cervix, lung or colon which are reversible with folic acid supplementation (*Heimburger DC: Localized deficiencies of folic acid in aerodigestive tissues. Ann NY Acad Sci 669:87-95, 1992*).

Vitamin B_{12} deficiency causes folate deficiency by causing folic acid to be trapped as methylfolate, which is unavailable to the body. A deficiency of the amino acid methionine has a similar effect. Oral contraceptives or deficiencies of vitamins B_3 or C also prevent adequate utilization.

Comments

Folic acid itself does not occur in food or human tissue unless taken as a dietary supplement, and it is physiologically inactive until it has been reduced to dihydrofolic acid. Folic acid is in fact the parent molecule for a number of derivatives known collectively as folates. The main circulating folate is known as 5-methyl tetrahydrofolate, but the active forms inside cells are known as polyglutamates.

Supplementation

In research studies, folic acid supplements have been found to:

- Prevent spina bifida in the unborn
- Treat megaloblastic, aplastic and sickle cell anaemias (if folic acid is deficient)
- Reduce levels of harmful homocysteine (which is linked with heart disease and osteoporosis)
- Reverse cervical dysplasia (pre-cancerous condition of the cervix)
- Treat depression and schizophrenia

Preferred form and suggested intake

B vitamins should not normally be taken singly, since they work together as a team and good nutrition is about avoiding imbalances. A B complex supplement providing 200–400 mcg of folic acid is enough for most purposes.

Cautions

Megadoses of folic acid as given by many doctors to pregnant women (often 4,000 mcg or more) are unnecessary and may reduce zinc absorption.

Folic acid supplements given to patients who may be developing a vitamin B_{12} deficiency may obscure a correct diagnosis and delay the appropriate treatment.

Food additives

Chemicals added during the processing of food to help preserve them, to assist in their manufacture, or to improve their taste, texture or appearance. Some categories of food additives include: colourings (E100–180), preservatives (E200–297), antioxidants (E300–321), emulsifiers, stabilizers and thickeners (E322–495), acids, bases and related materials (E500–529), anti-caking agents (E530–585), flavour-enhancers and sweeteners (E620–640), glazing agents (E900–914), flour treatments and bleaching agents (E920–928), packing gases (E941–948), sweeteners (E950–967), and miscellaneous (E999–1518).

E numbers are the numbers allocated by the European Union for approved products.

Flavourings form the largest group of food additives, but government controls over these substances are often lacking because of the very small quantities used. Sometimes just a few molecules are needed to obtain a powerful flavouring effect.

Many individuals and consumer groups are concerned about the widespread use of artificial food additives. Large numbers of people are known to be sensitive to these chemicals. For instance, sulphur-based preservatives may trigger asthma attacks, and digestive disturbances, and colourings have been linked with hyperactivity in children. One of the greatest concerns is the possible 'cocktail effect' of consuming numerous additives in combination. Government regulations only require the testing of additives singly, not in combination, and the safety testing is usually left to the additive manufacturing company itself.

Food families

Foods are related to each other when they belong to the same species or 'family'. Some individuals can be allergic or intolerant to a whole family of foods rather than just one member of that family, and this is thought to be because members of the same plant family often share the same chemical components, particularly mildly toxic chemicals (toxic ingredients found in plants are known as secondary plant metabolites) which are designed to protect the plant from over-consumption by predators.

Names of some common plant food families and their members

Anacardiaceae: cashew, mango, pistachio
Betulaceae: hazelnuts
Caricaceae: papaya
Chenopodiaceae: beetroot, spinach, sugar beet
Compositae: artichokes (globe and jerusalem), chamomile, chicory, dandelion, endive, lettuce, safflower, salsify, sunflower, tarragon
Convolvulaceae: sweet potato
Cruciferae: Brussels sprouts, broccoli, cabbage, cauliflower, Chinese cabbage, horseradish, kale, kohlrabi, mustard, radish, rape, swede, turnip and watercress.
Cucurbitaceae: cucumber, courgette, marrow, melon, pumpkin, squash, watermelon
Cycadaceae: sago
Dioscoreaceae: yam
Ebenaceae: persimmon
Ericaceae: bilberry, blueberry, cranberry, huckleberry, sloe
Euphorbiaceae: cassava, tapioca
Fugaeceae: sweet chestnut
Fungi: mushrooms, yeast
Gramineae: bamboo shoots, barley, sweetcorn, millet, oats, rice, rye, sugar cane, wheat
Juglandaceae: butter nut, hickory nut, walnut
Lablatae: balm, basil, mint, marjoram, oregano, peppermint, spearmint, rosemary, sage, thyme
Leguminosae: beans, lentils, liquorice, peas, peanuts
Liliaceae: asparagus, chives, garlic, leek, onion, shallot
Musaceae: banana, plantain
Oleaceae: olive oil
Polygonaceae: buckwheat, rhubarb
Rosaceae: apple, apricot, blackberry, cherry, loganberry, nectarine, peach, pear, plum, prune, raspberry, rosehip, strawberry
Rubiaceae: coffee
Rutaceae: grapefruit, lemon, lime, mandarin, orange, tangerine
Saxifragaceae: gooseberry, blackcurrant, redcurrant
Solanaceae: aubergine, cayenne, chillie, paprika, pepper, pimento, potato, tobacco, tomato
Theaceae: Indian tea
Torreya: nutmeg, mace, brazil nut
Umbelliferae: angelica, aniseed, caraway, carrots, celeriac, celery, coriander, dill, fennel, parsley, parsnips, samphire
Vitaceae: grape

Food intolerance (see Allergy)

Food poisoning

Food poisoning is defined as an acute illness, which usually includes one or more gastrointestinal symptoms, caused by the recent consumption of food or drink.

Although food poisoning can occur as a result of substances like heavy metals, pollutants or natural plant toxins, most people think of it as microbiological in origin – caused by bacteria, viruses and protozoa. Micro-organisms can cause food poisoning in two ways, by directly invading the intestinal wall (e.g. Salmonella), or by producing a toxin. This toxin may be produced by living micro-organisms in the gut, or may be in food already. If the food has been cooked after it was infected, the micro-organisms may have been destroyed, but their toxins can remain and still cause symptoms of food poisoning.

If food poisoning occurs within a few hours after consumption of the offending food, this tends to suggest that it is toxic in origin. Symptoms of Salmonella infection take 12–36 hours to appear, and campylobacter can take up to 5 days. Salmonella species can invade the blood, causing fever and even meningitis and multiple abscesses. Food contaminated with the toxins of *Clostridium botulinus* (the botulism agent) may cause no gastrointestinal symptoms at all, and botulism is often fatal because it is not diagnosed in time. Symptoms of botulism, which include fatigue, swallowing difficulties and double vision, may take 18 hours to 1 week to appear.

Gastroenteritis is often caused by *E coli* (a common cause of travellers' diarrhoea and infant diarrhoea) and *Giardia lamblia*. However, these are not normally food-borne but water-borne organisms. Campylobacter causes fever, bloody diarrhoea, abdominal pain and nausea. Listeria, sometimes found in soft cheeses, can be fatal to an unborn child if eaten by a pregnant woman.

It is usually not possible to tell from the taste or smell of food whether it could cause food poisoning. Food allergy may occasionally cause identical symptoms to those of food poisoning.

Formula feeds

Also known as infant formulas, these are commercial substitutes for breast milk, used in the first year of life, and resemble human breast milk as closely as possible. Formula feeds can be based on cows milk, goat's milk or soya milk.

Fortification

The addition of vitamins, minerals or amino acids to a food, in addition to those normally found in a food, for instance iodine in salt. Fortification is sometimes required by law for foods which replace a staple food. For instance vitamins A and D are added to margarine because margarine may be used instead of butter, a source of vitamins A and D.

Restoring some of the original nutrient content in foods which have been depleted by processing – for instance adding B vitamins and iron to white flour – is known as restoration. Restoration is often imposed by law for staple foods.

Artificially adding more of a nutrient to a food than it would normally contain is known as enrichment. Examples are vitamin C-enriched fruit juice and vitamin-enriched milk powder.

Free radicals
(also see Antioxidants)

Also known as free oxidizing radicals, these are oxygen molecules with an electron 'missing' from their outer orbit. They seek to steal electrons from any molecules with which they come into contact, thus oxidizing and destabilizing them. A single oxidizing reaction can initiate many others, resulting in a cascade of free radical formation rather like an atomic explosion.

Ultraviolet light, sunlight, X-rays or any form of high-energy ionizing radiation causes the formation of free radicals by knocking electrons out of orbit. Nuclear radiation is deadly because it generates massive numbers of free radicals. Within the body, the consumption of alcohol and tobacco greatly increases free radical activity, as do pollution, infection, overexertion, excessive amounts of iron and copper, excessive physical exercise, poor nutrition and stress.

Although free radicals are produced by a number of normal metabolic processes in the body (for instance they are by-products of normal energy production processes, liver detoxification or immune system attacks against bacteria and other microorganisms) if the amount of oxidation which occurs in human body tissues overwhelms the body's antioxidant capacity (its capacity to quench the oxidative reactions) this results in *oxidative stress* to the body's cells, and consequent damage.

Within the cell all components are susceptible to free radical attack. In particular the lipids which constitute the cell membrane are highly susceptible, especially those lipids which contain unsaturated double bonds (see *Fats* for explanation of double bonds). Free radical attack on these lipids leads to the formation of poisonous peroxides, hydroperoxides and aldehydes. The membrane proteins in cells, which are involved in the transport of ions and in maintaining the balance of nutrients inside and outside cells, are also vulnerable to free radical attack. Thus free radicals can, by disrupting at least two essential components of the cell membrane, alter its structure and function, leading to membrane instability, alteration of membrane-dependent enzymes, and abnormal proportions of nutrients and fluid inside and outside cells. Impairment of the calcium-magnesium pump by free radical damage results in an increased influx of calcium into the cell, which activates arterial contraction mechanisms, reduces blood flow and can in itself destroy sensitive cells such as those in the brain and nervous system.

Free radicals also cause inflammation. For instance if they find their way into the fluid which bathes the joints in our body, causing this fluid to lose its lubricating quality and promoting irritation, chronic inflammation and the destruction of cartilage can occur in the form of arthritis. Chronic fatigue can result from free radical damage to the membranes of mitochondria, the portion of the cell where energy is produced. Toxic compounds can be produced which result in the decreased reproduction of mitochondria and a consequent reduction in their numbers.

The superoxide (O_2-) free radical is particularly common in mammals, and is a potent initiator of cell damage. One of the body's best defences against this free radical is the antioxidant enzyme superoxide dismutase. When the superoxide radical is captured, hydrogen peroxide is created, and must be removed by another antioxidant enzyme, either catalase or glutathione peroxidase. It is thought that deficiencies of SOD and catalase are especially common in all types of arthritis. Among the flavonoids, quercetin, myricetin and rutin are the most powerful inhibitors of the superoxide ion.

Peroxides (RCOO·), which are known as 'reactive oxygen species' and readily disintegrate into free radicals, are formed when lipids (fats) are oxidized. Cell membranes are highly susceptible to them. Peroxides are linked with heart disease, damage to liver function, premature ageing, and skin diseases such as skin cancers, age spots and psoriasis as well as premature wrinkling. Since the liver consists of nearly 50 per cent fatty tissue, it is very vulnerable to peroxides. The antioxidant enzyme glutathione peroxidase, which consists of the amino acid glutathione and the trace element selenium, combats peroxides. The heating and reheating of cooking oils in particular promotes the generation of damaging peroxides.

Another highly reactive form of oxygen, which consists of single atoms rather than molecules, is singlet oxygen. Beta-carotene and lycopene are effective scavengers of singlet oxygen. The hypochlorite ion (OCl-), formed by the oxidation of chloride ions, is also a powerful oxidizing agent, and requires adequate amounts of the amino acid taurine to control and scavenge it. Individuals with a taurine deficiency may become especially sensitive to aldehydes, bleach and chlorine, and free amino acids in their body may become toxic aldehydes. For this reason infant formula feeds should always be enriched with taurine at least to the levels found in human breast milk.

Probably the most dangerous of all free radicals is the hydroxyl (OH·) radical – the main toxin generated by exposure to radiation. Hydroxyl radicals are also formed during exercise, especially in closed rooms or in a polluted environment. Chemicals and toxins stored in our fatty tissue are released as we 'burn off' fat by means of exercise or dieting, and these toxins then generate the formation of hydroxyl radicals. A particularly important substance involved in combating hydroxyl radicals is an antioxidant known as melatonin (*which see*). The nutrients methionine, glutathione and selenium also play an important role.

Nutrients such as vitamin E, beta-carotene and flavonoids play an important part in deactivating free radicals. Without sufficient antioxidant nutrients and enzymes, oxidative stress can lead to cancers and heart disease as well as premature ageing and many associated disease processes.

Fructo-oligosaccharides
(see Probiotics)

Fructose, (see Carbohydrates)

G

GABA
(Gamma-amino butyric acid)

Although not strictly speaking an amino acid, GABA is often classified with the amino acids. It functions as the most widely distributed inhibitory neurotransmitter (*which see*) in the brain. The manufacture of GABA is regulated by vitamin B_6. Benzodiazepine tranquillizer drugs (such as Valium) produce their anti-anxiety and muscle-relaxant effects by activating the neurons (nerve cells) and receptor sites which respond to GABA.

GABA is almost always deficient in clinical and experimental seizure disorders. It is involved in the regulation of mechanisms related to blood pressure, therefore stimulants of GABA receptors are considered useful in combating hypertension.

Availability: GABA is not readily available as a dietary supplement, but supplementation with the amino acid taurine (*which see*) increases the breakdown of glutamate to GABA.

Galactose
(see Sugars)

Gamma linolenic acid (GLA)
(also see Fats)

A polyunsaturated fatty acid which is an intermediate in the conversion of linoleic acid to prostaglandins. Some individuals are thought to perform this conversion inefficiently, and may therefore benefit from supplementation with GLA, which is rarely found in food. Nutrients needed for the conversion process include magnesium, zinc, biotin and vitamin B_6. Deficiencies of any of these nutrients may result in a GLA deficiency in the body.

Symptoms of GLA deficiency may include dry skin, extreme thirst (where no apparent cause can be found on medical investigation), hyperactivity in children, premenstrual syndrome and eczema.

The richest food sources of GLA include human breast milk, borage seed oil, evening primrose oil and blackcurrant seed oil. The seed oils are readily available in health food shops for use as dietary supplements.

Gamma oryzanol

A phytosterol (cholesterol-like substance) found in rice bran oil and consisting of ferulic acid esters of triterpene alcohols. Gamma-oryzanol is partially metabolized to ferulic acid in the intestine but is primarily (though poorly) absorbed intact. It is sold as an intestinal health supplement. Japanese research studies claim that it has been successfully used against diseases as diverse as peptic and duodenal ulcers, psychosomatic complaints, hypercholesterolaemia, and menopausal symptoms.

Availability: From nutritional therapists.

Garcinia cambogia

This is another name for tamarind, a fruit used in Indian cookery and food preservation. It contains the substance (-)hydroxycitrate, which is related to citric acid and is sold in supplement form as an aid to weight loss. (-)Hydroxycitrate is thought to be able to partially inhibit an enzyme required for the conversion of blood glucose into fat, which results in higher glycogen (stored carbohydrate) levels instead. High levels of glycogen in the blood can help to suppress the appetite and glycogen is readily used as an energy source.

There is a shortage of human studies carried out on (-)hydroxycitrate as a weight-loss aid. Individuals who have tried it obtain a varied response. It may be of most use in curbing an excess sugar consumption since sugar consumption results in early satiety if (-)hydroxycitrate supplements are taken previously.

Availability: From health food stores.

Garlic

Herb

Garlic is used as both a culinary and medicinal herb. Numerous research studies have confirmed its anti-bacterial, anti-parasitic, anti-blood-clotting, cholesterol-lowering, triglyceride-lowering and blood pressure-lowering effects.

Garlic contains a substance known as alliin. When garlic is chopped or crushed, alliin comes into contact with the enzyme allinase, to produce the odorous and medicinally active substance allicin. Allicin is unstable and is lost when garlic is cooked, distilled or chopped and left to stand for a few days. Without allicin, garlic loses its anti-microbial properties, although some experts believe that it may still retain some of its other effects. Others disagree. For instance, according to renowned German herbalist Rudolph Fritz Weiss MD, if the smell is reduced, so is the medicinal action.

Some authorities have proposed that commercial garlic preparations should be measured in terms of their 'allicin-releasing potential'. Garlic products produced by heat or solvent extraction processes contain alliin but are devoid of allinase and therefore have no allicin-releasing potential. On the other hand, dried garlic powder contains both alliin and allinase, therefore it does have allicin-releasing potential.

Allicin, the active principle, enters the bloodstream when ingested, soon reaching all parts of the body. Elimination is mainly via the lungs and skin, which is why the breath and sweat have the characteristic smell of garlic. As it pervades the lungs, garlic sterilizes the alveoli and bronchial tree of the lungs, so is helpful against bronchitic infections. It also has expectorant properties, and is sometimes added to cough medications.

Garlic has been used effectively to treat dysentery, typhoid, cholera, bacterial food poisoning, and worm infestations. Weiss describes it as particularly useful after amoebic dysentery when the bowels are still irritable, finding that it helps to heal the bowel with its significantly anti-bacterial, antispasmodic and antidyspeptic properties.

Some research has found that garlic improves the ability of the pancreas to produce insulin. Some components of garlic may also inhibit the growth of malignant (cancerous) cells. One of the most exciting recent studies in garlic research is that reported at a 1989 Aids conference. Ten HIV-positive patients with severely low natural killer cell activity, abnormal helper-to-suppressor T-cell ratios (both these parameters are indicators of advanced Aids, probably with short life expectancy) and opportunistic infections such as cryptosporidial diarrhoea were given 5 grams daily for six weeks and then 10 grams daily for six weeks of an aged garlic extract. Three patients died before the trial ended, but seven of the 10 experienced a return to normal natural killer cell activity by the end of the 12 weeks. Chronic diarrhoea and candidiasis also improved. (*Int Conf AIDS [Canada] 5:466, 1989. ISBN 0-662-56670-X*). Various trials have shown garlic to be effective against cryptococcus, crytosporidia, herpes, mycobacteria and pneumocystis – all common infectious agents in Aids.

Kyolic garlic is garlic which has been subjected to a 'cold-ageing' process for 20 months. This process promotes the breakdown of alliin, the parent sulphur compound in garlic, into components which are odourless and chemically more stable. The therapeutic effects of kyolic garlic have mainly been researched (and found effective) in studies on the heart and circulation, and it is not known whether this form of garlic retains all the therapeutic properties of fresh garlic.

Suggested therapeutic intake: 1–3 cloves of fresh, raw garlic daily, chopped and swallowed with water or lemon juice. Or garlic products as advised by a practitioner.

Gelatin

Protein derived from collagen and obtained by boiling bones, hooves, tendons, etc. in water. Commonly used in cookery. One third of gelatin consists of the amino acid glycine (*which see*).

Gene

A discrete unit of DNA, carrying instructions for the proteins which make up the structures and functions of all living organisms. Genes ensure that the right proteins are made in the correct place, at the right time and in the appropriate amount. This strict control is necessary for the integrated and balanced functioning of complex biological structures and processes.

Genetic engineering

The isolation, cutting, joining and transfer of single or multiple genes between unrelated organisms. As a result, combinations of genes are produced that would never occur naturally. Natural species barriers can be circumvented, producing, for example, 'transgenic' tomatoes and strawberries containing the 'anti-freeze' gene from an arctic fish, to allow greater tolerance to frost. Transgenic so-called super salmon are being produced, with genes from the arctic sea flounder which allow the salmon to grow six times larger and 10 times faster. Already on the market are soya beans containing a bacterial gene to confer pesticide resistance. An engineered insect virus possessing the scorpion toxin gene is being tested for spraying on crops as a broad-spectrum pesticide. Hundreds more projects are poised for commercialization in the next few years.

Genetic engineering is said to promise disease- and pesticide-resistant crops and animals, crops which can grow in poor climatic and soil conditions, and tastier food with better nutritional value. Critics argue that transgenic crops and animals are experimental life forms with unpredictable long-term effects on human health and the environment. For instance, a transgenic bacterium developed to overproduce the amino acid tryptophan for use in dietary supplements caused 37 deaths and more than a thousand cases of the rare blood disorder eosinophilia myalgia syndrome in 1989. Field trials in Scotland and Denmark using transgenic, herbicide-resistant oil-seed rape have cross-pollinated with wild Brassica species, generating herbicide-resistant super-weeds. To allow consumers the opportunity to reject transgenic foods such as soya beans, used in some 60 per cent of processed food products, environmental organizations are campaigning for the segregation and labelling of such foods.

Genistein (see Soya products and Oestrogen)

Gentian

Herb

Gentian is known as the most important of all the European 'bitter' herbs. These are herbs containing bitter-tasting substances which act as digestive stimulants, stimulating gastric secretion and motility and promoting gastric tone, thus enabling food to be more easily digested. Gentian is active the moment that it is absorbed by the mucous membrane of the mouth. It may be beneficial in anorexia.

In the Chinese classification system, gentian is a 'cold bitter' which means that it is best applied in conditions of excessive vitality and avoided in any conditions involving coldness, such as depressed circulation or low metabolic rate, frequent urination or chronic respiratory congestion.

Germanium

Trace element

There is no known function for germanium in the human body, and it is therefore described by scientists as a 'contaminant' in foods such as garlic, which is rich in germanium.

Because of reports that germanium could stimulate the immune system and may be of benefit for Aids sufferers, germanium was for a short time in the late 1980s available as a dietary supplement in two forms: germanium sesquioxide (also known as organic germanium or Ge-132) and germanium lactate citrate. Germanium dioxide, which is known to be toxic, was not sold as a dietary supplement – at least not by reputable suppliers. Unfortunately a number of individuals in Japan did obtain and consume germanium dioxide preparations, and suffered permanent kidney damage. As a result germanium received a very bad press, and there was widespread withdrawal of all germanium supplements. A search of the scientific literature reveals that some individuals who had taken the supposedly non-toxic forms of germanium also suffered kidney damage. It is still not known whether these forms are indeed non-toxic or whether the products in question were contaminated with germanium dioxide. Experts confirm that it may be virtually impossible to manufacture a completely uncontaminated product.

Gerson diet

A diet developed by the late Max Gerson MD for the treatment of cancers and other degenerative or chronic diseases. (*See Therapeutic diets*)

Ginger

Herb

Ginger is known as a 'hot bitter' herb, which promotes gastric acidity and aids digestion. It is a useful herb for many stomach conditions, and a great deal of research has been conducted into its potential benefits. In one study rheumatoid arthritis sufferers using ginger experienced a reduction in joint pain and an improvement in joint mobility. Ginger has also been used successfully against motion (travel) sickness. In animal studies, ginger has been used to reduce blood sugar in diabetic rats, and to reduce blood cholesterol levels in animals fed a cholesterol-rich diet. In Chinese medicine, ginger is considered to be a warming circulatory stimulant which can also remove catarrh and help bronchitic conditions, as well as help to prevent painful menstrual periods.

Ginkgo biloba

Herb

Ginkgo biloba is one of the most widely researched medicinal herbs and has been found most effective for improving capillary strength and circulation. Its beneficial effects on the blood circulation in the brain makes it potentially very useful in Alzheimer's disease and stroke prevention.

Clinical and laboratory tests have shown *Ginkgo biloba* extract to have significant benefit in the treatment of Raynaud's disease, asthma, chronic cerebral and circulatory problems, senile dementia, tinnitus, macular degeneration and glaucoma. Ginkgo is also a potent antioxidant. It has a stabilizing effect on cell membranes by preventing lipid peroxidation and modulating calcium influx. In a recent study on Chernobyl salvage workers exposed to radiation, *Ginkgo biloba* supplements reduced the 'clastogenic factors' (markers of damage to DNA) which had been found in these workers and are commonly present after exposure to radiation.

Ginkgo's effects are due to its high flavonoid content, including quercetin, kaempferol and proanthocyanidins, as well as to its terpenoids such as ginkgolides.

Availability: *Ginkgo biloba* products are widely available in health food shops.

Ginseng (Korean)

Herb

Also known as Panax ginseng, this is one of the oldest medicinal herbs in the Far East. Considerable research has been carried out into ginseng. It is used short term as a tonic to treat fatigue, low blood pressure, general and nervous weakness and mild depression, and long term to improve well-being in the elderly.

Research studies have demonstrated the following benefits for ginseng:

- Ability to normalize high or low blood pressure in some individuals
- Improvements in liver detoxification function
- Improvement in overall well-being (including appetite, mood and sleep)

- Improvement in physical endurance, mental ability and concentration
- Improvements in serum total cholesterol levels
- Reduction of insulin requirements in diabetics

Ginseng appears to act as an adaptogen, that is to say it has neither an excessively stimulating nor a sedating effect, but is capable of acting in either direction depending on the individual's needs.

In Chinese medicine, ginseng is used to increase deficient *chi* (a type of energy which has been likened to the elusive 'life force'), with symptoms of debility, irritability, poor circulation and prolapse of the lower abdomen. Its beneficial effects in the elderly may be related to its ability to maintain the adrenal cortex in an optimally functioning condition.

Ginseng should not be taken by individuals with cardiovascular disease or by women with an unstable menstrual cycle.

Availability: Panax ginseng is readily available in health food shops.

Ginseng (Siberian)

Herb

Also known as *Eleutherococcus*, this is used as a 'harmonizing' tonic. Like Panax ginseng, *Eleutherococcus* is considered to be an adaptogen – adapting its effects to the individual's needs. This herb has undergone much study by scientists in the former USSR. It has been found to provide the following benefits:

- Ability to improve capillary resistance
- Ability to perform physical work
- Ability to withstand motion sickness
- Adaptation to a high temperature environment

- Improvement in acute craniocerebral trauma
- Improvement in acute pyelonephritis
- Improvement in atherosclerosis
- Improvement in chronic bronchitis
- Improvement in diabetes mellitus
- Improvement in oxygen metabolism (i.e. oxygen uptake, oxygen pulse, total work and exhaustion time)
- Improvement in rheumatic heart disease
- Improvement in speed and quality of work
- Normalizing of high or low blood pressure
- Stimulation of the white cells of the immune system, especially the T-lymphocyte cell count

Availability: *Eleutherococcus* is most easily available through nutritional and herbal practitioners.

GLA (see Gamma-linolenic acid)

Glandulars

This is a term used for dietary supplements consisting of dried, powdered, usually raw animal glands and other organs such as ovaries, adrenals, thyroid and pancreas. The active hormone is removed before the product is made into a supplement. Glandular supplements are used to help combat weakness or underactivity of the human glands in question, by providing the closest possible match of raw materials for repair purposes. Advocates of glandular therapy believe that it is the specific nucleic acid (RNA and DNA) content of glandular products which accounts for their treatment successes. If so, this must be reconciled with the commonly held scientific view that nucleic acids do not survive the digestive process.

Availability: Not readily available in UK health food shops. May be prescribed by some nutritional therapists or other natural practitioners.

Glauber's salts

This is another name for crystals of sodium sulphate, which are often used for their laxative effect in a similar way to Epsom salts (*which see*).

Glucagon (see Blood sugar)

Gluconates (see Chelates)

Gluconeogenesis

The formation of glucose from sources such as lactate, amino acids and the glycerol portion of fats. Gluconeogenesis takes place in the liver when glycogen (stored glucose) is depleted, in order to help maintain blood sugar levels.

Glucosamine sulphate

Glucosamine is a type of nutrient known as an 'amino sugar'. It is converted into larger molecules that go to make up connective tissue. Clinical trials and studies have shown that when taken as a dietary supplement, glucosamine combined with sulphate can help to prevent the breakdown of cartilage which occurs in osteoarthritis. Glucosamine sulphate is taken up by joint tissue, stimulates the production of glycoaminoglycans (the building blocks of cartilage), and can reduce joint pain, tenderness and swelling, allowing joint movement to increase. The supplement is often given with vitamin C and the amino acid tyrosine to optimize its action. (*Also see Section II, Osteoarthritis*.)

Availability: From health food shops and nutritional therapists.

Glucose (see Carbohydrates)

Glucose Tolerance Factor (GTF) (see Chromium)

Glucuronic acid

A substance derived from glucose, which can combine with chemical and bacterial toxins and convert them to a form ready for excretion.

Glutamic acid

Amino acid

Glutamic acid or glutamate can be manufactured by the body. It is a precursor of proline, ornithine, arginine and polyamines. It functions as a stimulatory neurotransmitter (*which see*) and can also be converted by the body into the inhibitory neurotransmitter GABA and the amino acid glutamine, which participates in the production of DNA. Glutamic acid is found in particularly high levels in the brain, for instance in the nerves of the hippocampus, its memory centre.

Researchers working with epileptic patients have found that most epileptics have decreased taurine, GABA and glycine, with increased aspartic acid and glutamic acid. An explanation for this imbalance may be that glutamic acid is not being properly converted to GABA in these patients. The vitamin B_6-dependent enzyme glutamate decarboxylase makes GABA from glutamic acid. Vitamin B_6 deficiency is known to be associated with seizures and convulsions.

'Chinese restaurant syndrome', the symptoms of which include headache, nausea, weakness, flushing and sweating after eating Chinese food, may be due to a high content of monosodium glutamate – a sodium salt of glutamic acid – in the food. Those who suffer from this syndrome may also have reduced levels of glutamate decarboxylate. It has been proposed that this syndrome can be prevented with vitamin B_6 supplementation.

Glutamine

Amino acid

Glutamine is not found in food. It is primarily a brain fuel which can take the place of glucose. It is particularly abundant in the substantia nigra and thalamus of the brain, as well as in the blood, where its concentration is three to four times greater than all other amino acids. It is 10 to 15 times more concentrated in the cerebrospinal fluid than in the blood. In fasting or starvation states, when glycogen stores have been exhausted, large amounts of glutamine (and alanine) are released from muscle tissue and serve to shuttle amino acid nitrogen and carbon to other tissues. The carbon may be converted to glucose by the liver and made available for energy production (*which see*).

In the 1960s an experiment was carried out supplementing 15 grams a day of L-glutamine to alcoholics. Compared with placebo, this was found to produce a significant improvement in control over alcohol consumption, but follow-up studies are lacking.

Glutamine also performs a major role in DNA synthesis. An influx of large amounts of glutamine may stimulate muscle protein synthesis. 60 per cent of the ammonia produced in the kidney tubules to buffer excessive urinary acidity comes from the breakdown of glutamine.

Availability of supplements: From health food stores.

Glutathione

Amino acid

Glutathione, produced from the amino acid cysteine, is the body's primary defence against oxidative (free radical) damage within cells. Exposure to toxic chemicals stimulates the secretion of glutathione from the liver into the plasma. Once in the plasma, glutathione complexes (conjugates) with the toxins. The resultant conjugate is then converted to mercapturic acid, which can be excreted by the kidneys. Glutathione also deactivates hydrogen peroxide and other peroxides. Many individuals with chemical sensitivity are deficient in glutathione.

Glutathione is also needed for the production of prostaglandins (*which see*) and it is a coenzyme for the breakdown of insulin in the liver and kidney.

Glutathione can be taken as a dietary supplement, in which case its most effective chemical form is known as *reduced* glutathione. (*Also see Detoxification*.)

Availability: Glutathione is available from health food shops. Reduced glutathione is available from nutritional therapists.

Glutathione peroxidase
(see Antioxidants and Free radicals)

Gluten

A protein found in many grains (cereals) including wheat, oats, rye and barley, but not rice, buckwheat and millet. Maize (corn) is usually promoted as gluten-free, whereas in fact gluten is an important by-product of maize. Individuals who are severely allergic to gluten are diagnosed with a condition known as coeliac disease, or gluten-sensitive enteropathy.

Gluten is a very tough, sticky substance, capable of encapsulating smaller molecules such as sugar, fats and salts. In individuals with a leaky or over-permeable gut (*see Leaky gut syndrome*) gluten can be absorbed intact through the gut wall into the bloodstream, to be transported to and deposited in the liver, spleen, pancreas, joints or other organs and tissues, where it becomes embedded and interferes with good function. According to Dr Nadya Coates, writing in her book *A Matter of Life*, gluten is present in the bodies of modern people to such a degree that in some instances it can make up one fifth of the total body weight, and may form part of abnormal growths such as fibroids. This is

because many Westerners eat such large quantities of wheat in the form of bread, pasta, biscuits, cakes, etc. Wheat is our major source of gluten, and modern varieties of wheat have been bred to yield much larger amounts of gluten than ever before. Gluten assists the raising process in bread-making, allowing the use of less flour to make the same volume of bread.

Gluten sensitivity has been linked with multiple sclerosis, rheumatoid arthritis and schizophrenia. Many individuals are allergic to gluten, or their digestive system has difficulty with handling it.

Glycaemic index

A measure of a food's effect on blood sugar (*which see*) levels. Foods with a low glycaemic index resulting in the slow absorption of sugars from the diet, a modest rise in blood glucose, and a smooth return to normal are considered desirable. Foods with a high glycaemic index result in the fast absorption of sugars and a surge in blood glucose levels. This is particularly undesirable for diabetics. In individuals with a tendency to reactive hypoglycaemia (*which see*), such foods eaten in excess may result in a subsequent surge in insulin levels leading to rebound low blood sugar within a few hours after eating.

A table of foods with their glycaemic index is shown on page 96.

Glycerine (glycerol)

Glycerine or glycerol forms about 5–10 per cent by weight of most triglycerides (fats). Fats are composed of a glycerol 'backbone' attached to three fatty acid molecules. Glycerol is also a component of lecithin.

Some foods with a high glycaemic index	Some foods with a moderate glycaemic index	Some foods with a low glycaemic index
Bananas	Buckwheat	Apples
Beetroot	Canned beans (unless sugar-	Black-eyed beans
Bread (wholemeal and	free)	Butter beans
white)	Chocolate	Chick peas
Broad beans (fresh)	Digestive and oatmeal	Fructose
Carrots	biscuits	Grapefruit
Corn chips and cornflakes	Oranges and orange juice	Grapes
Honey	Pasta	Haricot (white) beans
Instant potato	Peas	Ice-cream (except low fat)
Low-fat ice-cream	Potato crisps (fried)	Kidney beans
Millet	Pumpernickel	Lentils
Puffed wheat	Rich Tea biscuits	Milk
Muesli	Spaghetti	Nuts
Raisins	Sugar (sucrose)	Oatmeal
Rice (both brown and white)	Sweetcorn	Pears
Rice cakes	Sweet potato	Soya beans
Rye and wheat crackers	Yams	Yoghurt
Shredded wheat		

Glycine
(also see Detoxification)

Amino acid

Glycine is the simplest of the amino acids, and can be synthesized by the body from the amino acids serine or threonine. Like taurine and GABA it acts as a major inhibitory neurotransmitter (*which see*) and is highly concentrated in the brain, particularly in the areas that are involved in Parkinson's disease. Glycine is rapidly broken down in the body.

Glycine is a glycogenic amino acid – it is capable of building up glycogen, or stored carbohydrate. It assists in the manufacture of DNA, glycerol and phospholipids, cholesterol conjugates, collagen and glutathione. Glycine can be converted to pyruvate and thus act as fuel for energy production (*which see*). It is essential for glycine conjugation – one of the key liver detoxification pathways. Glycine is a potent stimulator for the secretion of glucagon, which raises blood sugar levels, and when supplemented in large amounts can also raise growth hormone levels. Low glycine levels are often found in manic-depressive and epileptic patients, who may respond to supplementation since glycine is an inhibitory neurotransmitter.

Glycine supplementation can increase the clearance of uric acid by the kidneys, and may be a useful aid to the treatment of gout. It is essential for wound healing, and may be added, along with zinc, to ointments and creams for this purpose. Glycine, in combination with alanine and glutamic acid, has been used to improve the symptoms of benign prostate hypertrophy (prostate enlargement).

One third of the protein gelatin consists of glycine. Gelatin is therefore a cheap and useful source of this amino acid.

Glycogen

The storage form of carbohydrate within the body. Glycogen is mostly stored in the liver (where it is used to maintain the blood sugar level between meals) and in the muscle cells (where it is used as a source of energy). Higher amounts of muscle glycogen can be induced by feeding a high-carbohydrate diet after heavy exercise which depletes muscle glycogen stores.

Glycolysis (see Energy production)

Glycoproteins

Proteins attached to oligosaccharides. They form part of many substances and components of the human body, including cell walls, collagen, bone matrix, mucous secretions, hormones, enzymes and nutrient transport mechanisms.

Goitrogens

Naturally-occurring substances found in some foods, which in large amounts can inhibit the body's production of thyroid hormone. Some of these foods are: cabbage, peanuts and soya products.

Golden seal

Herb

A herb originally used by Native Americans for indigestion, local inflammations, liver disorders and to improve the appetite, golden seal is one of the most useful herbs in the modern repertoire. It is a drying, anticatarrhal herb, with both a gentle laxative and astringent effect, making it particularly useful for intestinal conditions involving excess mucus and inflammation. Nutritional therapists include it in programmes which combat problems such as mucus colitis, dysbiosis (which see) and gut inflammation, leaky gut syndrome, diarrhoea, poor appetite and poor liver function. Medical herbalists may also use it in programmes to treat premenstrual, menstrual or menopausal problems linked with stagnation. However, golden seal should be avoided in pregnancy as it is a uterine stimulant. It is also contraindicated in high blood pressure.

A broad spectrum of anti-microbial activity against bacteria, fungi and parasites has been reported for berberine, one of the constituents of golden seal. This would account for its effectiveness against many types of infective diarrhoea. Berberine can also stimulate bile secretion and ease gallbladder congestion.

In the Chinese classification system, golden seal is a 'cold bitter' which means that it is best applied in conditions of excessive vitality and avoided in any conditions involving coldness, such as depressed circulation or low metabolic rate, frequent urination or chronic respiratory congestion.

Availability: Through specialist herb shops, nutritional therapists and herbalists.

Gotu kola

Herb

This herb is said to have relaxing qualities and to be restorative for the nervous system. It is sometimes added to herbal and nutritional formulations for hypoglycaemia (low blood sugar) since in one clinical study it was shown to increase the mean concentration of blood sugar. Gotu kola may improve the blood circulation in the lower limbs and improve vein tonicity.

Availability: Through specialist outlets and herbalists.

Grapefruit seed extract

Herb

This is a bitter substance used by natural medicine practitioners for its broad-spectrum anti-bacterial and anti-parasitic properties. It is very poorly absorbed from the intestines, hence is useful in helping to treat dysbiosis (*which see*).

Availability: Mainly from specialist outlets and nutritional therapists.

Green tea

Herb

When black tea is produced, the oxidation of its polyphenols is promoted. Green tea is prepared with a process that prevents this oxidation. It is consumed primarily in China, Japan and a few countries in North Africa and the Middle East.

Fresh green leaf tea is particularly rich in antioxidants known as polyphenols, one type of which – catechins – may constitute up to 30 per cent of the dry leaf weight. Small amounts of caffeine, theobromine and theophylline are also present. Polyphenols are also found in red wine and it is thought that they account for the apparent ability of red wine to protect against heart disease. Green tea has been found to have some anti-carcinogenic action in animal studies.

Green-lipped mussel extract

Also known as New Zealand green-lipped mussel extract, this is a substance extracted from this species of mussel which seems to have anti-arthritic properties for many individuals. A number of clinical trials have obtained positive results. It is not yet known how the mussel extract works on arthritis, and there appear to be three groups of responders: those who find that the product has a sustained positive effect after only one course of capsules; those who find the product effective but need to take it on a long-term basis, and those who do not find it effective at all.

Availability: Widely available in health food stores.

GTF
(see Glucose Tolerance Factor)

Guarana

Herb

Guarana is a South American herb which is often taken in capsule form as a tonic. Its active ingredient is known as guaranine. Although pharmacists believe that guaranine is identical to caffeine because analytical procedures cannot distinguish between the two substances, an alternative view is that guaranine is in fact 8-methyl caffeine, closely related to caffeine, but with different properties.

According to researcher Brian Hildreth (now deceased), the use of heat in the analytical procedure could even convert guaranine to caffeine.

A placebo-controlled study carried out on human volunteers, comparing the effects of guarana and caffeine found that guarana improved the speed of reaction time and accuracy in a test of hand/eye co-ordination, whereas caffeine had a detrimental effect on the performance of this task. Compared with caffeine, guarana resulted in greater alertness, calm and sociability.

H

Haem

A red, iron-containing pigment found in haemoglobin, which binds and carries oxygen in the red blood cells, releasing it to tissues which can exchange it for carbon dioxide. Each molecule of haem can carry one molecule of oxygen.

Haemoglobin

A protein-iron compound in the red cells of the blood which carries oxygen to the cells from the lungs and carbon dioxide away from the cells to the lungs. More than 100 different types of haemoglobin have been identified, and are referred to as haemoglobin A, C, S, D, E, G and so on.

In the lungs, haemoglobin binds with oxygen to form oxyhaemoglobin which is carried to the tissues by the arteries. In the peripheral tissues of the body and other areas of low oxygen concentration, the oxygen is replaced with carbon dioxide to form carboxyhaemoglobin. The carboxyhaemoglobin is then released in the lungs for excretion via the breath.

Hair mineral analysis

The chemical analysis of the mineral content of hair, for calcium, magnesium, iron, chromium and many other nutritional elements, as well as toxic (heavy) metals such as mercury, lead and cadmium. Research has shown that for many elements hair more closely reflects body mineral stores than does blood or urine, particularly in cases of toxic metal accumulation, since hair growth is a vehicle for the excretion of these metals. Although hair will often show toxicity when blood and urine will not, it is more difficult to interpret the significance of levels of nutritional minerals in hair. For instance a high calcium level in the hair does not necessarily mean that there are high calcium levels in the blood. High zinc levels in the hair can be indicative of a zinc excess or a zinc deficiency in the body. For these reasons, hair analysis must be interpreted by a skilled professional and preferably used in conjunction with other tests.

Stringent conditions are required for the collection and handling of the hair samples, to avoid contamination. Only hair growing close to the scalp should be collected and analysed, since only this part of the hair will reflect recent conditions in the body.

Hay diet

A diet which avoids the consumption of starch and protein in the same meal. Also known as Food Combining. (*See Therapeutic diets*)

HDLs (see Lipoproteins)

Heavy metals

Technically metals with a specific gravity five or more times than of water, such as cadmium, mercury and lead, but usually taken to mean toxic heavy metals which the body excretes with difficulty. It is not widely known that as well as aiding the absorption of calcium, magnesium and other nutritional minerals, vitamin D can also aid the absorption of heavy metals. Conversely, lead, cadmium and aluminium block the synthesis of active vitamin D by the kidneys.

Heme (see Haem)

Hemoglobin (see Haemoglobin)

Hesperidin (see Flavonoids)

Histamine

A neurotransmitter (*which see*) derived from the breakdown of the amino acid histidine. Histamine effects include capillary dilation, reduced blood pressure, and increased stomach acid production. Histamine is stored in mast cells, from which it is released in allergic reactions, producing symptoms such as skin redness, swelling, or constriction of the bronchi in the lungs (asthma).

Histidine

Amino acid

Adults and children are able to synthesize histidine from glutamic acid and possibly biotin, but infants (babies) are not. Major food sources of histidine are meat and dairy produce. Very little histidine is found in most cereals and vegetables. Histidine is thought to help in copper transport and to have a mild anti-inflammatory effect because of the way it combines in the blood with copper.

Histidine is the precursor of histamine, which triggers orgasm when released from the mast cells in the genitals and is also involved in allergic reactions. High levels of histamine promote orgasm in both males and females.

Rheumatoid arthritis sufferers have low blood histidine levels – possibly due to too-rapid removal of histidine from their blood. Promising results have been achieved by supplementing histidine to these patients, particularly those most seriously affected. Histidine seems to improve their grip strength and walking ability.

Histidine supplements should be avoided by women with heavy menstrual bleeding, and individuals subject to depression.

Suggested dosage for rheumatoid arthritis: histidine 4 grams a day in divided doses.

Vegetarian sources: Weight for weight, soya protein concentrate, peanuts, tofu and sunflower seeds are as rich in histidine as animal proteins.

Homocysteine

Amino acid

A sulphur-containing amino acid formed as a breakdown product of the essential amino acid methionine. Homocysteine should exist only briefly before being converted to the harmless cystathione by means of the vitamin B_6-dependent enzyme, cystathionine synthetase, and then to cysteine. This process requires adequate levels of methionine. If the process (known as trans-sulphuration) does not occur efficiently, raised blood levels of homocysteine can occur. These are associated with atherogenesis (clogging of arteries with cholesterol deposits) because homocysteine is easily oxidized and can therefore damage cell structures, blood lipids and artery walls, as well as eye lenses, bones and joints.

Full-blown defects in the cystathione synthetase gene give rise to a condition known as homozygous homocystinuria, which affects about one in 200,000 people and involves the accumulation of homocysteine inside cells and the dumping of homocysteine into the bloodstream. It is an extremely serious condition, associated with early death from atherosclerosis.

Heterozygous homocystinuria (excess homocysteine in the urine) or homocystinaemia (excess homocysteine in the blood) affects about one in 200 people. In these individuals cystathione synthetase is functional, but inefficient, resulting in raised blood levels of homocysteine.

Homocysteine can also be removed from the blood by conversion to methionine, using the enzyme methionine synthase in a process known as remethylation. This process is dependent on the B vitamins folic acid and vitamin B_{12}, and deficiencies of these nutrients can therefore also result in homocystinaemia. In fact elevated serum homocysteine levels are often used as a marker for functional folic acid and vitamin B_{12} deficiencies. In a follow-up to the famous Framingham study on heart disease, 12 per cent of the survivors had clear signs of vitamin B_{12} deficiency. Folic acid (*which see*) is normally found in fresh fruit and vegetables and is very easily destroyed by storage and cooking. Many individuals have severely restricted intakes of good food sources of folic acid and are likely to be deficient in this nutrient.

Research into the treatment of heterozygous homocystinaemia using supplementation with vitamins B_6, B_{12} and folic acid is showing promise, and tests are now available to determine an individual's requirements for these nutrients by measuring lymphocyte (white blood cell) growth responses.

Hops

Herb

Hops are particularly used to combat sleeplessness, and can be taken orally or placed in a pillow under the head at night to encourage sleep. The bitterness of hops when ingested orally also makes them a gastric stimulant.

Another indication for the use of hops is to reduce sexual arousal in men, in order to combat premature ejaculation or 'wet dreams'.

A study carried out using hops in combination with uva-ursi (*which see*) and vitamin E found improved irritable bladder and urinary incontinence in 772 out of 915 patients.

Availability: From specialist outlets and herbalists.

Hormones

Substances produced in one part of the body (often called a 'gland') which regulate the activity of an organ or group of cells in another part of the body.

Also see Endocrine system and individual hormones.

The major hormones and their effects

Gland	Hormone	Controls
Anterior pituitary	Growth hormone	Growth and metabolism
	Thyroid-stimulating hormone	Thyroid gland
	Adrenocorticotropic hormone (ACTH)	Adrenal cortex
	Gonadotropic hormones (follicle-stimulating hormone and luteinizing hormone)	Gonads (reproductive glands)
Posterior pituitary	Oxytocin	Milk 'let-down'. Uterine motility
	Antidiuretic hormone	Water excretion by the kidneys
Adrenal cortex	Cortisol	Metabolism. Stress response.
	Androgens	Male characteristics. Sex drive in men and women
	Aldosterone	Excretion of sodium and potassium by the kidneys
Adrenal medulla	Adrenaline	Metabolism. Stress response
	Noradrenaline	Metabolism. Stress response
Thyroid	Thyroxine and triiodothyronine Calcitonin	Energy, metabolism and growth
Parathyroid glands	Parathyroid hormone	Calcium and phosphate balance in blood
Pancreas	Insulin Glucagon Somatostatin	Metabolism. Blood sugar control
Ovaries	Oestrogen and progesterone	Reproductive system in women. Female characteristics
Testes	Testosterone	Reproductive system in males. Male characteristics
Pineal	Melatonin	Diurnal rhythms (sleep and waking)

Horsetail

Herb

Horsetail is principally used for its content of water-soluble, colloidal silica. It is therefore primarily a treatment for connective tissue problems and internal bleeding, but also has diuretic properties and may help to remove excess lead from the body. The plant should be boiled in water for three hours with a little sugar to extract the silica.

One of the most important uses of horsetail is as a urinary astringent, helping to reduce irritation of the bladder sphincter and therefore combating frequent urination. This astringent effect is thought to be particularly helpful against the problems associated with prostate enlargement in men.

Availability: From specialist outlets and herbalists.

Hydrazine sulphate

A man-made material which, it is theorized, can deprive tumours of the energy they need to grow, thus combating cancer. It is thought to work best against breast cancer, sarcomas, neuroblastoma, laryngeal cancer and Hodgkin's disease, but there has been little research to support this. Some studies of terminal cancer patients have claimed to show an inhibition of the cancer wasting syndrome known as cachexia. Hydrazine sulphate must not be used with alcohol or barbiturates.

Availability: Only available from specialist suppliers.

Hydrochloric acid

Composed of hydrogen and chloride atoms, hydrochloric acid is produced by the gastric glands in the stomach to aid protein digestion by 'uncoiling' proteins, preparing them for the later stages of digestion. The strong acidity of the stomach prevents bacterial growth and kills most bacteria ingested with food.

Hydrogen peroxide

A free radical (*which see*) initiator which must be removed by an antioxidant enzyme, either catalase or glutathione peroxidase. Hydrogen peroxide solution is also used as a disinfectant and bleach and, in some alternative circles, as a controversial oral treatment for candidiasis. However, most natural medicine practitioners feel that the claims made for this treatment are difficult to verify and they are not prepared to take the risks associated with the deliberate introduction of large amounts of free radicals into the body.

Hydrogenated fats (see Fats)

Hydroxyl radical
(see Free radicals)

Hydroxyproline

Amino acid

Hydroxyproline can be synthesized by the body from proline, using ascorbic acid (vitamin C) as the major cofactor. The primary role of this amino acid is in bone and connective tissue. It is highly concentrated throughout the body, except in cerebrospinal fluid.

Hyperglycaemia
(also see Blood sugar)

Literally means 'excess sugar in the blood'. Hyperglycaemia is characteristic of the disease diabetes.

Hypoallergenic diet
(see Therapeutic diets)

Hypochlorhydria
(see Achlorhydria)

Hypoglycaemia
(also see Blood sugar)

Literally means 'low blood sugar'. Hypoglycaemia is normally prevented by hormonal blood sugar control mechanisms. It is when these mechanisms fail that blood sugar drops too low. In diabetics, hypoglycaemia may occur when insulin or blood sugar-reducing drugs are present in the blood in excessive amounts.

Reactive (rebound) hypoglycaemia may occur a few hours after a susceptible individual has consumed sugary food or drinks, especially on an empty stomach. The sugar enters the bloodstream rapidly, stimulating a correspondingly rapid release of insulin. The more rapidly insulin is released, the more likely the pancreas is to 'overshoot the mark' and produce too much. Since the function of insulin is to remove sugar (glucose) from the blood into the cells, too much insulin can leave the blood containing too little sugar, and this may result in a number of unpleasant symptoms. These typically affect the brain, which is the first organ to be affected by a lack of glucose.

Some possible symptoms of hypoglycaemia

Fainting	Trembling and shaking
Fatigue	Aggressive outbursts
Headaches	Depression
Sleepiness	Dizziness

Hypoglycaemia can also occur when insulin begins to become defective – larger and larger quantities are needed to perform its function of removing sugar from the blood. The body may try to compensate for this by producing a state of chronic hyperinsulinaemia (excess insulin in the blood), leading to hypoglycaemic symptoms. As the condition worsens, it may develop into maturity-onset diabetes, where insulin becomes too weak to reduce blood sugar, and hyperglycaemia (chronic excessive blood sugar) results. This 'weakness' of insulin may be due to nutritional deficiencies such as B vitamins, chromium and zinc and can often be reversed with help from a professional nutritional therapist.

I

Iatrogenic

An iatrogenic illness is one caused by medical personnel or medical treatment or procedures. Adverse drug reactions are common causes of iatrogenic illness. The most outstanding example of modern times is probably SMON – subacute myelo-optic neuropathy, a condition which affected thousands of Japanese people from 1959 to 1973 causing internal bleeding, diarrhoea, nerve damage, paralysis, and many deaths. During all this time, doctors were intent on seeking an infectious cause despite the absence of any indicators that the disease was communicable. The epidemic only came to a halt when it was accidentally discovered that the anti-diarrhoea drug clioquinol (Entero-viaform) was entirely responsible for the disease. What doctors did not realize was that clioquinol could cause diarrhoea as well as treat it. The more they dosed their patients with the drug, the worse the symptoms became, which were then treated with higher and higher doses of the drug, to the point of severe toxicity and frequently death.

Similarly there is an increasing following in medical circles for the hypothesis that toxic anti-viral drugs are causing immune system damage mistakenly attributed to the HIV virus. The reasoning is that many HIV-positive individuals who have not taken anti-Aids medication have not gone on to develop Aids. This, and the fact that injecting the HIV virus into test animals does not appear to produce any Aids-like syndrome, suggests that HIV itself is quite harmless and has nothing to do with Aids. Many experts have secretly doubted the connection for a long time. It may be that the severe immune system depletion which occurs in HIV-positive individuals only occurs if they have been given anti-HIV drugs, and is solely due to these drugs, which are known to be very toxic.

According to the Aids dissidents, the statistics attributed to African Aids may also have little to do with the HIV virus, and may instead be the result of diseases from which Africans have always suffered, except that when HIV antibodies are present, death from these diseases is now classified as Aids-related death.

A 1992 study by Social Audit in the UK estimated that 10,000 hospital admissions a year – one in six hospital patients – are due to side-effects from prescribed medicines.

Ileum

The lower portion of the small intestine.

Immune system

The immune system protects the body from outside harmful influences by creating barriers and defence mechanisms. The skin and mucous membranes are the first of these barriers. The stomach contains powerful acid to kill bacteria and other micro-organisms that may be ingested with food. The friendly bacteria in the intestines serve to prevent overgrowth with more harmful species. The liver neutralizes toxins absorbed in food, air and drink, and the white blood cells and antibodies serve to detect, destroy and ingest harmful micro-organisms which penetrate into the blood-stream and tissues.

Immunoglobulins

Any one of five types of antibody present in the body. In response to specific antigens (*which see*) immunoglobulins are formed in the bone marrow, spleen and most lymphoid tissues and may be used as markers indicating an allergic reaction. The immunoglobulins are known as IgA, IgD, IgE, IgG and IgM. IgE reactions are taken to be indicators of classical allergy, and the modern ELISA test measures IgM as an indicator of food intolerance.

Inosine

A component of DNA which is sometimes taken as a dietary supplement. It has been used in the treatment of congestive heart failure and angina, and is under investigation as an anti-cancer and anti-viral agent.
Availability: Not easily available.

Inositol

Vitamin-like substance

FUNCTIONS
Component of cell plasma membranes
Lipotropic (helps to remove fat from the liver)
Fat metabolism
May be involved in neurotransmitter (*which see*) function

GOOD FOOD SOURCES
Beans
Citrus fruit
Grapefruit juice
Lecithin
Liver
Wheat germ
Whole grains

Deficiency symptoms

No known specific symptoms of deficiency.

Preventing deficiency

As with all other nutrients, a wide variety of foods, preferably for the most part unrefined, is the best health protection. It would be difficult to develop an inositol deficiency without also developing a number of other deficiencies.

Comments

Inositol is found in cereals (particularly the bran portion) and vegetables in the form of phytic acid, a combination of inositol with phosphorus.

Supplementation

In research studies, inositol supplements have been found to:

- Improve diabetic neuropathy
- Reduce symptoms of clinical depression and anxiety

Preferred form and suggested intake

The usual form of inositol supplementation is lecithin, which contains large amounts of inositol. Lecithin can be bought in granules and sprinkled on food or in hot drinks. The usual dosage is 1–2 tablespoons per day.

Cautions

There is no known unsafe dosage of lecithin.

Insulin (see Blood sugar)

International Units (IU)

International Units are a measurement system for the biological activity of vitamins A, D and E (and formerly some of the other vitamins too). Many products, particularly those in the higher dosage range, are still sold in International Units because consumers are accustomed to this system. However scientists no longer use International Units, and prefer to measure vitamins by weight.

1 iu vitamin A = 0.3 micrograms

1 iu vitamin D = 0.025 micrograms

1 iu vitamin E = 0.7 milligrams if the vitamin is in the usual supplement form of d-alpha tocopherol. Other forms of vitamin E have different equivalences.

Intrinsic factor

A protein secreted by the stomach which forms a complex with vitamin B_{12} in the diet, thus enabling this vitamin to be absorbed. A lack of intrinsic factor can lead to pernicious anaemia (severe vitamin B_{12} deficiency).

Inulin (see Probiotics)

Iodine

Trace element
UK RNI 140 mcg
US RDA 150 mcg

FUNCTIONS

Thyroid hormone production
Iodine is also actively concentrated from the blood by the gastric mucosa, salivary glands, the choroid plexus of the brain, and the lactating mammary glands, suggesting further functions as yet unknown.

GOOD FOOD SOURCES

Dairy produce
Fish and seafood
Pineapple
Raisins
Seaweed (e.g. kelp)
Exceptionally large quantities of iodine are found in the artificial food additive erythrosine (E127), which is used as a red colouring for cocktail and glace cherries. A high consumption of these foods is not advised if they contain this additive.

Deficiency symptoms

- Enlargement of the thyroid gland in the neck (goitre)

- Deficiency may cause excess oestrogen production (a risk factor for breast, uterine and ovarian cancers) by stimulating the sex glands in women
- Deficiency may cause fibrocystic breast disease
- Deficiency may cause neurological impairment associated with hearing loss
- Deficiency reduces the activity of some white blood cells
- Populations with a higher intake of iodine-containing foods (such as Japan) may have a lower incidence of breast cancer

Preventing deficiency

Many parts of the world lack iodine in their soil, and in these areas goitre and cretinism (a congenital condition involving dwarfism and mental retardation) are endemic. According to a 1987 study, the evidence suggests that multiple sclerosis, motor neurone disease, cancers of the thyroid and nervous system, Parkinson's disease and Alzheimer's disease are also associated with iodine deficiency. Rats on experimental iodine-deficient diets show many of the metabolic changes associated with these diseases. (*Foster HD: Disease family trees: the possible roles of iodine in goitre, cretinism, multiple sclerosis, amyotrophic lateral sclerosis, Alzheimer's and Parkinson's diseases and cancers of the thyroid, nervous system and skin. Med Hypotheses 24(3):249-63, 1987.*)

Comments

Goitrogens, certain chemicals found in turnips, cabbage, soya beans and peanuts, interfere with iodine uptake by the thyroid, but this is only likely to be a problem for individuals with a borderline iodine intake.

Supplementation

In research studies, iodine supplements have been found to:

- Treat goitre
- Improve fibrocystic breast disease (certain specific forms of iodine only)

Preferred form and suggested intake
Seaweed products such as kelp. Supplement manufacturers also use potassium iodide in multi-nutrient formulas. Do not consume iodine from your medicine chest – in this form it is poisonous.

Cautions
Excess dietary iodine may cause acne, goitre, thyroid suppression or hyperthyroidism.

Iron

Trace element
UK RNI 14.8 mg (women), 8.7 mg (men)
US RDA 15 mg (women), 10 mg (men)

> **FUNCTIONS**
> Cell proliferation
> Component of many enzymes
> Function of T cells and leucocyte microbiocidal activity
> Needed for cytochrome detoxification enzymes in the liver
> Oxygen supply to cells
> Present in electron transport system which produces energy
> Present in enzyme catalase which combats peroxide free radicals
> Production and disposal of free radicals

Black sausage

Cocoa powder and dark chocolate

Liver

Molasses

Parsley

Pulses

Red meat

Shellfish

Some types of cheap wine

Some green vegetables

Deficiency signs and symptoms

- Anaemia (weakness, anorexia, depression, confusion, dizziness, fatigability, pallor, breathlessness, palpitations and sometimes cold sensitivity, constipation and gastrointestinal complaints)
- Growth impairment
- Increased susceptibility to infection
- Pica (consumption of earth, ice, paint and other non-food items)
- Reduced bone density
- Scholastic underachievement (due to impairment of mental faculties)
- Severe iron deficiency can cause food malabsorption, possibly by a decrease in iron-dependent enzymes in intestinal mucosal cells
- Some forms of deafness

Preventing deficiency

The bioavailability of iron in vegetables (but not meats) is increased by consuming vitamin C-containing foods in the same meal. It can be seriously reduced by the simultaneous consumption of phytic acid (found in raw whole grains and bran), tea or coffee, antacids, or large quantities of calcium. The consumption of tea or coffee within one hour of a meal can reduce iron absorption by up to 80 per cent, according to researchers. Achlorhydria (which see) can also impair iron absorption. Blood loss, as in injury, heavy menstruation or blood donation causes heavy iron losses. Contrary to popular belief, spinach is not a good source of iron as it contains oxalate, which reduces the availability of the iron. Among green vegetables, broccoli may be a better source of iron.

According to the medical literature, approximately 500 to 600 million of the world's population are believed to have iron deficiency anaemia (Cook JD: The liabilities of iron deficiency. Blood 68(4):803-9, 1986).

Comments

Iron is the most abundant trace element in the human and animal body. Dietary iron occurs in two forms: haem iron (found in meat and animal produce) and the less easily absorbed non-haem iron found in plant foods.

Supplementation

In research studies, iron supplements have been found to:

- Improve detoxification ability in some individuals
- Improve some forms of hearing loss
- Reduce period pain (dysmenorrhoea) in anaemic women
- Treat anaemia
- Treat restless leg syndrome

Preferred form and suggested intake

Ferric forms of iron (see the formula on the pack) destroy vitamin E, while ferrous forms do not have this effect. Some commonly used forms of iron include iron amino acid chelates, ferrous gluconate, ferrous lactate and ferrous sulphate. Ferrous sulphate is often used for its cheapness but is a gastrointestinal irritant and not well absorbed.

Cautions

Owing to the frequency with which doctors prescribe iron supplements, there have been a number of incidents of children's accidental poisoning with iron supplements that resemble sweets. All dietary supplements should be kept safely out of children's reach, and products with child-proof caps used wherever possible.

High levels of iron supplementation may lead to zinc malabsorption and depletion.

Haemochromatosis is a serious iron overload condition which may be due to a genetic disorder and can lead to cirrhosis of the liver, diabetes, and hyperpigmentation of the skin, with irregular heartbeats, joint pains and cardiac failure. It is very unwise to take iron supplements unless they are needed.

Iron is a free radical promoter, especially if vitamin E levels are low.

Ischaemia

A condition characterized by a decreased supply of oxygen to a part of the body. For instance, angina is a manifestation of ischaemic heart disease – a lack of blood supply to the heart muscle, usually due to a blockage of the coronary artery which supplies that muscle tissue. The symptoms of angina are due to the heart muscle trying to labour without adequate oxygen.

Isoleucine

Amino acid

Isoleucine is one of the branched chain amino acids (*which see*). It cannot be made by the human body, and is particularly involved in stress, energy and muscle metabolism.

The Brain Bio Center in the US has found that chronic schizophrenics may have reduced levels of isoleucine and that supplementation with isoleucine can reverse their psychosis, particularly if given in combination with very large amounts of vitamin B$_3$.

Vegetarian sources: Weight for weight, soya protein concentrate, soya flour, tofu, peanuts, almonds, pumpkin seeds and sunflower seeds are as rich in isoleucine as animal proteins.

Availability of supplements: Usually available only in combined BCAA products.

Isomers

Molecules that have the same formula but their structures are arranged differently. For instance, an amino acid may have two isomers – a D form and an L form, as in L-phenylalanine and D-phenylalanine. Essential fatty acids may exist as *cis* isomers or *trans* isomers: e.g. cis-linoleic acid or trans-linoleic acid. (*See Fats*)

Itai-itai disease

A disease occurring in Japan which is probably associated with a high intake of the toxic metal cadmium from eating rice grown on land irrigated with cadmium-contaminated water. Symptoms include kidney and gastrointestinal damage, with bone softening. The disease particularly affects older women.

IU (see International Units)

J

Jejunum

The middle section of the small intestine. This is the section which absorbs most of the substances in the diet.

Jojoba

An acorn-like fruit with a history of medicinal use by Native Americans. The nuts may be roasted and eaten, or made into a coffee-like drink. Jojoba oil is widely used in cosmetics, and has a high content of myristic acid, which is also found in nutmeg and mace and may have anti-inflammatory effects.

Juniper berries

Herb

The main indications for juniper berry treatment are chronic arthritis or gout, rheumatism and tendonitis, and the herb may be taken internally or applied externally to affected areas. Juniper has a diuretic effect, and should not be used for more than six weeks in succession as it may irritate the kidneys. It may also stimulate uterine contractions and thus cause miscarriage in pregnant women (hence the reputation of gin for being used in attempts to induce abortion – gin is flavoured with juniper berries). However, the risk of abortion is not very great; gin is largely ineffective for this purpose.

Availability: Commonly available from herb and spice suppliers.

K

Vitamin K (Phylloquinone or Menaquinone)

Vitamin (fat-soluble)
UK RNI None
US RDA 80 mcg

FUNCTIONS

Production of four proteins involved in blood clotting
Involved in bone calcification and mineralization

GOOD FOOD SOURCES

Alfalfa
Broccoli
Brussels sprouts
Cabbage and other leafy green vegetables
Cauliflower
Green tea
Liver
Meats
Soybean, rapeseed and olive oils
Tomatoes
Whole grains

Deficiency signs and symptoms

- Bleeding and haemorrhage
- Increased urinary calcium excretion
- Osteoporosis

Preventing deficiency

Vitamin K can be synthesized by Bacteroides bacteria in the small intestine so it is not essential to obtain all vitamin K from the diet unless these bacteria have been depleted by taking antibiotics. Bacterial synthesis alone is not sufficient to meet all the body's needs. Vitamin K produced by bacteria in the colon is not absorbed.

Since vitamin K is fat-soluble, the presence of chronic diarrhoea, or any defect in fat digestion and absorption, or a deficiency of fat or oil in the diet, could result in depletion of vitamin K levels. About 60–70 per cent of dietary vitamin K is excreted daily, so a daily intake of vitamin K-rich foods is advisable. The long-term use of aspirin-based medication increases vitamin K requirements.

Comments

The plant form of vitamin K is known as phylloquinone (sometimes known as vitamin K_1). Intestinal bacteria synthesize a family of compounds with vitamin K activity known as menaquinones (vitamin K_2). Liver stores of vitamin K are small, and mainly consist of menaquinones. Bone contains substantial concentrations of both phylloquinone and menaquinones.

Vitamin K is often given routinely to newborn, especially premature, babies to prevent haemorrhagic disease of the newborn. Newborn infants have a low vitamin K level due to the lack of gut bacteria in the first few days of life. Proteins found in bone tissue – known as osteocalcin, bone Gla protein and matrix Gla protein – are dependent on adequate vitamin K levels, which may explain why supplementation with this nutrient helps to reverse osteoporosis.

Supplementation

In research studies, vitamin K supplements have been found to:

• Accelerate healing of bone fractures
• Increase bone formation in post-menopausal osteoporotic women
• Reduce urinary calcium excretion

Preferred form and suggested intake

Vitamin K supplements are not normally available since for most purposes more than adequate amounts of the vitamin can be obtained from vegetables.

Kelp

A seaweed (*Ascophylum nodosum*) which is often taken as a dietary supplement for its high iodine content (about 500 mcg per gram). It is also a good source of other minerals.

Availability: In tablet form from health food shops.

Ketone bodies

A term used for the three substances acetoacetic acid, beta-hydroxybutyric acid and acetone, which are products of incomplete fatty acid oxidation and are formed when fat is used as an energy source by the body. Being water-soluble, ketones can be used by most cells as an alternative to glucose.

An abnormal accumulation of ketone bodies is known as ketosis. When severe, ketosis is known as ketoacidosis, because the body becomes over-acidified due to the acidity of two of the ketone bodies.

Conditions leading to ketosis are fasting or starvation, a shortage of carbohydrate, or uncontrolled diabetes mellitus which results in the body's inability to utilize carbohydrate as an energy source. In all these cases the body is forced to use fat as an alternative energy source, and free fatty acids in the circulation are converted to ketone bodies in the liver. Ketone production increases gradually during fasting or carbohydrate deprivation, reaching its maximum by about 10 days.

Ketosis (see Ketone bodies)

Kidneys

The kidneys consist of small funnel-like units called nephrons which filter blood under high pressure, removing water, urea, salts and other soluble wastes from blood plasma, and eliminating them as urine. All the blood in the body passes through the kidneys about 20 times every hour.

The kidneys also play an important role in the activation of vitamin D.

Koji

An Oriental enzyme made from the mould *Aspergillus oryzae* and used in the preparation of miso (*which see*).

Availability: From macrobiotic suppliers.

Kombu

A type of seaweed ('sea vegetable') used in Japanese and macrobiotic cookery, kombu is rich in protein and minerals and greatly increases the nutritional value of a meal. It can also serve to tenderize beans.

Availability: Health food shops and macrobiotic suppliers.

Kombucha

Sometimes known as the Manchurian mushroom, kombucha is a yeast culture with a rubbery texture which has a symbiotic (mutually helpful) relationship with certain bacteria. Kombucha thrives on sugar and tea, which it converts to glucose, fructose, vitamin C and B vitamins, glucuronic acid, lactic acid and other substances thought to have health-giving properties.

Availability: Specialist suppliers.

Krebs cycle (see Energy production)

Kuzu

A pure white starch extracted from the root of a Japanese vine, and used as a thickener (like arrowroot) in macrobiotic cookery. It is claimed to be more nutritious than other, similar starch thickeners.

Availability: Macrobiotic suppliers.

Kwashiorkor

A type of protein-energy malnutrition. (*See Nutritional deficiencies*)

Kyolic garlic (also see Garlic)

Garlic which has been subjected to a 'cold-ageing' process for 20 months. This process promotes the breakdown of alliin, the parent sulphur compound in garlic, into components which are odourless and chemically more stable. Although its therapeutic effects on the heart and circulation have been researched, it is not known whether kyolic garlic retains all the therapeutic properties of fresh garlic.

L

Lactase

A digestive enzyme required to split the sugar lactose into glucose and galactose (*also see Carbohydrates*).

Lactic acid

An acid formed by the fermentation of milk sugar. In the human body, lactic acid is formed in the muscles from glucose when the oxygen supply is inadequate, and causes the characteristic burning pain associated with muscular over-exertion. Lactic acid can be converted back to glucose by the liver.

Lactic acid bacteria
(see Probiotics)

Lactobacilli (see Probiotics)

Lactose
(see Carbohydrates)

Laetrile

Also known as amygdalin and 'vitamin B_{17}' (it is not a vitamin), the term laetrile was first introduced by Dr Ernst Krebs Sr in 1952. It is extracted from apricot kernels and has been used as an alternative cancer therapy. Amygdalins are chemical compounds consisting of two molecules of sugar, one molecule of benzaldehyde and one molecule of cyanide bound tightly together. As reported by Dr Richard Passwater in his book *Cancer and its Nutritional Therapies*, studies have shown an almost 100 per cent inhibition of cancer by apricot kernels in a strain of mice particularly susceptible to breast cancer. This effect has been attributed to the cyanide content, which is thought to be released from amygdalin by the action of an enzyme beta-glycosidase. It is theorized that because more of this enzyme is secreted by cancer cells than by normal cells, and because cancer cells may have much less of another enzyme, rhodanese, which in normal cells can detoxify cyanide, the cyanide destroys cancer cells more easily.

Many human cancer sufferers who have used laetrile therapy report great benefits, although others do not. Most of the scientific studies have shown no clear benefit. The orthodox scientific community has pointed out that laetrile forms cyanide on digestion, by the action of gut bacteria, and that oral consumption is therefore potentially highly dangerous. Laetrile taken by injection has less risk of toxicity.

Availability: From some specialist alternative cancer clinics.

Lapacho

Herb

Lapacho (also known as taheebo or Pau D'Arco) tea has anti-fungal and possibly anti-cancer properties and is made from the bark of a South American tree. Although most of the commercial variety now comes from Brazil, it is said that the authentic, more medicinally active, lapacho only comes from north eastern Argentina. Lapacho contains a quinone known as lapachol, which is thought to form active derivatives when the bark is made into a tea or into the alcoholic extracts (elixirs) which are popular in South American cancer clinics.

Availability: Not easily available. May need to be obtained from a specialist supplier.

LDL (see Cholesterol)

Lead

Toxic element

A common pollutant, lead belongs to the group of so-called heavy metals which tend to accumulate in the body. The major source of lead is fall-out from petrol (gasoline) vehicle exhausts, which is both inhaled into the lungs and washed by the rain into drains, rivers and lakes, forming a danger to wildlife. Another significant source can be lead water pipes or lead-soldered joints in water pipes, particularly in soft-water areas. Soft water is slightly acidic and capable of dissolving lead. Individuals who are deficient in iron and calcium may absorb more lead than others from food and drink. Most Westerners now have a body burden of lead some 500 to 1,000 times greater than would have been the norm before widespread lead pollution began. According to experts, this is enough to adversely affect the nervous system of each and every one of us, and in particular to lower our threshold for the expression of anger, hostility and aggression.

Other sources of lead include:

- Bonemeal supplements (lead absorbed into the human or animal body accumulates in bone)
- Canned foods where cans are sealed with lead solder
- Cigarettes
- Game shot with lead pellets
- Lead-glazed pottery
- Milk from animals grazing on lead-contaminated grass
- Old house paint (lead is banned from modern paint)
- Plants grown in urban areas or berries by the roadside
- Roadside dust and dirt (animals may be particularly affected)
- Some hair colour restorers

Lead exerts its toxic effects by interfering with the normal function of physiologically important minerals and trace elements. For instance, the chemistry of lead resembles calcium so greatly that if calcium is in short supply and there is plenty of lead available, then lead can be absorbed instead of calcium both from the gastrointestinal tract (if ingested) and from the bloodstream into cellular systems.

The problem is that lead cannot perform the same tasks as calcium, so it disrupts the function of the cellular systems which are attempting to use it, and these effectively become calcium-deficient. Also, as described by Professor Derek Bryce-Smith in 1983, lead interferes with the synthesis of neurotransmitters (essential messenger substances used by the brain and nervous system) and can produce a false neurotransmitter called ALA, which competes with the real neurotransmitter GABA. GABA is needed to prevent the nervous system from becoming overactive. An individual whose GABA receptors are instead picking up ALA may develop a lack of inhibitory control. It is not difficult to see why high lead levels in the body are linked with hyperactivity and learning difficulties in children (*see Section II*), and aggressive or sociopathic behaviour in adults.

Mild lead toxicity exerts its most damaging effects on the unborn foetus and on children, leading to stillbirths, low birthweights, developmental abnormalities and learning and behavioural disorders. Research has found a link between lead and hyperactivity/attention-deficit disorder in children, and also that children with a high body burden of lead may have a lower IQ. The organic lead from petrol exhaust fumes has the most toxic effect on the nervous system.

Early symptoms of severe chronic lead toxicity include lack of appetite, constipation, headache, weakness, anaemia and a blue or black line along the gums. This may progress to vomiting, poor co-ordination, unsteady gait, visual disturbances and kidney failure.

Leaky gut syndrome

Apart from its functions as a digestive/absorptive organ, the small intestine also acts as a barrier to permeation of dietary and bacterial products with toxic properties. These include viable bacteria, bacterial cell wall polymers, chemotactic peptides, bacterial antigens capable of inducing antibodies, and bacterial and dietary antigens which can form systemic immune complexes.

If the integrity of the gut becomes impaired, this may result in the enhanced uptake of inflammatory macromolecules and pathogenic bacteria. Some of the factors which may damage the gut wall include: chronic allergic inflammation, chronic irritation due to non-steroidal anti-inflammatory drugs, chronic irritation due to dysbiosis (*which see*), parasites, or to the continual presence of excessive amounts of undigested food, and penetration by the mycelial form of *Candida albicans*. Alcoholism, cancer chemotherapy and Aids are also associated with increased gut permeability, leading to 'leaky gut syndrome'.

The symptoms of this condition may be non-specific: swelling and bloating of the abdomen, symptoms of an increased toxic load on the liver, such as the development of food allergies and chemical sensitivities, and increasing symptoms of nutritional deficiency as nutrient absorption worsens. (Paradoxically, while permeability to large molecules may increase due to the increased porosity of intercellular junctional complexes, permeability to small molecules decreases due to atrophy of the microvilli). According to the scientific literature, increased gut permeability appears to correlate with a number of frequently seen clinical disorders, including:

- Allergic disorders
- Ankylosing spondylitis
- Chronic dermatological conditions
- Coeliac disease
- Crohn's disease
- Food allergy
- Inflammatory bowel disease

- Inflammatory joint disease
- Rheumatoid arthritis
- Schizophrenia

The permeation of water-soluble molecules through the intestinal mucosa can occur either through cells (transcellular uptake) or between cells (paracellular uptake). Small molecules such as glucose and mannitol readily penetrate cells and passively diffuse through them. Larger molecules such as disaccharides (e.g. lactulose, sucrose) are normally excluded by cells. Leaky gut syndrome can therefore be diagnosed by measuring the ability of mannitol and lactulose to permeate the intestinal mucosa. Mannitol serves as a marker of transcellular uptake, and lactulose, being only slightly absorbed, serves as a marker for mucosal integrity. To perform the test, the patient mixes pre-measured amounts of lactulose and mannitol and drinks the challenge substance. The test – which is available through nutritional therapists – measures the amount of lactulose and mannitol recovered in a six-hour urine sample. Low levels of mannitol and lactulose indicate malabsorption. Elevated levels of lactulose and mannitol are indicative of general increased permeability and leaky gut syndrome. An elevated lactulose/-mannitol ratio indicates that the effective pore size of the gut mucosa has increased, allowing larger molecules to access the bloodstream, where they are capable of provoking allergic reactions.

Iron deficiency anaemia may cause leaky gut syndrome in babies and young children. (*Berant M et al.: Effect of iron deficiency on small intestinal permeability in infants and young children. J Pediatr Gastroenterol Nutr 14(1):17-20, 1992.*)

Lecithin

A number of types of lecithin are found in human cell membranes, particularly those of the liver, nerve tissue and semen. Lecithins are a type of phospholipid (*which see*). Like fats, they consist of a backbone of glycerol – but instead of having three fatty acids attached to it, the glycerol has only two fatty acids plus a phosphate group and a choline molecule. Lecithin is synthesized by the liver.

The fatty acids in lecithin and other phospholipids make it soluble in fat, and the phosphate-containing group makes it also soluble in water. Lecithin in cell membranes therefore enables fat-soluble substances, including vitamins and hormones, to pass easily in and out of cells. Lecithin also acts as an emulsifier, helping to keep fats suspended in the blood and body fluids.

Lecithin is synthesized by the food industry, where it is widely used as an emulsifier in products such as mayonnaise. It is also available as a food supplement, usually as granules or in capsules. Although the gut enzyme lecithinase probably breaks down most dietary lecithin before it reaches the body fluids, lecithin supplements – also known as phosphatidylcholine – usually contain large amounts of the nutrients choline and inositol, and are generally a safe and economical way to supplement them.

Good food sources of lecithin include liver, meats, fish, eggs, wheat, peanuts and soya beans. The calorific value of lecithin is similar to that of fats, at about 9 kcal per gram.

Availability: Widely available in health food shops.

Lectins

Toxic substances found in pulses (legumes) which are removed by boiling these foods for at least 10 minutes or by pressure-cooking them until soft. Lectins can cause severe food poisoning, with vomiting and diarrhoea.

Lentinan (see Shiitake)

Leucine

Amino acid

Leucine is one of the branched chain amino acids (*which see*). It cannot be made by the human body, and is particularly involved in stress, energy and muscle metabolism. Leucine is a purely 'ketogenic' amino acid – that is to say it is metabolized through fat pathways.

This amino acid is particularly good at stimulating protein synthesis. It also inhibits protein breakdown, and can substitute for glucose, providing an alternative, and perhaps superior, energy source for the body. Because of its ability to maintain blood sugar levels, some doctors believe that leucine, with other nutrients, may be a more ideal energy source than glucose in intravenous feeding solutions, particularly as branched chain amino acids (BCAAs) decrease the rate of breakdown and utilization of other amino acids.

A high intake of leucine can decrease brain serotonin and dopamine concentrations and, by increasing the excretion of vitamin B_3 in the urine, can worsen the psychotic symptoms of pellagra, the vitamin B_3 deficiency disease which has been likened to schizophrenia. Leucine is more highly concentrated in foods than other amino acids. Milk and pork are particularly good sources.

Vegetarian sources: Weight for weight, soya protein concentrate, soya flour, peanuts, tofu, almonds and pumpkin seeds are as rich in leucine as animal proteins.

Availability of supplements: Usually available only in combined BCAA products.

Leukotrienes

Leukotrienes are eicosanoids – hormone-like compounds derived from fatty acids, which regulate blood pressure, clotting and other body functions. Leukotrienes occur naturally in white blood cells and are potent constrictors of smooth muscle, blood vessels and small airways in the lungs. These actions may cause pain, swelling, wheezing and other symptoms associated with allergic reactions. (*Also see Prostaglandins.*)

Linoleic acid (see Fats)

Linseeds (see Flax seeds)

Lipase (see Digestion)

Lipids

Another term for fats (*which see*).

Lipofuscin

Brown pigments produced by the oxidation of fats, which accumulate with age, especially in the brain. Antioxidant nutrients such as vitamin E and selenium are thought to be able to inhibit the formation of lipofuscin deposits, which may account for the 'age spots' or 'liver spots' seen in the skin of elderly people.

Lipoic acid

Also known as thioctic acid. Loosely classified with the B complex group of vitamins, lipoic acid is a sulphur-containing fatty acid found in liver and yeast and synthesized by the body. It is involved in the chemistry of energy production (*which see*) and has been recently identified as an important antioxidant which scavenges the free radicals: superoxide radicals, hydroxyl radicals, hypochlorous acid, peroxyl radicals and singlet oxygen. It also protects cell membranes by interacting with vitamin C and the amino acid glutathione, which may result in recycling vitamin E. Lipoic acid is an important treatment for some types of liver disease and in poisoning by toxic mushrooms.

Recent research has also identified benefit from lipoic acid supplementation in the prevention and treatment of the following clinical conditions:

- Cataract formation
- Diabetic insulin resistance
- Diabetic neuropathy
- Glaucoma
- Neurodegeneration
- Radiation injury

In *in vitro* studies, lipoic acid supplements have also been found to protect nerve cells against injury caused by cyanide, glutamate or iron ions. The active form of lipoic acid is probably its reduced form dihydrolipoic acid.

Availability: Available from some health food shops and through practitioners.

Lipoproteins

Complexes of fat and protein which enable fats to be transported in blood plasma. (*See Cholesterol*)

Lipotropic factors

Substances (methionine, choline, inositol and betaine) which can help to prevent the excessive accumulation of fat in the liver. Lipotropics assist the liver with producing lecithin, thus in turn helping to prevent cholesterol from forming harmful deposits.

Liquorice

Herb

Widely used as a flavouring agent, the root of the liquorice plant also has a number of medicinal uses, the most well known of which is probably its soothing and healing effect on the digestive system. Liquorice is usually made into a tea or taken as capsules. If taken in large amounts or for lengthy time periods it can cause fluid retention, potassium depletion and raised blood pressure. The 'deglycyrrhizined' form (a form of liquorice from which the substance known as glycyrrhizin, which is responsible for these side-effects, has been extracted) is thought to be safer, but this form may lack some of the therapeutic benefits of whole liquorice extract.

Other well tried and tested medicinal uses for liquorice include:

- Adrenal tonic
- Anti-allergic effect
- Anti-inflammatory
- Anti-microbial activity, particularly against *Candida albicans*, hepatitis B and *Staphylococcus aureus*
- Cortisone-like activity
- Detoxification
- Expectorant
- Helps those coming off steroid drugs
- Mild laxative
- Oestrogen-balancing effect
- Protection of gastric mucosa against ulceration

Most of the above effects have been confirmed by scientific investigation.

The Chinese form of liquorice (*Glycyrrhiza uralensis*) is used as an energy tonic, particularly for the stomach and small intestine.

Avoid liquorice if you suffer from high blood pressure or take digoxin-based drugs.

Availability: Widely available in health food shops and from practitioners.

Listeria (see Food poisoning)

Liver

The liver performs a large number of functions in the human body, including detoxification, digestion, metabolism of carbohydrates, protein, fats and alcohol, inactivation of hormones, synthesis of proteins, urea, ketone bodies, glucose, lecithin, bile and cholesterol, the conversion of vitamins to their active form and storage of fat-soluble vitamins, folic acid and glycogen.

Consumed as a food, liver is a rich source of vitamin A, B vitamins and all minerals and trace elements. Pregnant women are cautioned against consuming liver from intensively-reared animals, since these are given large amounts of vitamin A as a growth promoter. The liver of such animals may contain 20 times as much vitamin A as organically-reared animals, causing a potential risk of birth defects if over-consumed in pregnancy.

Lutein (see Carotenoids)

Lycopene (see Carotenoids)

Lysine

Amino acid

Lysine cannot be synthesized in the human body and must be obtained from the diet. It is highly concentrated in muscle tissue, and is primarily metabolized to acetyl CoA, a critical nutrient in energy production. Lysine is also the precursor for carnitine, an important amino acid for fat transport and the conversion of fat to energy. Other roles include regulating calcium absorption, collagen production (using vitamin C and iron), production of the amino acids citrulline and homoarginine (needed for protein metabolism), and production of the neurotransmitter pipecolic acid.

Lysine supplements (about 1 gram per day) are extensively used to treat herpes virus infections. They work best in conjunction with zinc and vitamin C supplements, and a high-lysine low-arginine diet, since the amino acid arginine shares a cell transport system with lysine and may therefore be antagonistic. Lysine can be very low in many vegetarian diets, since grains such as wheat are poor sources of lysine while being rich in arginine. Rich food sources of lysine include meat, dairy products, fish, cabbage, lentils and other pulses. (*Also see Therapeutic Diets: Anti-herpes diet*.)

Vegetarian sources: Weight for weight, soya protein concentrate, soya flour, tofu and freeze-dried parsley are as rich in lysine as animal proteins.

Availability of supplements: Widely available in health food shops.

M

Macrobiotics

A Japanese philosophy which sees ill-health as the result of an imbalance between the two Oriental energy principles known as yin and yang and uses diet to help correct the imbalance. Certain foods are classified as yin foods and others as yang foods. Both the foods themselves as well as their preparation methods and factors such as whether they have been frozen, baked, ground or mixed with water are believed to affect their yin and yang qualities.

Macrobiotarians advocate avoiding extremes of yin and yang in their diet, and use only whole, natural, vegan foods and, rarely, a little fish. The central focus of the macrobiotic diet is usually brown rice and other whole grains (up to 70 per cent of the diet) and the diet also includes specialist Japanese foods and condiments such as miso, seaweeds ('sea vegetables') and salted white radish.

Balance and control of calcium, potassium and sodium ions

Bone development (more than 60 per cent is found in bone)

Calcium balance

Can substitute for manganese (*which see*) in many instances

Co-factor for vitamins B_1 and B_6

Energy production

Helps bind calcium to tooth enamel

Methionine metabolism

Muscle contraction and relaxation

Nerve impulse transmission

Protein synthesis, growth and repair

Removal of excess ammonia and sulphuric acid from the body

GOOD FOOD SOURCES
Bitter chocolate
Leafy green vegetables
Nuts and seeds
Soya beans
Whole grains (particularly oats)

Magnesium

Mineral
UK RNI 300 mg
US RDA 350 mg

FUNCTIONS
Anti-diabetic: release of insulin, maintenance of pancreatic insulin production cells, and maintenance of affinity and number of insulin receptors

---

Deficiency signs and symptoms

- Anaemia
- Anorexia
- Back pain (some types)
- Chronic fatigue
- Chronic muscle pains
- Convulsions and epileptic fits
- Difficulty in relaxing muscles
- Difficulty swallowing
- Flickering eyelids and facial tics

- Fluid retention
- High or low blood pressure
- Hyperactivity in children
- Hypoglycaemia
- Increased risk of heart attack
- Insomnia
- Irregular heartbeats
- Kidney stones
- Late-onset diabetes
- Loss of bone density
- Muscle jerks and spasms
- Muscle weakness and tremors
- Nervousness and anxiety
- Palpitations
- Period pains
- Poor circulation
- Potassium depletion
- Premenstrual syndrome
- Reduced ability to detoxify
- Sodium accumulation inside the cell
- Tendency to 'startle' too easily

Preventing deficiency

On testing for nutritional deficiencies, doctors in the UK find magnesium (and zinc) deficiency more frequently than any other minerals. The diet of many people is low in magnesium-rich foods. In addition, several studies have shown that a diet high in calcium and phosphorus can render magnesium less bioavailable and thus aggravate a potential deficiency. Wholemeal flour contains three times as much magnesium as white flour, therefore this and other whole grains such as oatmeal should be regularly consumed, along with nuts, sesame seeds and dark green leafy vegetables, preferably on a daily basis.

Coffee consumption has been associated with the increased excretion of magnesium and other minerals. Magnesium status can be compromised by chronic diarrhoea, over-use of enemas or laxatives, and by the contraceptive pill. Magnesium is also severely depleted both by stress and by strenuous exercise. Dietary imbalances such as a high intake of fat and/or calcium can intensify magnesium inadequacy, say one group of researchers, especially under conditions of stress. Low magnesium status increases the release of stress hormones which in turn depletes tissue magnesium levels. These hormones also stimulate the liberation of fatty acids, which then complex with magnesium, reducing its bioavailability. Thus, say the researchers, all stress, whether exertion, exercise, heat, cold, trauma, pain, anxiety, excitement or even asthma attacks, increases the need for magnesium. (*Seelig M S: Consequences of magnesium deficiency on the enhancement of stress reactions; preventive and therapeutic implications [a review]. J Am Coll Nutr 13(5):429-46, 1994. Also Casoni I et al.: Changes of magnesium concentrations in endurance athletes. Int J Sports Med 11(3): 234-7, 1990.*)

In some cases of functional magnesium deficiency, such as in chronic fatigue states, there may be adequate levels of magnesium in the blood serum but the magnesium fails to be adequately absorbed into the cells. In such cases vitamin B_6 supplementation may assist in the transport of magnesium across the cell membrane. In one study, all members of a group of nine premenopausal women were found to have low red blood cell magnesium levels while only three had low plasma levels. After receiving 100 mg vitamin B_6 twice a day their red cell magnesium levels rose significantly, and doubled after four weeks of therapy. (*Abraham GE et al.: Effects of vitamin B_6 on plasma and red blood cell magnesium levels in premenopausal women. Ann Clin Lab Sci 11(4):333-6, 1981*).

Comments

Oestrogen enhances the utilization of magnesium and its uptake by soft tissues and bone. This may explain why young women are resistant to heart disease and osteoporosis. However, these effects of oestrogen may be harmful when oestrogen is high (as in the contraceptive pill and hormone replacement therapy) and magnesium levels are low. The resulting calcium/-magnesium imbalance can favour blood clotting and thrombosis. (*Seelig M S: Interrelationship of magnesium and estrogen in cardiovascular and bone disorders, eclampsia, migraine and premenstrual syndrome. J Am Coll Nutr 12(4):442-58, 1993.*) High levels of magnesium can block the binding of calcium on to cell membranes and block calcium channels in nerve cells.

Supplementation

In research studies, magnesium supplements have been found to:

- Enhance strength gains during athletic training
- Improve chronic fatigue
- Improve circulation in peripheral vascular disease
- Improve energy levels
- Improve fibromyalgia
- Improve glaucoma
- Improve glucose tolerance in late-onset diabetes
- Improve mitral valve prolapse
- Improve mood
- Improve osteoporosis
- Improve pulmonary function in asthma patients
- Prevent angina attacks
- Prevent kidney stones
- Reduce cardiac arrhythmias
- Reduce noise-induced hearing loss
- Reduce high blood pressure
- Reduce myopathy associated with magnesium deficiency
- Reduce premenstrual symptoms and period pain
- Reduce reactive hypoglycaemia
- Reduce total cholesterol and raise HDL cholesterol
- Relieve insomnia
- Relieve migraine
- Reverse gum disease
- Treat eclampsia and pregnancy-induced high blood pressure

Preferred form and suggested intake

Good forms of magnesium supplements are magnesium citrate and magnesium taurate. Inorganic forms such as magnesium oxide or carbonate and dolomite are much less bioavailable. Combined calcium/magnesium supplements are often sold in a ratio containing twice as much calcium as magnesium. These products are probably not suitable for those trying to correct a magnesium deficiency.

Cautions

Since the body rejects excess magnesium, supplementation with this mineral is generally very safe, with the exception of individuals with kidney insufficiency.

Manganese

Trace element

Estimated lowest acceptable intake: 1.4 mg/day (UK)
Estimated acceptable range of intake: 2.5–5 mg/day (US)

Deficiency symptoms

- Bone fragility
- Dermatitis
- Disturbed carbohydrate metabolism
- Heavy menstrual periods
- Hypocholesterolaemia
- Impaired blood sugar control
- Joint and spinal cartilage degeneration
- Lower seizure threshold in epileptics
- Possible impairment of sex hormones
- Some types of schizophrenia

Preventing deficiency

Milling removes manganese from whole grains. Diets high in refined flour, sugar and milk can easily be manganese deficient, especially for non tea-drinkers. In the UK the major source of manganese is from tea.

A daily intake of manganese-rich foods is important, as manganese is readily excreted. Its intestinal absorption is hindered by calcium, phosphate, iron and phytate (found in bran). Some spices (ginger, black pepper, cloves, bay leaves) are rich in manganese, although the amounts involved are too small to provide a significant intake.

Supplementation

In research studies, manganese supplements have been found to:

- Reduce epileptic seizures
- Enhance natural killer cell and macrophage activity

Preferred form and suggested intake
Manganese deficiency is probably caused by poor diet, which would also give rise to other mineral deficiencies. The best form of manganese supplementation is therefore in the form of a multimineral preparation providing about 5 mg of manganese. Citrate has been found to aid manganese absorption, and minerals in citrate form are generally available.

Cautions
Manganese is one of the least toxic of all elements because it is poorly absorbed and readily excreted. The only reports of manganese toxicity have been in relation to occupational exposure to large amounts of manganese inhaled through the lungs.

Marshmallow

Herb

Marshmallow root soaked in cold water is a remedy rich in mucilage which is used internally to soothe inflammation or ulceration in the digestive tract, and externally to treat burns and wounds. Many individuals find it helpful in relieving the symptoms of hiatus hernia. Marshmallow is also used as a remedy against coughs and catarrh.

Garden hollyhock flowers can be used as an alternative to marshmallow.

Some animal studies suggest that diabetics on blood-sugar reducing medications should exercise caution with this herb as it may reduce blood sugar.

Availability: From specialist suppliers and herbalists.

Megavitamin therapy

The therapeutic use of vitamins in exceptionally large doses. Some examples of megavitamin therapy are 3,000 mg niacin against schizophrenia, 10 grams a day of vitamin C to treat the common cold, 4 mg folic acid to prevent spina bifida, 800 mg vitamin E to prevent heart attack, and 5,000 mcg vitamin B_{12} to treat pernicious anaemia.

The rationale for using niacin megadoses is that individuals who have suffered from an insufficiency of a particular nutrient may develop a 'dependency' state in which their deficiency symptoms cannot be relieved by a normal dietary intake of that nutrient, or even a moderately raised intake. This phenomenon was observed in former pellagra sufferers in the US, who sometimes needed as much as 600 mg of vitamin B_3 to remain symptom-free. This is 50 times the amount of the vitamin needed to prevent pellagra in individuals who have never had it.

Vitamin C megadoses are probably more commonly used than any other, and there is much research to support their use. Folic acid megadoses are used only by doctors. Where prescribed to prevent spina bifida the rationale for such large doses is purely that these were the doses used in clinical trials. Nutritional therapists point out that the need for these high doses has not been scientifically established, and may in fact be harmful since very high doses of folic acid can interfere with the body's ability to use zinc. The borderline zinc levels found in many pregnant women could put them and their babies at risk of deficiency.

The term megavitamin therapy is often misapplied. It should not be used when only moderately large ('higher-range') supplementation is applied, such as in the correction of common deficiency states. (*See Nutritional deficiencies*.)

Contrary to popular belief, there is much scientific research into the value and safety of megavitamin therapy.

Melatonin

A breakdown product of the amino acid tryptophan, which is produced in the pineal gland, the gut and several other sites in the body. Until recently the only known function of melatonin was assumed to be its role in circadian regulation (sleep and waking cycles) – it is often taken by those suffering from jet lag to help adjust their cycles.

More recently, melatonin has been found to act as a powerful antioxidant (*which see*) and free radical scavenger. Research has shown it to be five times better than glutathione at neutralizing the hydroxyl radical, and twice as effective as vitamin E in inactivating the peroxyl radical. Melatonin also stimulates the antioxidant enzyme glutathione peroxidase and inhibits the nitric oxide synthase enzyme which forms the free radical nitric oxide. Experimental rats pretreated with melatonin are several times more likely to survive exposure to the toxic herbicide paraquat than untreated rats, which suggests that melatonin is highly protective against poisoning. It is described as a highly versatile antioxidant which, because it is both water- and fat-soluble, is not restricted to certain compartments of the cell but is present throughout it: in the membrane, cytosol and nucleus. Researchers believe that the most significant protective effect of melatonin is in the brain, which, due to its heavy consumption of oxygen, is particularly vulnerable to oxidative damage. Since diseases such as parkinsonism, motor neurone disease and Alzheimer's disease are linked with oxidative stress, an increased intake of melatonin may be valuable in helping to prevent them. Research has shown some success in using melatonin supplements against breast cancer.

A more recently discovered function of melatonin is its role in the immune system. If melatonin production is experimentally inhibited, a state of immunosuppression is produced which disappears when melatonin is restored. Melatonin is now being researched as a treatment for immune deficiency and against cancers.

Melatonin is not only found in the animal kingdom, it also occurs in small amounts in foods such as bananas, tomatoes and cereals, in amounts sufficient to influence physiological processes.

Menadione (see Vitamin K)

Menaquinone (see Vitamin K)

Mercury

Toxic element

One of the group of so-called heavy metals which accumulate in the body, mercury has been described as one of the most toxic substances known to man, particularly the organic forms of mercury such as methylmercury and ethylmercury. These forms are created by micro-organisms in the sea and lakes, from inorganic mercury salts which have been discharged in industrial effluent. Fish consume the plankton which contain these toxic forms of mercury, and humans can be poisoned by the fish, especially the larger varieties such as tuna, which can accumulate quite large quantities of mercury from eating many smaller fish. In 1953, when mercury was accidentally discharged into Minamata Bay in Japan, 46 people died after eating mercury-contaminated fish. Poisoning by organic mercury has also occurred in Iraq, Guatemala and Pakistan, when people consumed grains which had been dressed with mercury fungicides. These grains were not intended for human consumption but for planting. Humans also suffered mercury poisoning after eating animals which had been fed with such grains.

Other sources of mercury include:

- Accidental breaking of thermometers, discarded batteries and mercury vapour lamps
- Amalgam in silver tooth fillings
- Coal burning
- Fungicides sold for use on lawns and gardens
- A wide variety of industrial processes
- Medicines such as calomel talc
- Some ethnic cosmetics and medicines

As shown by studies on animals given amalgam tooth fillings, mercury mainly accumulates in the kidneys; the minute amounts of mercury which come out of the teeth during chewing and are then swallowed, can in time result in a loss of 50 per cent of kidney function. (*Drasch G et al.: Quecksilberkonzentration in der Nierenrinde. 6th International Trace Element Symposium, Leipzig, 1989.*)

A large number of enzymes in the body can be inactivated by mercury, and toxicity symptoms can include insomnia, dizziness, chronic fatigue and weakness, depression, tremors, nervousness, poor co-ordination and dermatitis. Mercury alters protein structure, rendering it unusable. It interferes with sulphur binding sites and can therefore impair insulin synthesis and haemoglobin function. These symptoms may progress to kidney damage and brain damage. Insanity is a typical sign of severe mercury poisoning. The mental illness known as 'general paralysis of the insane' or tertiary syphilis, was very common before the advent of modern treatments for syphilis, and is now known to have probably been caused by poisoning due to the old-fashioned anti-syphilis treatments which were based on mercury, antimony and arsenic.

Some individuals can develop a sensitivity to mercury which makes them susceptible to it in different ways. Many cases of auto-immune diseases such as multiple sclerosis, diabetes and systemic lupus erythematosus have responded to the removal of mercury amalgams from teeth. An increasingly common condition known as multiple allergy syndrome (in which the sufferer is allergic to many different foods and other substances) may also respond to the removal of mercury amalgams. These successes may be explained by the fact that the mercury acts as a constant source of stress to the body's detoxification system, which may recover and work normally once this stress has been removed.

Dentists are at particular risk of mercury poisoning, since they are exposed to mercury vapour, which when inhaled through the nose quickly reaches the brain. The trace element selenium helps to protect against mercury's toxic effects.

Metabolic rate

The amount of energy released or expended in a given unit of time.

Metabolism

The chemical processes which take place in living organisms. Metabolism can be anabolic (turning smaller molecules into larger ones) or catabolic (breaking larger molecules down into smaller ones). Metabolism results in growth, energy production, waste elimination and many other functions.

Methionine

Amino acid

Methionine is one of the sulphur amino acids. It cannot be synthesized by the human body, and must be obtained from the diet. It plays an important role as a precursor for the synthesis of other sulphur amino acids (cysteine and taurine), and donates sulphur and other compounds required for the synthesis of many other substances such as choline, creatine, adrenaline and carnitine. Without adequate daily amounts of dietary methionine the body cannot produce sufficient adrenal and other hormones.

Methionine is a component of the body's natural painkillers encephalin and endorphin, and has sometimes been used as a painkilling treatment. It is also essential in regulating the availability of folic acid. A methionine-deficient diet can cause folic acid deficiency as this B vitamin becomes trapped in the liver in an inactive form.

The Brain Bio Center in the US uses methionine to treat one type of schizophrenia, classified as the 'high histamine' type, which is associated with severe depression and suicidal tendencies. L-methionine is thought to alleviate this condition by lowering blood histamine, and in some cases of depression has been described as more effective than conventional drugs. On the other hand, excessive supplementation with methionine can aggravate psychotic symptoms in other types of schizophrenia where individuals suffer from folic acid deficiency. Researchers have also used methionine supplements in parkinsonism, and claim to obtain results comparable to those of conventional treatments.

Along with vitamin B_6, methionine is essential for the metabolism of homocysteine. If allowed to build up in the blood, homocysteine can encourage the build-up of cholesterol deposits in arteries.

In the brain, methionine is metabolized to s-adenosyl-methionine (SAM).

Vegetarian sources: Weight for weight, brazil nuts, sunflower seeds and sesame seeds are as rich in methionine as animal proteins. Vegans should take particular care to obtain enough methionine. Pulses (including many soya products) are a poor source of this amino acid.

Availability of supplements: Methionine supplements are readily available in health food shops.

Methylxanthines

A family of substances: caffeine, theophylline and theobromine, which are derived from xanthine, are found in tea, coffee, cola and chocolate, and have pronounced physiological effects on the body.

Caffeine stimulates the central nervous system, while theophylline and theobromine stimulate the heart. Theophylline is also available as an anti-asthma drug.

There is some evidence that the consumption of methylxanthines is associated with breast lumps and cysts. Women who have ceased consuming methylxanthine-containing foods have experienced a reversal of this condition.

Micronutrients

Substances required in the diet in amounts measurable in milligrams or smaller units. These substances include vitamins, minerals and trace elements.

Milk

The natural food of infants, milk is a good source of protein, fatty acids, vitamins and some minerals. However, cow's (and other animals') milk is not a suitable substitute for human breast milk before weaning, so special formula feeds must be fed to young babies. Some authorities believe that cow's milk should not be fed to infants below one year of age because an immature digestive system may be unable to digest it sufficiently. The improper digestion of any food can lead to the development of an allergy.

Other authorities believe that cow's milk and dairy produce are not suitable foods for children or adults because other mammals do not continue to consume milk after weaning. A large percentage of the world's population is lactose-intolerant – they cannot digest the sugar lactose found in milk, and develop diarrhoea if they try to drink it.

Cow's milk allergy is one of the most common food intolerances and can be responsible for a wide range of symptoms from migraine to sinusitis, eczema and irritable bowel syndrome. The promotion of milk drinking by workers in the public health sector is intended to ensure that those who know and understand little about healthy eating and who may eat, and may feed their children, an otherwise poor diet, will at least be assured of a good range of vital nutrients if they consume milk daily.

Those eating a well-balanced wholefood diet rich in nuts, seeds, whole grains and leafy vegetables do not normally need to consume milk and dairy produce in order to obtain sufficient calcium.

Mineral water

Natural spring water containing small amounts of dissolved minerals such as iron sulphide and sodium bicarbonate.

Miso

A Japanese food made from soya beans (and sometimes grains such as rice or barley) and sea salt fermented for 18 months to three years with the koji culture. Koji produces enzymes which break down the starches, oils and protein of the beans into easily assimilated simple sugars, fatty acids and amino acids. The fermentation process is also said to produce vitamin B_{12}, but analysts have found only 0–0.02 mcg B_{12} in miso samples.

Miso is said to be excellent for people with weak digestive systems and, for those who have been taking antibiotics, to help repopulate the gut with friendly bacteria.

Miso is sold as a dark brown paste which should be diluted with hot water and used as soup or stock. It has a pleasant savoury flavour similar to stock made from yeast extract. Traditional miso soup consists of miso dissolved in hot water and flavoured with spring onion and a little wakame seaweed. Instant miso soup can be bought in packets in powdered form.

Availability: From health food shops and macrobiotic suppliers.

Molybdenum

Trace element
Estimated range of acceptable intake: 50–400 mcg/day (UK)
150–500 mcg/day (US)

FUNCTIONS
Aldehyde detoxification
DNA metabolism
Haemoglobin production
Iron metabolism
Sulphate production
Sulphite inactivation
Methionine and cysteine metabolism
Taurine synthesis
Uric acid production

GOOD FOOD SOURCES
Beans (especially butterbeans)
Buckwheat
Lentils
Liver and other organ meats
Split peas
Whole grains

Deficiency signs and symptoms

- Aggravation of symptoms in sulphite-sensitive asthmatics
- Associated with cancer of the oesophagus
- Eye lens dislocation
- Gouty arthritis
- Low levels of inorganic sulphate in urine
- Mental retardation and neurological problems caused by sulphite toxicity and/or inadequate amounts of inorganic sulphate for the formation of sulphated compounds present in the brain
- Poor growth
- Sexual impotence
- Tooth decay
- Very low levels of uric acid in serum and urine

Preventing deficiency

The use of whole grain rather than white flour products is as important to prevent molybdenum deficiency as it is for most vitamins and minerals. You should ensure a daily intake of the molybdenum-rich foods listed above.

A high intake of copper or of sulphate (e.g. ferrous sulphate iron supplements or magnesium sulphate – better known as Epsom salts) can impede the absorption of molybdenum and increase its excretion.

Comments

Molybdenum is required for the three important enzymes: xanthine oxidase (needed for purine metabolism), aldehyde oxidase (needed for the conversion of aldehydes [see *acetaldehyde*] to acids), and sulphite oxidase (needed for sulphur amino acid metabolism and the production of inorganic sulphate).

Supplementation

Very little research appears to have been carried out. One small study has found that molybdenum supplementation resulted in reduced 'aches and pains' in a group of arthritis and joint pain sufferers.

Preferred form and suggested intake

Unless you are under the care of a nutritional therapist it is advisable to take molybdenum as part of a multi-nutrient formula containing approximately 100–200 mcg molybdenum, since little is known about the use of this supplement. Excess molybdenum can interfere with some aspects of detoxification, promote gout, and deplete iron and copper in the body.

Monoamines

Neurotransmitters (*which see*) formed from amino acids. The most common monoamines are dopamine, adrenaline, noradrenaline, serotonin and histamine.

Monosaccharides
(see Carbohydrates)

Monosodium glutamate

A food additive used as a flavour enhancer and widely used in Chinese cookery. Some individuals who appear to be sensitive to monosodium glutamate have reported symptoms of headache, nausea, sweating and weakness, described as 'Chinese restaurant syndrome'.

Monounsaturated fats (see Fats)

Mucopolysaccharides

Polysaccharides (complex carbohydrates) which occur in combination with protein in body secretions and tissues. They are responsible for the viscosity of mucus secretions. Mucopolysaccharides may be found in cartilage, cornea, skin, blood and heart valves, for instance. Some of the different varieties of mucopolysaccharide include chondroitin sulphate, heparin and dermatan sulphate.

Mycotoxins

Toxins produced by fungi found in food. Some mycotoxins are highly poisonous and may be carcinogenic, particularly the variety known as aflatoxins which may contaminate peanuts, nuts and grains grown in warm, moist conditions.

Muesli

A cereal dish originating in Switzerland and generally consisting of raw oatmeal or porridge oats which have been soaked in milk or water overnight or for several hours. Muesli may be mixed with fresh or dried fruit, nuts and other whole grains, and served with milk or fruit juice. This dish has been commercialized and widely adopted by other countries, where the essential soaking process may be omitted in error. Due to its raw grain content, unsoaked muesli contains pancreatic enzyme inhibitors which make it relatively indigestible and potentially stressful to individuals with a weak digestion. Cooking or soaking the grains inactivates these natural chemicals.

N-acetyl cysteine (NAC)

An antioxidant, free radical scavenger and essential precursor for glutathione biosynthesis. Given orally or intravenously, NAC is an effective detoxifying agent against a variety of toxic compounds, including residues of toxic drugs after cancer chemotherapy, and is the treatment of choice in paracetamol (acetaminophen) overdose.

NAC forms glutathione, cystine, cysteine, L-methionine and mixed disulphides in the body. Supplementation results in elevated levels of reduced glutathione (the most active form of glutathione – *which see*) in the liver, plasma and bronchial tract. NAC is therefore an extremely useful product to assist with liver detoxification. It also has a pronounced mucolytic (mucus-dissolving) action and in research studies has been found effective against bronchitis. (*Also see Detoxification.*)

Availability: From nutritional therapists.

N-acetyl glucosamine (NAG)

This is a particularly important nutrient directly involved in repairing the superficial layers of the gut mucosa – that is to say those layers which come directly into contact with the intestinal contents. NAG belongs to a class of compounds called amino sugars, which are formed from a sugar and an amino acid and are essential components of all body tissues.

NAG is synthesized from glucosamine (*which see*). It is a substrate (raw material) for metabolic transformation to larger molecules that go to make up connective tissue. Like vitamin C, NAG is extremely important in the renewal of all structures which depend on collagen, including the gut mucosa.

Some data suggest that the conversion of glucosamine to NAG in the gut epithelium may be genetically less efficient in some individuals. In particular it has been known for some time that salicylates (found in aspirin and many aspirin-based painkillers) as well as alcohol can inhibit this conversion. For this reason it may be given by practitioners in supplement form.

Availability: From nutritional therapists.

NAC (see N-acetyl cysteine)

NAG
(see N-Acetyl glucosamine)

Naturopathy

Often used as a synonym for natural medicine, naturopathy is a philosophy rather than a treatment modality. Practitioners trained in colleges of naturopathy work on the basis that the body is a self-healing organism given the right conditions. They use diet and other therapies such as hydrotherapy (the external application of hot and cold water), herbalism and osteopathy to help obtain these conditions.

Neuron

A nerve cell. Neurons have a cell body fringed with outgrowths known as dendrites and containing a nucleus. Extending from the cell body sometimes several feet in length are one or more axons insulated by a myelin sheath and ending in axon terminals. Grey in colour, large clusters of neuronal cell bodies in the brain are sometimes known as 'grey matter' and the axons, due to the white colour of myelin, as 'white matter'. Motor neurons are those which transmit nerve impulses from the brain and spinal cord to the muscles and glandular tissue.

Nerve impulses are passed in accordance with electrochemical processes involving sodium, calcium and potassium ions and neurotransmitters (*which see*).

Neurotransmitter

A substance which modifies or helps to transmit nerve impulses between neurons. Up to 10,000 neurotransmitters can be stored in a neuron's 'synaptic knobs'. When a nerve impulse reaches a nerve terminal, voltage-sensitive calcium channels open, allowing calcium to diffuse into the terminal. This stimulates the release of neurotransmitter molecules into the space (synapse) between this neuron and the next connecting neuron. The neurotransmitters then bind to specific receptors.

Neurotransmitters can have 'excitatory' or 'inhibitory' effects which in turn depend on the type of receptor to which the neurotransmitter attaches. An excitatory neurotransmitter-receptor combination causes membrane channels to open, which are permeable to sodium, potassium and other small, positively charged ions. This slightly depolarizes the neuron, bringing it closer to the threshold at which it will 'fire', or send impulses to further neurons.

An inhibitory neurotransmitter-receptor effect opens potassium or chloride channels, and this lessens the likelihood of the cell firing.

Some substances which act as neurotransmitters include: acetylcholine, GABA, dopamine, adrenaline, noradrenaline, serotonin, histamine, the amino acids glycine, glutamate and aspartate, and the opioid substances known as endorphins and encephalins.

Niacinamide (see Vitamin B₃)

Nickel

It is not known whether nickel is an essential element for humans, but traces of it are found in all tissues and especially in skin, bone marrow, RNA and DNA. Although dietary nickel is not thought to be toxic, more toxic forms of nickel can be absorbed into the body as a result of contamination from cooking utensils, food processing equipment and cigarette smoke. In tobacco smoke nickel can combine with carbon monoxide to form the carcinogen nickel carbonyl. Increased skin levels of nickel have been found in individuals with psoriasis and eczema. Increased blood levels have been found in those with lung cancer and hyperthyroidism, and after trauma such as heart attack or even labour. Hair mineral analysis is a useful method for determining nickel toxicity.

Rats maintained on a nickel-deficient diet develop anaemia as a result of reduced iron absorption.

Grains, pulses, soya products and vegetables are good sources of nickel.

Nicotinic acid (see Vitamin B₃)

Nitrates

Sodium and potassium nitrate are widely used as preservatives for meat and meat products such as bacon, ham and salami. However, this does not constitute a significant source of nitrate. Much larger amounts are found in vegetables grown with nitrate fertilizer, for instance spinach and beets, and in water originating from nitrate-treated soil. 80–90 per cent of the nitrate circulating in the human body is produced by the body itself, by a process which is not yet understood.

Nitrates readily convert to nitrites, which can form the carcinogenic nitrosamines (*which see*).

Nitrites

Sodium and potassium nitrite are widely used as preservatives for meat and meat products such as bacon, ham and salami. They also occur in plant foods which have been grown with nitrate fertilizer. Nitrite preservatives are prohibited from use in baby foods since in large amounts nitrites can oxidize haemoglobin to methaemoglobin in red blood cells. This oxidized haemoglobin can no longer bind oxygen. The result may be the dangerous condition known as methaemoglobinaemia or 'blue baby syndrome'.

Nitrites readily combine with amines found in food to produce the potent carcinogens nitrosamines. This process is more likely to occur in a hypochlorhydric individual (one with abnormally low levels of stomach acid) and when the meal does not also contain vitamins C and E (e.g. as found in fruit, fresh vegetables, nuts and whole grains).

Nitrogen balance

An individual is in proper nitrogen balance when the intake of nitrogen (from protein) in the diet equals the output of nitrogen in the urine and faeces. A negative nitrogen balance, which may occur in protein deficiency, fasting, starvation and wasting diseases, is indicative of tissue loss. A positive nitrogen balance indicates that the body is forming tissue.

Nitrosamines

Carcinogenic (cancer-causing) substances formed in the digestive tract from nitrites and amines in food. (*Also see Nitrates* and *Nitrites*.)

Noradrenaline
(see Catecholamines)

Nori

A type of seaweed widely used in cookery. In Japan, rice is wrapped up in sheets of nori to make sushi. In Wales this seaweed is known as *laver*, and is mixed with oatmeal and fried to make laverbread.

Nucleic acids

Two complex compounds known as DNA (deoxyribonucleic acid) and RNA (ribonucleic acid) which contain purines, pyrimidines, sugars and phosphoric acid, and are involved in the determination and transmission of genetic characteristics.

Molecules of DNA contain instructions coded into their molecular structure for the synthesis of cell proteins, ensuring that cells will reproduce correctly. Genes are those parts of a DNA molecule which contain the information determining how proteins will be formed. One DNA molecule contains many genes.

The transfer of information from DNA in the cell nucleus to the site of protein synthesis is carried out by RNA. RNA synthesis is in turn determined by DNA.

One of the richest sources of nucleic acids in animals is the thymus gland. 12 per cent of dried yeast consists of nucleic acids.

It is widely believed that nucleic acids found in the diet or taken as dietary supplements are broken down in the intestines and that their components are not available for the synthesis of RNA and DNA in the human body.

Nutrient density

Nutrient per 100 g/energy (calorie count) per 100 g

RDA for nutrient/RDA of energy

According to conventional nutritionists, foods with a nutrient density of less than one are poor sources of this nutrient; a value of more than one is satisfactory. Nutrient-poor foods are often described as 'empty calories' foods – those consisting of mainly fat, sugar and refined starch. Nutrient-dense foods are usually those described as 'nutritious' in ordinary terminology: wholefoods, fruit, vegetables, fish, nuts, etc. However, scientists use the term 'nutritious' to refer to all foods, even those with a very poor content of vitamins and minerals. This is because sugar, fat and refined starch are also nutrients.

Nutrients

Components of the diet which are essential to life and health. Nutrients are classified as macronutrients (carbohydrates, fat and protein, dietary fibre and essential fatty acids) and micronutrients (vitamins, minerals and trace elements).

Nutritional deficiencies

An individual whose intake of a nutrient is insufficient for his or her needs is described as suffering from a nutritional deficiency. Deficiencies can be overt or sub-clinical. Overt deficiencies are often given specific names, as follows:

The anaemias

Nutritional anaemias occur when the oxygen-carrying capacity of the blood is reduced due to a deficiency of one or more of the nutrients required for red blood cell formation. Symptoms of anaemia may include fatigue, breathlessness on exertion, dizziness and pallor.

Iron deficiency anaemia is the most common type of anaemia. Other nutritional anaemias include folic acid, vitamin B_2, vitamin B_6 (often associated with taking the contraceptive pill), vitamin B_{12}, vitamins C and E, copper, zinc and protein, in which deficiencies of these nutrients result in inadequate red blood cell formation.

Macrocytic anaemia, characterized by reduced numbers of abnormally large, malformed red blood cells, is caused by vitamin B_{12} and folic acid deficiencies.

Pernicious anaemia, caused by a failure to absorb vitamin B_{12} (often because of a lack of intrinsic factor – *which see*) is a type of macrocytic anaemia.

Beri-beri

A disease resulting from prolonged, severe vitamin B_1 (thiamine) deficiency. This disease used to be particularly common in the far east due to the consumption of polished rice. Early signs and symptoms of beri-beri include anorexia, indigestion, constipation, malaise, calf muscle tenderness, palpitations and 'pins and needles' in the legs. More advanced cases develop into either of two sets of symptoms, referred to as 'wet' or 'dry' beri-beri. Wet beri-beri signs and symptoms include oedema, heart insufficiency, digestive disorders, emaciation, tense, painful calf muscles, high blood pressure and decreased urine volume. Dry beri-beri signs and symptoms include memory loss, disorientation and nystagmus.

Kwashiorkor

A type of severe protein-energy malnutrition commonly found in the third world, especially in children. The signs and symptoms are oedema, failure to thrive and grow, apathy, impaired mental development, dermatosis, reduced immunity, sparse hair, and vitamin deficiencies (particularly vitamin A).

Marasmus

Similar to kwashiorkor, but used to describe protein-energy malnutrition in infants or in children who have adapted to the deficiency by retarded growth, thus avoiding some of the kwashiorkor symptoms. The signs and symptoms are sparse hair, wasting of body fat and muscles with shrunken, wizened appearance, and anaemia.

Osteomalacia

Sometimes known as adult rickets, this is a softening of the bones, accompanied by weakness, fracture, pain, anorexia and weight loss, caused by a lack of vitamin D, calcium or phosphorus, leading to problems with bone mineralization.

Pellagra

A disease resulting from prolonged, severe vitamin B_3 (niacin) deficiency. Pellagra occurred mainly where people used corn as a staple of their diet without processing it with lime (as Mexican people do) to render the niacin bioavailable. Parts of the world where pellagra used to be endemic were Spain, Italy and the southern states of the US. Signs and symptoms of pellagra include muscular weakness, anorexia, indigestion, cracked pigmented scaly dermatitis on parts of the skin exposed to sunlight, tremors, sore red tongue, confusion, disorientation and neuritis.

Rickets

A disease of children, associated with malformation of the bones due to dietary vitamin D deficiency or lack of exposure to sunlight (required to allow the body to synthesize its own vitamin D). In rickets the bones are not strong and rigid enough to support body weight and stresses, resulting in knock-knees, bow legs, pigeon breast and skull deformity. In adulthood, softening of the bones due to vitamin D deficiency is known as osteomalacia.

Scurvy

Vitamin C deficiency disease. Signs and symptoms include weakness, poor appetite and growth, anaemia, swollen, inflamed gums, loosened teeth, small haemorrhages under the skin and severe infections. Wounds may fail to heal, and scars may break open.

Sub-clinical deficiencies

The effects of nutritional deficiency can be experienced anywhere on a scale from overt deficiency disease to mild hypofunction of the immune, endocrine, nervous or other systems. Commonly used blood tests may fail to identify a problem since the blood is subject to what is known as 'homoeostatic control', that is to say blood nutrient levels are always more or less constant. They have to be kept constant because excessive variations could be dangerous. For instance, if blood calcium levels are getting low the body could develop a dangerous condition known as 'tetany', leading to convulsions. So the blood borrows calcium from the bones, hoping to put it back later. If the calcium shortage continues, more and more calcium will be 'borrowed' from the bones. The blood will continue to show normal calcium readings, but the bones will become demineralized and osteoporotic.

The same applies to most nutrients, and organs or structures other than the bones may be involved. As Adelle Davis, a nutritionist writing in the 1960s remarked:

The first stage of a dietary deficiency occurs when there is failure of supply – either because food is mishandled, the diet is poorly selected, or the individual, for one of many reasons…has increased his needs. Failure of supply may also be initiated or aggravated by difficulties in the digestion, the absorption, or transport of nutrients within the body. Other difficulties may be created by a breakdown in enzyme systems.

Once supply has failed for any of these reasons, there will be a drop in the blood levels of the nutrient. The blood now draws upon the tissues and when that process comes to an end, it borrows from the organ reserves. Note: Although you are well on your way towards trouble at this point, the blood levels of nutrients reveal nothing abnormal, because of the borrowing the body initiates to achieve more equitable distribution of an inadequate supply.

Then functional disability begins – indigestion, nervousness, irritability, a tendency to weep without provocation, a shortening of the memory and attention spans, difficulty in concentration, insomnia, and bad dreams – for which the doctor's X-ray, blood tests, urine analysis, stethoscope and blood-pressure instruments will find no physical justification…

(*Eating Right for You*, Adelle Davis 1967)

Only if tissue and organ reserves become so depleted that the deficiency begins to show up in the blood, will a condition such as 'scurvy' or 'beri-beri' be diagnosed. About 30 people a year in Britain die from these diseases, according to a 1991 Government survey.

Meanwhile, in people who never reach this drastic endpoint because their deficiency is not absolute, what damage is occurring to their ability to make hormones, corpuscles, enzymes and other substances needed for good health? Drained of the raw materials they need to make these substances, how can the organs function efficiently? Organ biopsies (small samples of tissue) would show a deficiency state more clearly than a blood sample, but would be extremely impractical.

While the initial symptoms of sub-clinical nutritional deficiency may be minor, such as fatigue, weakness, poor skin condition, lowered immunity, mood changes and other symptoms mentioned above, damage and disturbance to metabolic functions as a result of the deficiency are potentially very serious. For instance, a lack of antioxidant nutrients or those needed to metabolize magnesium, methionine or molybdenum may result in an increased level of highly toxic intermediates such as acetaldehyde which are produced by the liver in the course of its detoxification functions. The accumulation of such substances has been linked with the development of diseases such as parkinsonism and motor neurone disease. But because such diseases take many years to develop, no connection with nutritional deficiencies is suspected by conventional medical practitioners.

An inadequate zinc intake can lead to a decreased production of stomach acid and digestive enzymes, and thus ever worsening nutritional deficiencies due to impaired digestion and absorption. Zinc and many other nutrients are needed for countless tasks such as tissue repair, hormone and enzyme production and normal immunity. A very considerable body of scientific literature exists describing beneficial results of studies giving dietary supplements to individuals with a variety of clinical illnesses. Surprisingly, it is sometimes assumed that these positive results have nothing to do with the correction of nutritional deficiency. In fact the nutritional status of the test subjects is sometimes not measured in advance of the studies to ascertain whether there is any difference in results between those with a low or a normal status of the nutrient in question.

It is generally recognized that certain groups of the population are especially vulnerable to develop nutritional deficiencies: pregnant or lactating women, those on weight-loss diets, children and adolescents, and the elderly.

Causes of nutritional deficiency

These can be divided into six main categories:

1. Inadequate intake
2. Inadequate digestion
3. Inadequate absorption
4. Inadequate cellular assimilation (absorption into cells and tissues of the body)
5. Increased needs
6. Increased losses

Causes of inadequate intake

These include poverty, starvation, famine, poor food selection, bad cooking methods, weight-loss diets, ignorance, food fads (particularly in children), dental problems (leading to the selection of only those foods which are easy to chew), apathy (particularly in the elderly), anorexia, and a reduced sense of taste. Deficiencies of a number of nutrients such as zinc and B vitamins may lead to anorexia. Zinc deficiency in particular can result in a reduced sense of taste which leads to faddy eating as sufferers unconsciously learn to select only foods with a strong taste such as highly salted or sweetened foods and strong cheese.

Causes of inadequate digestion

These include poor chewing, and a reduced production of gastric acid, bile and pancreatic and gut enzymes. These secretions are in turn dependent on the availability of a number of nutrients such as zinc, amino acids and B vitamins. However, protein cannot be broken down to amino acids, nor vitamins and minerals extracted from food without sufficient gastric acid and digestive enzymes.

Causes of inadequate absorption

Nutrients are absorbed through the villi and microvilli located on the walls of the small intestine. The absorption mechanisms may be complex – dependent on carrier molecules which transport the nutrients through the epithelium into the bloodstream on the other side. Other nutrients diffuse through the epithelium.

Nutrients which have not been digested into sufficiently small particles cannot be absorbed through the gut wall. Likewise any inflammation of the gut wall, such as that caused by food allergy, dysbiosis (*which see*) or other sources of irritation, and also increased gut permeability (*see Leaky gut syndrome*) may cause the gut wall to become dysfunctional and compromise its absorption ability.

Chronic diarrhoea also causes malabsorption, since the contents of the intestine pass through too quickly for proper absorption to take place. Parasitic infestations (e.g. worms) can result in severe malabsorption. In particular tape-worm utilizes vitamin B_{12}, making it unavailable for absorption. Tea, coffee and phytic acid (found in bran) can bind minerals such as zinc and iron in the intestine, making them unavailable for absorption.

Causes of inadequate cellular assimilation

Once nutrients enter the bloodstream, they have to be taken up by the cellular systems which use them. One of the principal problems which can occur with this process is that some toxins commonly present in the body appear to be very similar to essential nutrients. For instance, the chemistry of lead resembles calcium so greatly that if calcium is in short supply and there is plenty of lead available, then lead can be absorbed instead of calcium both from the gastrointestinal tract (if ingested) and from the bloodstream into cellular systems.

The problem is that lead cannot perform the same tasks as calcium, so it disrupts the function of the systems which are attempting to use it, and these effectively become calcium-deficient. Countless other toxins can have similar disruptive effects on metabolism and function. They need not be present in large quantities to have these effects.

It is also possible that the mechanisms which pump specific nutrients from the blood into the cells can become damaged by toxins, nutritional deficiencies, or even viruses or other micro-organisms. Symptoms may then occur which suggest that these nutrients are deficient even when large amounts of them are present in the bloodstream. In the illness known as ME (myalgic encephalomyelitis) or chronic fatigue syndrome, for example, sufferers have muscle pain thought to be due to chronic muscular spasm, a common symptom of magnesium deficiency. Magnesium supplementation appears to make little difference to sufferers in the short term, but magnesium injections, which flood the cell with very large amounts of magnesium, appear to offer temporary relief. It is thought that in these cases some damage may have occurred to magnesium uptake mechanisms, perhaps by unknown toxins.

The contraceptive pill is one of the many medications which disrupts normal nutrient status in the blood and cells and results in increased requirements. Nutrients most often affected include vitamin B_6, folic acid, vitamins C and E and zinc.

When deficiency symptoms seem to occur in the absence of any dietary inadequacy, this is known as a 'functional' deficiency. *See individual nutrients for deficiency symptoms associated with them.*

Causes of increased needs

The ordinary rules of genetic diversity dictate that some individuals will have higher requirements for certain nutrients than others. In addition, smoking, certain medications, heavy exercise, stress, alcohol consumption, pregnancy, breast-feeding, infections and rapid growth are all factors which increase our nutritional requirements.

Experience with the nutritional treatment of many individuals suffering from mental illness suggests that a prolonged nutritional deficiency state can lead to exceptionally raised baseline requirements for certain nutrients, particularly vitamins B_3, B_6 and zinc. These exceptionally raised requirements have been termed 'vitamin dependency' states. Many individuals are not free of symptoms such as hallucinations and severe depression unless these dependency states are acknowledged and appropriately treated. For instance, doctors treating pellagra victims in the 1930s observed that some sufferers could only remain symptom-free by taking 600 mg a day of vitamin B_3. This is 50 times the amount needed to prevent the disease in those who have never had it. As reported by psychiatrist Dr Abram Hoffer, the treatment of many veterans who suffered arthritis and residual psychiatric symptoms after being detained for lengthy periods in Japanese prisoner-of-war camps in World War II was not fully successful until they were given 1 or more grams a day of vitamin B_3.

Causes of increased losses

These include menstruation, heavy prolonged physical work or exercise, diarrhoea, use of diuretics, and hot climates causing heavy sweating.

Laboratory tests for nutritional deficiencies

The measurement of blood levels of nutrients, although widely used in conventional medicine, is not usually sensitive enough to detect sub-clinical deficiencies. Other methods may be more appropriate, depending on the nutrient. Such methods may be 'functional' tests, that is to say instead of measuring the nutrient itself, the investigator measures levels of a metabolite (a product of metabolism) which is dependent on the nutrient for its production, before and after supplementation with the nutrient. Low levels of the metabolite before supplementation, followed by significant increases afterwards, can indicate a low 'activity' of the nutrient, and therefore a functional deficiency. *(See table overleaf.)*

Nutritional therapy

Nutritional therapists are complementary medicine practitioners who combat ill-health by the use of special diets and a wide variety of nutritional products to enhance or repair specific metabolic functions. They are trained in biochemistry, physiology, pathology, nutrition and the principles of naturopathy and complementary medicine.

Laboratory tests for nutritional deficiencies

Vitamin A   Vitamin A (retinol) and beta-carotene are usually measured in the serum. Isotope dilution assay with tetradeuterated vitamin A allows the estimation of total body reserves of vitamin A.

Vitamin B_1 Red blood cell thiamine diphosphate measurements may be more sensitive than the commonly used red blood cell transketolase activity test, since a transketolase effect is sometimes not observed even in severe vitamin B_1 deficiency states. Measuring the amount of this vitamin excreted in urine after taking an oral dose of it is also thought to be a reliable method.

Vitamin B_2 The measurement of the vitamin B_2-dependent enzyme glutathione reductase in red blood cells is thought to be the best available method, although several factors such as deficiencies of other nutrients or the age of the red blood cells may interfere with its accuracy.

Vitamin B_3 Red blood cell NAD levels are thought to be a good indicator of B_3 status. The measurement of the two metabolites N-methylnicotinamide and 2-pyr excreted in urine are also thought to be reliable.

Vitamin B_5 The measurement of coenzyme A activity, which is dependent on pantothenic acid, is thought to be the most reliable indicator.

Vitamin B_6 Measurement of red cell pyridoxal-5-phosphate (P5P) is thought to be more accurate than plasma pyridoxine. The most reliable functional test is thought to be measurement of the enzyme glutamate amino transferase.

Vitamin B_{12} Elevated urinary methylmalonic acid or homocysteine are indicative of vitamin B_{12} deficiency. The Schilling test is used to determine vitamin B_{12} absorption.

Biotin   Measurement of the enzyme pyruvate carboxylase in white blood cells before and after treatment of the cell preparation with excess biotin, together with measurement of 3-hydroxy and 2-hydroxyisovaleric acids in the serum.

Folic acid   Folate depletion in red blood cells occurs only in the later stages of deficiency, when megaloblastic anaemia may already be present. Micro-biological assays (which measure the extent of growth of folate-dependent bacteria cultured with a blood sample) are thought to be more sensitive than red cell levels.

Vitamin C   A saturation test may be used to diagnose scurvy: vitamin C is given in multiple small doses. Some hours later vitamin C excretion is measured in the urine. If urinary vitamin levels do not rise, scurvy is present. White cell vitamin C measurements are considered the best available method for assessing vitamin C reserves. Under most circumstances a simple serum vitamin C measurement will suffice.

Vitamin D   Measurement of 25-hydroxycholecalciferol in the plasma is thought to be the most reliable method to determine vitamin D reserves.

Vitamin E   A useful method to measure vitamin E status is to determine the fragility of red blood cells in the presence of hydrogen peroxide. (Vitamin E deficient red cells burst in the presence of hydrogen peroxide.) Platelet vitamin E levels are thought to be a good method of measuring the dietary intake of vitamin E.

Calcium	There is no reliable method for measuring calcium status. Serum calcium is almost always normal. Hair mineral analysis can provide some indication, but high hair calcium levels can reflect a low as well as high calcium status.
Chromium	Serum chromium levels are a good indicator of chromium status. Sweat chromium levels correlate well with serum levels. Hair chromium levels can be useful if the hair has received no cosmetic treatments.
Copper	Low serum copper levels are rare, even in the presence of deficiency. The measurement of the copper-dependent enzyme superoxide dismutase in red cells is thought to be the best index of copper status.
Iron	Measurements of serum ferritin (an iron storage protein) are thought to be a good indicator of iron status. Less expensive is the measurement of serum iron and serum iron-binding capacity (IBC). Low serum iron and high IBC are indicative of iron deficiency.
Magnesium	White blood cell magnesium levels are accepted as the definitive test for magnesium status. Measurements of urinary magnesium excretion over a 24-hour period after magnesium loading are also reliable. Red cell magnesium tests are cheaper but their usefulness is limited.
Manganese	Serum and sweat manganese levels are considered to be good indicators of manganese status.
Phosphorus	Serum inorganic phosphorus and urine phosphate measurements are normally used.
Potassium	Red cell potassium is a good indicator of potassium status.
Selenium	Levels of the selenium-dependent enzyme glutathione peroxidase in the blood are a sensitive indicator of selenium status. Red cell selenium measurements are also reliable.
Sodium	24-hour urinary sodium excretion is a useful indicator. Sodium deficiency is relatively rare.
Zinc	White blood cell zinc levels are accepted as the best indicator of zinc status. Sweat zinc levels can be equally sensitive, more so than hair or serum zinc. Also used are the zinc tolerance test, indicating zinc deficiency if plasma zinc does not significantly rise after zinc loading; and the zinc taste test, a fairly crude device in which a 0.1 per cent zinc sulphate solution is given by mouth, suggesting deficiency if the subject cannot taste it.
Amino acids	24-hour urinary measurements of amino acids, their metabolites, and the products of the amino acid pathways. Serum levels may also be appropriate.
Essential fatty acids (EFAs)	Levels in red cell membranes give a good indication of status. The results should be given as a 'profile', which allows imbalances between different fatty acids to be identified. These imbalances can indicate defects in enzymes such as delta-6-desaturase, required for EFA metabolism.

O

Octacosanol

A long-chain alcohol found in wheat germ oil and used as a dietary supplement to improve exercise tolerance and stamina, effects which are probably achieved by an improvement in oxygen utilization. Octacosanol supplementation may also reduce muscle pain after exercise. One small study has found some benefit against Parkinson's disease in a proportion of sufferers.

Experts recommend avoiding artificial octacosanol supplements and using only those extracted from wheat germ oil since these comprise a complex mixture of natural materials which may be required to reproduce the beneficial results obtained by the investigators.

Availability: From health food shops or mail order suppliers.

Octothiamine (see Vitamin B₁)

Oestrogen

The term oestrogen refers not to one hormone but to a group of hormones: oestradiol, oestrone and oestriol, which promote female characteristics and reproductive functions. Oestrogen is made in the ovaries in women, and in the adrenal cortex and peripheral body fat in both men and women. It is also made by the male testes.

During the first half of the menstrual cycle, oestrogen is produced in response to the stimulus provided by follicle stimulating hormone, and renders the female reproductive system ready for fertilization, implantation and nutrition of the early embryo. Female sex drive is not dependent on oestrogen but on male hormones (androgens) synthesized by the female adrenal glands. Poor adrenal function or removal of the adrenals can therefore greatly reduce the sex drive.

Small amounts of testosterone are produced by the ovaries, which then use enzymes to convert them to oestrogen. In the female body an excess of oestrogen (or of progesterone) promotes fluid retention, while an oestrogen deficiency causes hot flushes of menopause.

Pharmaceutical preparations of oestrogen are used in oral contraceptives and as 'hormone replacement therapy' (HRT) to relieve menopausal discomforts and treat osteoporosis. Oestrogens in oral contraceptives have an adverse effect on circulation, and have caused venous thrombosis in many Pill users. HRT is associated with dependency problems by suppressing the body's own natural oestrogen production. Discontinuing the medication can lead to withdrawal symptoms which are identical to the original hot flushes and other problems but more severe. This makes the patient reluctant ever to discontinue the treatment and she may require higher and higher doses to maintain a feeling of well-being. Both oral contraceptives and HRT are associated with a higher risk of some cancers.

Cow's milk is the most significant source of natural oestrogens in the Western diet. However, phyto-oestrogens (plant oestrogens also known as isoflavones) are found in many foods, including wheat, rice, soya products, oats, barley, carrots, potatoes, apples, cherries, plums and parsley, and in herbs such as sage leaf, hops and liquorice. Vegetable oils, including safflower, wheat germ, corn, linseed, peanut, olive, soya and coconut oils, may also be high in phyto-oestrogens. One of the most potent phyto-oestrogens, genistein, is found in soya products. High dietary levels of phyto-oestrogens have been found to have an oestrogen-balancing effect on female health. Both problems of excess oestrogen, such as breast cancer, and problems of inadequate oestrogen, such as hot flushes, are significantly reduced in populations with a high soya intake. Soya products also seem to be effective in preventing cancer of the prostate in men. A large body of scientific research now indicates that phyto-oestrogens are generally protective against cancer and reduce cholesterol levels.

In experimental animals, oestrogen has been shown to influence food intake. On days of the animal's cycle when oestrogen levels are high there is a decrease in food intake, likewise when animals are given oestrogen-like compounds in their diet.

An excess of oestrogen (in its oestradiol or oestrone rather than oestriol form) can promote tumours of the female reproductive system. In fact these cancers account for half of all cancers in women. Breast cancer is one of the major causes of mortality in the West. Many cases of breast cancer are hormone-dependent; that is to say, removal of the ovaries can, at least temporarily, check their growth. In populations with a high incidence of breast cancer, it has been found that women excrete a larger quantity of total oestrogens in their urine but a smaller quantity of oestriol than women in low-risk populations. The most active form of oestrogen, known as oestradiol, is normally metabolized to oestrone, and then to oestriol. Low oestriol levels suggest that the liver is not performing this metabolizing function adequately. The higher levels of circulating oestradiol may encourage tumour formation. Recent research shows that dietary broccoli may help the liver to metabolize oestrone more efficiently. In a study carried out on 16 men and women, 500 grams of broccoli a day added to their diet resulted in an increase in the cytochrome liver enzymes involved in oestrone metabolism. (*Kall MA et al.: Effects of dietary broccoli on human in vivo drug metabolizing enzymes: evaluation of caffeine, oestrone and chlorzoxazone metabolism. Carcinogenesis 17(4):793-9, 1996.*) High-fibre diets can also help to reduce blood oestrone and oestradiol levels (*Rose DP et al.: High-fibre diet reduces serum estrogen concentrations in premenopausal women. Am J Clin Nutr 54(3):520-5, 1991.*)

Excess body fat is associated with a higher incidence of female reproductive cancers, and obese women may have elevated oestrogen levels. Because adipose (fat) tissue is a major site of oestrogen synthesis even after the menopause, obese women may have a later menopause with fewer hot flushes and other symptoms.

Oestrogen and antibiotics

Normally over 60 per cent of circulating oestrogen is excreted into the intestines through the bile, to be deconjugated (broken down) by bacterial enzymes. Some of the oestrogen is reabsorbed and excreted in the urine. However, when antibiotics are used, oestrogen reabsorption drops, lower levels are found in the urine, and the quantity found in faeces may be up to 60 times greater than normal. Because of this excessive loss of oestrogen, antibiotics can lead to breakthrough bleeding in women.

Oleic acid (see Fats)

Olestra

A sucrose polyester (six or eight fatty acids attached to a sugar molecule) which is sold as an artificial fat. It can be used for cookery, but due to the large size of its molecules the body cannot absorb it. At the time of writing olestra is approved only in the US for use in potato crisps (chips) and snacks and has not yet been approved in the UK. Critics are particularly concerned about olestra's potential for stripping fat-soluble nutrients such as beta-carotene out of the gut contents, and for causing cramps, flatulence, bloating, loose stools, faecal urgency and 'anal leakage'. Because olestra cannot be absorbed by the intestines, it tends to pass straight through the gut, causing orange stains on underwear and tightly fitting clothes.

Oligosaccharides
(see Carbohydrates)

Olive oil

Used widely in Mediterranean cookery, olive oil is rich in the monounsaturated fatty acid oleic acid. When heated it forms fewer free radicals than most other vegetable oils,

because of its low polyunsaturated fatty acid content, and is therefore better suited for use in frying. Extra virgin olive oil is the oil from the first pressing of the olives, and has therefore been subjected to little heat (and therefore little free radical formation) during processing.

Omega-3 fatty acids (see Fats)

Organic food

Food grown without the use of artificial fertilizers or pesticides. Pests are controlled using techniques such as encouraging natural predators or growing other types of plants nearby which repel pests. Fertilizing is done with natural manures and composts.

Ornithine

Amino acid

Ornithine is a precursor of the amino acid arginine. Arginine may also be converted by the body to ornithine. Involved in the 'urea cycle' (*which see*), ornithine may be capable of stimulating the production of growth hormone if taken in very large amounts (more than 5 grams a day). It is probably not advisable to take more than 10 grams a day simply because there is no research into possible adverse effects at this level. No harmful effects have been reported from ornithine supplementation.

Availability: In health shops and some fitness centres.

Orotates

Mineral supplements chelated with orotic acid, a member of the vitamin B complex sometimes known as vitamin B_{13}. (*Also see Chelates*.)

Orthomolecular medicine

Literally 'medicine using the right molecules'. The term was coined by the late Linus Pauling PhD to describe nutritional me. cir e and particularly the use of higher-range dietary supplements in the treatment of disease.

Oxalates

Salts of oxalic acid, which is found in tea, rhubarb, spinach and cocoa. High levels of oxalate in the urine are associated with the formation of kidney stones. Speculation that vitamin C supplements may cause the formation of oxalate kidney stones has been disproved, since accurate testing methods show that vitamin C does not raise oxalate levels in the urine.

Oxides (see Bioavailability)

Ozone

Ozone is a type of reactive oxygen species (similar to a free radical) formed when nitrogen oxides and other components of car exhausts are exposed to sunlight. Ozone forms into photochemical smog. In high concentrations it is capable of causing severe damage to lung tissue. In lower doses it irritates the mucous membranes of the nose, mouth, throat and lungs, causing coughing and breathing difficulties.

P

PABA
(Para-aminobenzoic acid)

Vitamin-like substance

PABA is a constituent of folic acid and a member of the B complex family. Rich food sources include eggs, liver, molasses, yeast and wheat germ. PABA's functions in man are not known.

PABA is used as the active ingredient in some sunscreen lotions. In large oral doses PABA has been used as a treatment for vitiligo. PABA deficiency may cause prematurely grey hair.

Availability: Widely available in health food shops.

Palmitate

A compound of the fatty acid palmitic acid. Some dietary supplements, such as vitamin A, are sold as palmitates because this converts them to an ester form and stabilizes them.

Pancreatin

A concentrate of animal pancreatic enzymes, taken as an aid to digestion.

Pantethine
(see Vitamin B$_5$)

Papain

A protein-digesting enzyme found in the paw-paw (papaya) fruit, and taken as a digestive aid or used to tenderize meat.

Parathyroid hormone

Produced by the parathyroid glands located behind the thyroid gland, parathyroid hormone regulates calcium metabolism in the following four ways:

1. By increasing the mobilization of calcium (and phosphate) from bone into extracellular fluid
2. By stimulating the activation of vitamin D, which in turn increases the intestinal absorption of calcium (and phosphate)
3. By increasing the reabsorption of calcium by the kidneys, thus decreasing calcium excretion
4. By reducing the reabsorption of phosphate by the kidneys, thus increasing phosphate excretion and allowing the body to maintain higher levels of extracellular calcium

Parsley

Herb

While parsley leaves are used in cookery, the parsley fruit is used in herbal medicine as a powerful diuretic. Parsley leaf is a good source of the trace element vanadium and is rich in iron and vitamin C. When chewed after eating raw garlic, parsley is said to help control the odour.

Availability: Parsley fruit is not widely available except through medical herbalists, because of potential toxicity.

Pau D'Arco

Herb

Another name for lapacho (*which see*).

Pellagra
(see Nutritional deficiencies)

Peppermint

Herb

Used in both orthodox and complementary medicine to reduce colic, griping and flatulence and against diarrhoea, peppermint is a powerful antiseptic, anti-parasitic and astringent herb, with a relaxant effect on the digestive system and uterus. It has anti-emetic properties (prevention of vomiting), and promotes the flow of bile from the liver. Peppermint tea, made by infusing the leaves, is the preferred way to take it.

Applied externally in the form of a balm or oil, peppermint may be effective against tension headaches, and is very popular for this purpose in the Far East. Peppermint oil contains large amounts of menthol.

Availability: Peppermint tea is widely available in health food and grocery shops. Balms and oils containing peppermint (e.g. 'Essential Balm') are available from Oriental shops and some health food shops.

Pepsin (see Digestion)

Peptides (see Protein)

Peroxides (see Free radicals)

Pesticides

A collective name for the following types of chemicals:

- Insecticides (used to kill insects)
- Herbicides (used to kill weeds)
- Fungicides (used to kill fungi)

Insecticides
are used on growing crops and to treat stored grain. They are likely to be incorporated into plant tissue, which means that they cannot be washed off food before consumption. There are four main categories of insecticides: organochlorines, organophosphates, carbamates and pyrethroids.

Herbicides

There are at least 20 different types of herbicides, including the well-known paraquat. Some kill all types of plants, others are selective in their action. Some are applied to the growing plant, others are applied to the soil for the plant to absorb through its roots. Again, they cannot be washed off food.

Fungicides

are sprayed on plants, especially on fruits. They may be applied with paraffin to enhance the absorption of the chemical by the plant. Systemic fungicides are also used. There are more than seven chemical types of fungicide, some being based on poisonous heavy metals like mercury and arsenic. To suppress sprouting, the fungicide tecnazine is added to water in which potatoes are washed before sale. The run-off from these potato washing plants has caused ecological problems. Fungicides are also widely used in wood-preservative products.

Wherever we live we are likely to have pesticides in our blood. These poisonous substances are in our food, our water, and in the air. Governments reassure us that the amounts are insignificant, but in fact approximately one billion gallons of pesticide are sprayed on to our food in Britain alone every year. The rate of pesticide use is rising as insects soon become immune.

Spraydrift

This is the cloud of tiny pesticide droplets which floats away from the crop it is aimed at. Between 20 per cent and 50 per cent of the spray can drift away and blow into neighbouring gardens and towns. Spraydrift from as far away as Africa can end up in Europe and America. More locally, pesticide is sprayed on pavements and parks, used in gardens, as wood preservatives, on footpaths, road margins and in buildings. The chemicals soak into the water table, the underground water which ends up in our public water system. In the two years between 1985 and 1987 the limits for pesticide residues in public water were broken about 300 times in England and Wales.

The amount of pesticide which remains on our food is not great, but a 1983 UK survey revealed that just over a third of fruit and vegetables, together with foods such as bran, sausages, burgers and cheese, contained detectable residues. Apples and oranges are deliberately coated with a thin layer of pesticide-impregnated wax.

Higher levels of pesticide residue may be found in foods imported from the third world, because farmers there are often not properly trained in their use. Ill-health due to hazardous pesticide dumps in Africa is widespread according to *Pesticide News*, the journal of the UK's Pesticides Trust. Some countries receive large 'donations' of pesticides which they have not requested and do not need. Companies do this because it may be cheaper to get rid of chemicals which have been banned in their own country than to find methods of disposing of them locally.

Effects on health

The organochlorine insecticides (DDT-like compounds such as Lindane, Dieldrin and Aldrin) can produce tremors, twitching and convulsions, dizziness, hyperexcitability, sensitivity to noise, headaches and liver damage. Organo-phosphorus insecticides (such as Malathion, Dimethoate and Dichlorvos) also damage the nervous system. In fact nerve gases for use in chemical warfare are a by-product of research into these compounds. Symptoms of acute poisoning include tremors, dizziness, convulsions, flu-like symptoms, vomiting, lung failure and heart-block.

Thousands of people have suffered acute pesticide poisoning (symptoms or illness clearly linked with one or more incidents of pesticide exposure). But the burden of proof is always on the sufferer. Because of the technical difficulties of such proof, sufferers are rarely able to sue those responsible for their illness even though in some cases severe disability results.

Pesticide poisoning is often confused with other illnesses. Some chronic health problems such as asthma, epilepsy, repeated miscarriage or cancer are known to occur more frequently among those suffering long-term exposure to smaller amounts of pesticide, but this can never be legally proven. For instance, although a lot of pesticides are known carcinogens, many cannot be tested for in human body fluids. Even if they can be detected, it would be impossible to prove that it was one particular chemical which caused that person's illness when so many potentially cancer-causing substances are surrounding us all. Subtle effects can also include impaired mental performance, as shown in one study carried out on 146 sheep farmers regularly exposed to organophosphate sheep dip compared with 143 quarry workers who had not been exposed to organophosphates. The farmers performed significantly worse in tests to assess their ability to concentrate and to process information. The farmers were also more prone to psychiatric disorders. (*Stephens R et al.: Neuropsychological effects of long-term exposure to organophosphates in sheep dip. Lancet 345(8958):1135-9, 1995.*)

Anti-pesticide campaigners advise that the best way for the consumer to help in the battle to get these chemicals phased out is to buy organic food (*see Organic food*) and treat the extra expense as a donation to the fight against pesticides. As organic food becomes more widely produced, the price will come down.

Individuals most at risk of pesticide exposure

- Agricultural workers (especially sheep-dipping and crop-spraying)
- Greenhouse workers
- Pest control officers
- Those exposed to DIY and building materials such as wood, wallpaper and paint
- Those exposed to new carpets, textiles and furnishings
- Those exposed to wood and timber treated with fungicides and wood preservatives
- Those involved in the manufacturing, transport, storage and sale of pesticides
- Those living or working near fields, orchards, parks, airport runways, military establishments, etc. or in buildings which have been sprayed with pesticide
- Those working in buildings where pesticide is added to humidifier and air-conditioning systems

pH

Abbreviation for 'potential hydrogen', or a scale of 0 to 14 used to measure the hydrogen ion concentration of a solution. The lower the pH value, the greater the hydrogen ion concentration and the greater the acidity. Water, which is neither acid nor alkaline, has a pH of 7. pH values above 7 indicate increasing alkalinity. The blood is slightly alkaline at a pH of 7.4. Stomach juices are extremely acid at a pH of about 2. Pancreatic juices have a pH of about 8.

Phenylalanine

Amino acid

Phenylalanine is the raw material of the important amino acid tyrosine which in turn gives rise to the catecholamines (*which see*) dopamine, adrenaline and nora-drenaline. Phenylalanine cannot be synthe-sized by the body, and must be obtained from the diet. It is highly concentrated in the brain, and a deficiency can lead to a wide variety of changes in behaviour. The utilization of phenylalanine by the body requires adequate levels of iron, vitamins C, B_3 and B_6, and copper. Major food sources of phenylalanine are soya products, cheese, fish, meat, nuts, seeds and pulses. Phenylalanine is also an ingredient of the artificial sweetener known as aspartame (trade name *NutraSweet*).

As with most amino acids, phenylalanine is available in two isomer forms, the 'D' and 'L' forms. The 'D' form of amino acids is not usually found in nature and is not normally utilizable by the human body. However, a combination of D-phenylalanine and L-phenylalanine (known as DLPA) does appear to have some clinical value as a natural painkiller. It is thought to work by intensifying and prolonging the body's own natural painkillers, the endorphins, which are produced by the brain and resemble morphine. DLPA concentrates selectively on chronic, useless pain, and is claimed to be effective in 80–95 per cent of users. Users report that DLPA is not toxic, not addictive, does not become less effective in time, and pain relief can last far beyond the period in which DLPA is taken. In many people it works simultaneously as an anti-depres-sant. DLPA normally takes one to three weeks to start controlling pain.

Some individuals find that phenylalanine is effective in appetite control. It is thought to stimulate the release of an appetite-suppressing hormone called cholecys-tokinin from the wall of the small intestine, which is normally released when food has been consumed.

Dosages: for pain relief begin by taking 1 gram of DLPA before each meal until signif-icant pain relief occurs. If this does not happen within three weeks, double the dose and try again for another three weeks. If DLPA works for you, the dosage can be decreased once pain relief is obtained. Ensure that your intake of vitamins C and B_6 is adequate. For appetite control, take 500 mg L-phenylalanine before each meal.

Caution: individuals with phenylke-tonuria who have been given low-phenylala-nine diets by their medical advisers and instructed to avoid aspartame and pheny-lalanine should never take any form of phenylalanine supplements.

Vegetarian sources: weight for weight, soya protein concentrate, soya flour, tofu, peanuts, almonds, sesame seeds and sunflower seeds are as rich in phenylalanine as animal proteins.

Availability of supplements: Phenyl-alanine supplements are readily available in health food shops.

Phosphatidylcholine
(see Lecithin)

Phosphatidylserine

One of the five phospholipids (*which see*) which are essential for the structure and functioning of all the body's cells, phos-phatidylserine (PS) has several unique func-tions: it regulates the state of key proteins in cell membranes, facilitates membrane-to-membrane fusion, and activates the receptors on cell surfaces which enable the cell to respond to chemical messengers. A number of clinical trials have successfully used PS to combat age-related declines in memory, learning and concentration. These benefits are related to PS's special role in the function of nerve cell membranes.

Phospholipids

Lipids (fats) which contain phosphate and nitrogenous bases, such as phosphatidylcholine, phosphatidylserine and phosphatidylinositol. Phospholipids containing choline are known as lecithins, while those containing ethanolamine or serine are known as cephalins. Phospholipids are important structural components of cell membranes and lipoproteins, which hold the proteins and components of the cell membranes together and enable fat-soluble substances, including vitamins and hormones, to pass easily in and out of cells.

Phosphorus

Mineral
UK RNI 550 mg
US RDA 800 mg

FUNCTIONS

Phosphorus (as phosphate) is a major constituent of all living cells and is found in all natural foods, particularly those rich in protein and calcium. Most of the phosphate in the human body is found in bone, but it is also an important constituent of cell membranes and the nucleic acids RNA and DNA, and is essential for energy production.

GOOD FOOD SOURCES

Cheese
Meat and fish
Nuts
Soya products
Whole grains
Yeast

Deficiency symptoms

Phosphate deficiency in isolation is unlikely to occur in the Western world due to the widespread availability of this nutrient. However, some medical conditions can lead to low phosphate levels, causing problems such as osteomalacia, debility, weakness and mental confusion.

Comments

In the Western world, soft drinks and food additives may contribute excessive levels of phosphate to the diet, often more than 1,000 mg a day. Ideally, phosphate intake should be similar to that of calcium. If the phosphorus intake is disproportionately high, the secretion of parathyroid hormone is stimulated, which promotes phosphorus excretion and causes calcium to be mobilized from the bone to the blood. A long-term imbalance between phosphorus and calcium can in this way eventually lead to osteoporosis.

Phylloquinone (see Vitamin K)

Phytic acid

Also known as inositol hexaphosphate, phytic acid is found in cereal grains (particularly in the bran) and in pulses and soya products as well as in many other plant foods. It is capable of forming unabsorbable complexes known as phytates, with minerals such as calcium, iron and zinc, thus reducing the bioavailability of these nutrients. Under normal dietary circumstances these losses are probably not significant, but the regular consumption of unleavened flour products such as chapatis, or of much bran cereal may cause deficiency problems, especially in vegetarians. In the 1940s, Irish children who lived on mainly wholemeal flour products for several years without dairy produce developed rickets due to calcium deficiency. In Iran, where much unleavened bread is consumed and soil zinc levels are low, children frequently suffer from stunted growth.

When wholemeal flour is baked into bread, the enzyme phytase found in wheat and yeast, and the high temperatures used in breadmaking, serve to inactivate one third or more of the phytic acid content.

Phyto-oestrogens (see Oestrogen)

Phytosterols (see Sterols)

Picolinates

Chelates (*which see*) of minerals with picolinic acid, a natural chelating agent which the body makes from the amino acid tryptophan. Picolinates are a popular form of supplementation for chromium and zinc.

Pituitary gland

The pituitary gland lies at the base of the brain just below the hypothalamus, to which it is connected by a stalk containing nerve fibres and blood vessels. This gland consists of two separate lobes, known as the anterior and posterior pituitary glands, each with distinct and separate functions.

The *posterior pituitary* is really an outgrowth of the hypothalamus. It produces the two hormones oxytocin and antidiuretic hormone. The *anterior pituitary* is sometimes known as the body's 'master endocrine gland' because it produces six different hormones which control many body functions. These are growth hormone, thyroid-stimulating hormone, adrenocorticotropic hormone, prolactin, follicle-stimulating hormone and luteinizing hormone. (*See Hormones for their effects*)

Placebo

An inactive substance given as a dummy medicine. In so-called 'blind' or 'double-blind' (*which see*) clinical trials one group of patients is (unknowingly) given a placebo so that the expectation factor can be ruled out when assessing the effectiveness of the treatment being tested.

Polycyclic hydrocarbons

A class of carbon-containing pollutants which contain multiple benzene rings, such as benzopyrene and naphthalene. They are carcinogenic – capable of disrupting DNA. Formed as products of incomplete combustion, they are found in diesel smoke and on the surface of char-grilled and barbecued meats as meat fat drips onto the hot coals, causing smoke particles to rise and settle on the food.

Polyphenols

Also known as polyphenolic flavonoids, these are powerful antioxidants related to tannins and are found in green tea and red grapes (hence red wine is rich in them). They are powerful antioxidants. The processes used in the production of ordinary brown or black tea cause oxidation and therefore loss of these flavonoids.

Polyphosphates

Additives used in meat, poultry and fish products to increase their water content.

Polysaccharides
(see Carbohydrates)

Polyunsaturated fats (see Fats)

Potassium

Mineral
UK RNI 3,500 mg
US RDA 3,500 mg

FUNCTIONS
Acid-alkali balance
Carbon dioxide transport by red cells
Cell membrane function
Electrolyte (*which see*)
Enzyme activator, especially in energy production
Intracellular ion
Nerve and muscle function
Normal water balance
Protein synthesis
Stability of internal cell structure

GOOD FOOD SOURCES
Avocado pears
Bananas
Coffee
Dried fruit
Fruit juice
Molasses
Nuts
Potatoes
Salad vegetables
Soya flour
Tomato juice

Deficiency symptoms

- Acute muscular weakness
- Bloating
- Dizziness
- Drowsiness and confusion
- Intense thirst
- Low blood pressure
- 'Pins and needles'
- Vomiting

Preventing deficiency

Fresh fruits and vegetables should be consumed daily, and a low-sodium-high-potassium table salt should be used for seasoning food. Potassium can be displaced from the cells by high tissue acidity levels (*see Acid-alkaline balance*). It can also be depleted by the use of diuretic drugs and the long-term use of corticosteroid drugs. Diarrhoea and laxative abuse can cause important potassium losses in the faeces.

Comments

Concentrated potassium may cause bowel ulceration, therefore supplements are not recommended. Adequate quantities of potassium can be obtained from food sources such as fruit or tomato juices.

Pioneer cancer doctor Max Gerson postulated in the 1950s that one of the most important factors in cancer promotion was a lack of dietary potassium and an excess sodium intake. His treatment is based on correcting this balance with the use of large quantities of fresh fruit and vegetable juices.

Prebiotics (see Probiotics)

Pro-vitamins

Naturally-occurring substances such as beta-carotene, which the body can convert into vitamins.

Proanthocyanidins
(see Flavonoids)

Probiotics

Dietary supplements which provide bacteria and other factors to encourage a good balance of intestinal microflora. It has been estimated that over 400 bacterial species inhabit our digestive tract, amounting to three or more pounds in weight. Some of these species are 'symbiotic', or 'friendly', producing vitamins, short-chain fatty acids and other helpful substances, assisting bowel function, forming part of our immune defence system and preventing harmful species from taking up residence. Others are not so friendly. While not necessarily pathogenic (disease-causing) they are undesirable in large amounts because they produce endotoxins which can be absorbed into our bloodstream and significantly add to our toxic load.

Within a few days of birth, an infant's gastrointestinal tract is colonized by bacteria. Breast-feeding has been shown to favourably influence the balance of these bacteria. The main two types of friendly bacteria found in the gut are known as *Lactobacillus acidophilus* and *Bifidobacteria*; many probiotic supplements will provide a balance of these. In addition, *Lactobacillus bulgaricus* and *Streptococcus thermophilus* are also friendly, and are found in some yoghurt cultures. Some examples of undesirable putrefactive bacteria commonly found in the gut are *Clostridium* and *E coli*. The yeast *Candida albicans* is also highly undesirable in large amounts.

Antibiotics
The friendly bacteria are much more easily destroyed by antibiotics than their more undesirable cousins, so probiotic or prebiotic (*see below*) supplements or the frequent consumption of live acidophilus yoghurt is often recommended to ensure that the friendly species are replaced during oral antibiotic or herbal anti-bacterial

therapy, otherwise the gut may become overrun with undesirable species.

Sex hormones have an important relationship with the intestinal flora. Normally over 60 per cent of circulating oestrogen is excreted into the intestines through the bile, to be deconjugated by bacterial enzymes. Some of the oestrogen is reabsorbed and excreted in the urine. However, when antibiotics are used, oestrogen reabsorption drops, lower levels are found in the urine, and the quantity found in faeces may be up to 60 times greater than normal. Because of this excessive loss of oestrogen, antibiotics can lead to breakthrough bleeding in women.

A number of studies have shown that probiotic supplements are often a safe, effective treatment for infant diarrhoea.

Prebiotics

The friendly bacteria thrive on a type of fibre known as fructo-oligosaccharides (FOS) (also known as bifido growth factor [BGF] or vegetable inulin). This is found in certain vegetables such as jerusalem artichokes. When isolated and made into a commercial product, it has a sweet taste and dissolves in liquid. It can be added to food like sugar, although it is rather more expensive. Because the addition of FOS to the diet can result in a several-fold increase in friendly bacteria within a few days, these products are known as 'prebiotics'. However, they can also encourage the growth of harmful bacteria such as klebsiella.

Quality assurance

It is best to purchase probiotic products from a manufacturer who gives certain quality assurance guarantees and has a known reputation for quality in this area, since product quality can be extremely variable. On testing, it is not unknown for some products to contain no viable friendly bacteria at all, because of poor manufacturing

expertise, poor strain selection, or poor storage conditions. Probiotic products consist of delicate live organisms which require refrigeration or vacuum packing during storage. (*Also see Dysbiosis*.)

Progesterone

This female sex hormone is produced in the second half of the menstrual cycle (after ovulation) by the corpus luteum in the ovary. It prepares the uterus to receive a fertilized egg by stimulating the growth, blood supply and secretions of the endometrial cells of the uterus, and stimulates the mammary glands. Progesterone also stimulates the reabsorption of water, sodium and chloride ions by the kidneys, and this effect may be experienced as premenstrual fluid retention.

Some disorders of female health are attributed to an 'oestrogen overload' or to a progesterone deficiency, and there is an increasing tendency in the natural health movement to recommend rub-on progesterone creams to women with problems such as premenstrual syndrome, menopausal problems and osteoporosis. While this allopathic approach (similar to the use of oestrogen hormone replacement therapy) would never be tolerated if these creams were manufactured by the pharmaceutical industry, many practitioners have been persuaded that they are 'natural' because the active ingredient is extracted from plants. However, there is nothing natural about rub-on hormone treatments. Progesterone is secreted by the female body as and when it is needed, not on a permanent basis. The progesterone in such creams may take some months to permeate the body fat and to penetrate from here into the bloodstream. The long-term effects of saturating the body fat with these hormone treatments are unknown, but one likely effect is the development of a dependency state, as with artificial HRT. Hormone treatments suppress the body's own natural hormone production. Discontinuing the medication can lead to withdrawal symptoms which are identical to the original symptoms for which the medication was prescribed, but more severe. This makes the patient reluctant ever to discontinue the treatment and she may require higher and higher doses to maintain a feeling of well-being.

Oestrogen overload and progesterone deficiency problems are best treated by investigating their causes (such as poor liver clearance of oestrogen) and correcting any nutritional deficiencies such as zinc and vitamin E. Soya products are powerful oestrogen balancers, and many herbal combinations such as those containing *Agnus castus* and dong quai also have a beneficial balancing effect on female hormones.

Prolactin

A hormone produced by the anterior pituitary. Together with other hormones, it stimulates the development of the mammary glands. It is also involved in milk production.

Proline

Amino acid

Proline is synthesized from either L-glutamate or L-ornithine in the human body, and is used to make hydroxyproline which, with proline, is a major constituent of collagen.

Propionic acid

A short-chain fatty acid produced by the gut fermentation of dietary fibre.

Propolis

A resinous substance produced by bees and used to seal the hive, protecting the larvae from infection. Propolis is sold as an antiseptic health product in the form of lozenges used to soothe a sore throat, or in the form of a tincture which can be made into a gargle or antiseptic solution.

There is some scientific evidence that propolis solution aids in the healing of gastric ulcers. Its action here may be two-fold since gastric ulcers are now thought to be caused by infection with the *Helicobacter pylori* bacterium. Apart from a possible antibiotic effect against this bacterium, propolis is also a remarkably soothing agent when applied topically to mouth ulcers, and this effect may also contribute to its usefulness against gastric ulceration.

Prostacyclin

A type of prostaglandin (*which see*).

Prostaglandins

Short-acting hormone-like unsaturated fatty acids produced from precursor fatty acids found in the phospholipids of cell membranes. The enzymes prostaglandin synthetase and cyclo-oxygenase are required for this purpose. Together with similar substances known as prostacyclins, thromboxanes and leukotrienes, prostaglandins act locally and are involved in many body processes including blood clotting, blood pressure, pain, water balance, inflammation, uterine contractions, transmission of nerve impulses, immune assistance, hormone responses and the control of sodium, potassium and chloride ions across cell membranes. By controlling capillary permeability, the prostaglandins may promote the exchange of nutrients for waste products at this level.

The prostaglandins, prostacyclins, thromboxanes and leukotrienes should collectively be referred to as 'eicosanoids' or 'prostanoids' but the term prostaglandins is often used for all of them.

The body uses its enzymes to oxidize the precursor fatty acids in specific ways to make specific prostaglandin molecules. About 30 prostaglandins have been identified to date, and are categorized into three series (families) according to which fatty acid they are made from.

Series 1 and 2 prostaglandins are produced from linoleic acid, and have one and two double bonds, respectively. *Series 3 prostaglandins* are made from alpha-linolenic acid and have three double bonds. (*See Fats for information on fatty acid metabolism.*)

Linoleic acid is metabolized to DGLA, which can itself be metabolized to either series 1 prostaglandins, or to another fatty acid known as arachidonic acid. Series 2 prostaglandins are derived from arachidonic acid.

Alpha-linolenic acid is metabolized to EPA, which gives rise to series 3 prostaglandins.

Individual prostaglandins do not have names but are referred to as PG plus a letter of the alphabet and the number of the series they belong to.

Some prostaglandins and their functions

PGE1
- Prevents adhesiveness of blood platelets
- Helps prevent sodium retention by the kidneys thus preventing fluid retention
- Relaxes blood vessels, thus lowering blood pressure and improving circulation
- Reduces inflammation
- Promotes the action of insulin
- Promotes healthy nerve function
- Regulates calcium metabolism
- Enhances T-cell function in the immune system
- Prevents the release of arachidonic acid from cell membranes

PGE2
- Promotes platelet adhesiveness
- Promotes sodium retention
- Promotes inflammation

PGE3
PGI3
- Prevents the release of arachidonic acid from cell membranes, thus limiting the production of PGE2

Pollutant injury to cell membranes may result in altered responses to the normal formation of prostaglandins and other prostanoids.

The reputed anti-inflammatory properties of flavonoids such as quercetin, rutin, curcumin, silymarin and green tea polyphenols may be related to their ability to inhibit the enzymes cyclo-oxygenase and lipoxygenase, which are required for prostaglandin synthesis. The popular medication aspirin also works in the same way, which accounts for its effectiveness in treating problems such as headaches and joint pains caused by the over-production of pro-inflammatory prostaglandins from arachidonic acid.

Protease (see Digestion)

___

Protein

Most of the human body consists of protein in various forms: muscle tissue, hormones, enzymes, skin, hair, organs and the matrix of bone on which calcium is laid down. The different types of proteins are determined by the sequences and types of their building blocks, the amino acids (*which see*). Amino acids can be linked in a virtually infinite variety of sequences to form thousands of different proteins. The amino acids are joined together by peptide bonds. Short sequences of amino acids are known as 'peptides', longer sequences as 'polypeptides'. Polypeptides can be several hundred amino acids long.

Protein in the diet is digested into amino acids which are then absorbed into the bloodstream. A meal high in protein results in surges in the synthesis of liver and muscle protein in the body. Increased amounts of serum albumin (a type of blood protein) are formed. Excess amino acids are broken down ready to be converted to glucose or acetyl-CoA to be utilized for energy production (*which see*) or stored as glycogen and triglyceride. Albumin continues to circulate in the blood and is gradually broken down.

As the absorption of amino acids from the intestine begins to slow down after a meal, the synthesis of albumin and muscle protein also slows. As fasting begins, and glycogen stores are used up, the muscles begin to release amino acids for use in energy production. In long-term fasting, adaptations occur in protein, amino acid and overall fuel metabolism, reducing the need for muscle breakdown.

The breakdown of amino acids can also lead to ammonia production. Ammonia is converted to urea by the liver, and the urea is then excreted in the urine. If nutrients such as magnesium, needed for the conversion to urea, are deficient, and ammonia is not adequately broken down, one of its toxic effects is to interfere with the Krebs cycle of energy production (by depleting the supply of alpha-ketoglutarate). This can result in fatigue, headache, lethargy, irritability, and allergy-like reactions to high-protein foods.

Severe protein deficiency (mainly seen in the third world) is known as kwashiorkor. A lack of protein causes reduction of growth in children. Other protein deficiency effects include impairment of digestion, fluid retention (due to the liver's failure to synthesize serum albumin), muscle wasting and anaemia.

High-protein foods include meat, fish, eggs and other animal products, soya products, pulses and nuts. Vegetable proteins are often low in some amino acids. These are known as the 'limiting' amino acids, for instance lysine in grains and seeds, and methionine in pulses and soya products. This has given rise to a concept that vegans, who eat only plant foods, should carefully combine their foods to ensure that each meal provides a good balance of all essential amino acids. However, several human studies have shown that this is not necessary, at least in healthy volunteers eating calorie-adequate rice-based diets. Volunteers eating diets in which the protein was derived virtually only from rice, when compared with those eating both rice and chicken, showed no significant difference in nitrogen balance, indicating that their protein intake was sufficient. Rice as the sole source of their protein still provided between 1.5 and 4.5 times the World Health Organization (WHO) recommended amounts of all essential amino acids. The American Dietetic Association now confirms that, because amino acids obtained from food can combine with amino acids made in the body, it is not necessary for vegans or vegetarians to combine protein foods at each meal. The ADA furthermore states that soy protein has been shown to be nutritionally equivalent in protein value to proteins of animal origin and can thus serve as the sole source of protein intake if desired.

The adult minimum protein requirement is 45 grams a day for women and 55 grams a day for men. A highly excessive protein intake can lead to an over-acid condition of the body (*see Acid-alkaline balance*), excessive ammonia levels, and osteoporosis (by increasing calcium excretion).

Protein-energy malnutrition
(see Nutritional deficiencies)

Proteinates

Chelates (*which see*) of minerals with protein.

Psyllium husks

Sometimes known as 'flea seeds', the seeds of the *Plantago psyllium* plant have a husk which is widely used as a fibre supplement due to its water-absorbent properties.

Pulses

Seeds of the *Leguminosae* family, including beans, peas, peanuts and lentils. Pulses are good sources of B vitamins and are rich in protein, being the main protein source for strict vegetarians (vegans). They are, however, low in the vital sulphur amino acids, such as methionine, which can instead be obtained from rice, brazil nuts and sesame and sunflower seeds.

Pulses are rich in soluble fibre, and are very helpful in diets for the control of blood sugar. Most pulses except lentils and peanuts require soaking in water overnight before they can be cooked and must be boiled for 10 minutes or (pressure-cooked until soft) to break down highly toxic substances known as lectins.

Pumpkin seeds

Pumpkin seeds are particularly rich in zinc as well as essential fatty acids, and are therefore sometimes recommended for prostate problems in men, since these nutrients are frequently lacking in this condition. Other ingredients of pumpkin seeds may also have a therapeutic effect. One strain, used to make a preparation known in Germany as (Granu)Fink is found to be particularly effective, helping to increase bladder muscle tone, relax the sphincter mechanism and decongest the prostate. (*Also see Saw palmetto.*)

Purines

Nitrogenous compounds found in nucleic acids (*which see*), and produced as end products in the digestion of some dietary proteins. Purines are found in many foods, including caffeine, anchovies, sardines, fish roes, sweetbreads, liver and other organ meats, pulses and yeast extracts. Individuals who have difficulty in metabolizing purines may be prone to gout due to raised levels of uric acid in their blood. Such individuals are advised to avoid foods with a high purine content.

Pyridoxal-5-phosphate
(see Vitamin B$_6$)

Pyrimidines

Nitrogen-containing compounds found in nucleic acids (*which see*).

Q

Quercetin

A flavonoid found in onions, apple peel, cabbage, *Ginkgo biloba*, tea and red wine. Studies indicate that it can help to prevent cataract formation. Quercetin may also help allergy-related problems such as hay fever, asthma and eczema by stabilizing mast cell membranes, inhibiting histamine release (by inhibiting calcium channels in the mast cell membrane, thus preventing the influx of calcium and resultant mast cell degranulation) and decreasing the synthesis of pro-inflammatory prostaglandins. Quercetin is structurally related to the anti-allergic drug disodium chromoglycate. It can be synthesized by intestinal bacteria from rutin (*which see*).

Quinoa

A nutty South American seed which is sometimes cooked and eaten by food allergy sufferers as a substitute for rice or other grains to which they may be allergic.

R

Raw food diets

Raw food diets used to be very popular with naturopathic practitioners, and were often the mainstay of naturopathic treatments. Mainstream naturopathy has now moderated its views somewhat, and naturopaths who still rely mainly on this form of treatment are now known as Natural Hygienists.

Although many individuals feel that a raw food diet makes a substantial contribution to their sense of health and well-being, others do not. In particular the condition of individuals with chronic muscular weakness, severe fatigue and other debilitated conditions may deteriorate on such a diet. Cooking food breaks down and softens the tough, indigestible walls of plant cells, making the starch available for enzymes to work on in our intestines.

Oriental medicine does not advise individuals suffering from any of the conditions mentioned above, or with fluid retention or 'cold' conditions of the body, to eat more than a small amount of raw food. On the other hand, raw food diets may be extremely beneficial for individuals who suffer from hot, inflammatory conditions.

RDA
(see Dietary Reference Values)

Reishi mushroom

Known as one of the 'power mushrooms', records for the use of Reishi (Latin name *Ganoderma lucidum* or Chinese name *Ling zhi*) as a folk medicine to strengthen the heart and lungs go back to 2800 BC. Like the Shiitake mushroom (*which see*), one of Reishi's active ingredients is the complex polysaccharide lentinan. Other ingredients, cyclooctasulphur and the triterpene ganoderic acid, may also contribute to the therapeutic effects attributed to it against tumours, high blood pressure and chronic asthmatic bronchitis. Reishi is reputed to have a substantial anti-allergy effect by inhibiting histamine release.

Retinol (see Vitamin A)

Riboflavin (see Vitamin B₂)

Ribonucleic acid
(see Nucleic acids)

RNA (see Nucleic Acids)

RNI

Reference Nutrient Intake. Roughly equivalent to the former UK Recommended Daily Amount. (*See Dietary Reference Values*)

Rosemary

Herb

Originating from Mediterranean countries and widely used as an aromatic culinary herb, rosemary also has useful medicinal properties. The leaves yield an oil containing rosemary camphor, which has a tonic, anti-depressant, energizing effect on the nervous system and stimulates the circulation. To obtain these beneficial effects, the oil is often used in aromatherapy treatments, as it is absorbed when massaged into the skin.

Royal jelly

A substance made by bees to feed the queen bee. It contains B vitamins, protein, and some hormone-like substances. Those who sell royal jelly have made many claims for health benefits, but these are difficult to assess, particularly when royal jelly competes with other, less expensive and better-researched nutritional supplements.

Availability: Royal jelly is widely available in health food shops.

Rutin (see Flavonoids)

S

S-Adenosyl methionine (SAM)

Sometimes known as 'activated' methionine, this is made in the body from methionine with the aid of an enzyme, and provides methyl groups for the synthesis of a host of important biological compounds, including betaine, carnitine, choline, creatine, adrenaline, melatonin and nucleic acids.

Saccharin

The oldest of the artificial sweeteners, saccharin has been in use since before 1900 and is approved in more than 90 countries. It is claimed that saccharin does not accumulate in the body, is rapidly excreted in the urine, and passes through the digestive system unchanged. However, in the US saccharin must carry a health warning since it has been found to cause cancer in test animals. Studies on humans have found that heavy smokers who consume saccharin may have a slightly elevated risk of bladder cancer. There are concerns that the acceptable daily intake of saccharin may be regularly exceeded by individuals such as diabetics and children who make heavy use of artificially-sweetened products. (*Also see Aspartame*.)

Sage

Herb

Commonly used in cookery, sage (especially the purple variety) is also a valuable medicinal herb, particularly in the menopause, because it has oestrogenic properties. Sage also has antiseptic and anti-fungal properties, and can be used as a mouthwash. It is also reported to have memory-enhancing effects. (These may be due to its relaxant effects on peripheral blood vessels, allowing better circulation.) In Chinese medicine sage is classified as a herb with a cooling, drying effect on the body.

The consumption of sage is not advisable in pregnancy or during breast-feeding.

Salicylates

Compounds related to aspirin which occur naturally in many foods. Some individuals are sensitive (allergic) to salicylates. Many children suffering from hyperactivity or attention deficit disorder are thought to be susceptible, and the Feingold diet (*see Therapeutic diets*) has been developed to diagnose and treat these cases. The Feingold diet excludes artificial colourings and flavourings, as well as natural foods containing salicylates: almonds, apples, apricots, peaches, plums, prunes, oranges, tomatoes, tangerines, cucumber, blackberries, strawberries, raspberries, gooseberries, cherries, currants, grapes, raisins, cranberries, bilberries, mint, peppers, passion fruit and olives.

Salt (Sodium chloride)

Salt is used both as a condiment in cookery, and as a food additive and preservative. Foods high in salt include bacon, ham, salami, sausages, pork pies and other preserved meats, canned fish, smoked fish, soy sauce, yeast extract, many cheeses, salted butter, salted peanuts and other packet snacks, packet and canned soups and sauces, most bread, stock cubes and ready-cooked meals for reheating. The regular consumption of these foods, as well as the addition of salt at the table, can easily lead to an intake of 12–17 grams a day, whereas the World Health Organization recommends no more than 5 grams.

A high salt intake has been linked with high blood pressure and strokes by encouraging the body to retain water. However, not all individuals with high blood pressure respond to a low-salt diet – some are thought to be more salt-sensitive than others. Recent research also links a high salt intake with osteoporosis. Salt appears to increase the sensitivity of the bronchial tubes to histamine, and studies have shown that asthma is worsened by a high salt intake.

An individual's salt intake can be reduced by avoiding the above high-salt foods, by exercising caution with all foods not prepared at home (especially if they taste salty), and by using low-sodium salt or salt substitute (usually potassium chloride) in cooking and at the table.

Children who are faddy eaters and eat only sweet or highly salted foods may have an impaired sense of taste due to zinc deficiency, which is becoming increasingly common. In such cases all other foods taste too bland. Once the zinc deficiency has been corrected, the child's range of food intake may improve, particularly if highly flavoured foods are withheld.

Salt (i.e. sodium chloride) is not the only source of sodium in the diet, but most natural foods have only a small sodium content, the best sources being fresh fish, meat, eggs, celery, beetroot, carrots, radish, spinach and watercress. Sodium occurring in such foods is normally incorporated into living cells, and is therefore in organic form and may be handled differently by the body. As pointed out by Dr Nadya Coates in her book *A Matter of Life*, sodium chloride, in contact with water, breaks down in the body to hydrochloric acid and sodium hydroxide (caustic soda). The hydrochloric acid is removed from the blood and used in the digestion process. The sodium hydroxide remains as an irritant to the cells, and has to be neutralized with lactic acid. Severe sodium hydroxide irritation may be experienced as a burning sensation in the affected parts of the body, although the affected area may feel cold to the touch. Some authorities believe that the resultant damage to cells could act as a trigger for cancer. On the other hand, the organic sodium found in vegetables such as celery may help to keep inorganic sodium (from salt) in solution, thus aiding its elimination. (*Also see Sodium.*)

Saturated fat (see Fats)

Saw palmetto

Herb

Also known as *Serenoa repens*, saw palmetto has been traditionally used against prostate enlargement, and double-blind trials have confirmed that it is effective, inhibiting both processes which encourage prostate enlargement: the conversion of testosterone to the more active dihydrotestosterone, and the binding of dihydrotestosterone to androgen receptor sites. Other properties of saw palmetto which are thought to contribute to its effectiveness against prostate enlargement or prostatitis include its anti-oestrogenic activities and its urinary antiseptic and urinary tract antispasmodic (relaxant) properties. Saw palmetto is also used to treat cystitis, infections and catarrh of the genitourinary tract and other sex hormone disorders.

Scurvy

Severe vitamin C deficiency. Signs and symptoms include decreased urinary excretion of vitamin C, weakness, anaemia, poor appetite, swollen, inflamed gums, loosened teeth, haemorrhages under the skin, failure of wounds to heal, hypochondriasis and depression. Old scars may break open, and ribs or other bones may fracture. If not treated, death will follow.

Before the cause of scurvy was discovered, thousands of sailors died on long ocean voyages when fresh fruit and vegetables were not available. In 1757, Scottish naval doctor James Lind discovered that oranges and lemons could be used to treat scurvy. But it was not until 48 years later, in 1795, that the British Navy ordered lime juice rations to be given to its sailors to prevent the disease. The Merchant Navy did not follow suit until 1865, and meanwhile many sailors continued to die from scurvy.

Sub-clinical scurvy, or vitamin C deficiency without obvious symptoms, can lead to a weakening of the immune system, which depends on vitamin C. White blood cells deficient in this vitamin can be reduced in size, activity and numbers, thus predisposing the individual to infections and even cancers. (*Also see Vitamin C* and *Nutritional deficiencies*.)

Secondary plant metabolites

Natural toxins found in plant foods. These toxins are the defences used by plants to defend themselves against predators: bacteria and viruses, fungi, insects, humans and animals. Some of the toxic effects of secondary plant metabolites include interference with hormonal function, or with the activity of digestive enzymes or the absorption of nutrients, damage to blood vessels and interference with blood clotting and enzyme activity. Aminopropionitrile in chick peas can cause a type of poisoning called lathyrism, which affects the bones and blood vessels. Dioscorine in wild yams can cause paralysis of the central nervous system. Plants belonging to the deadly nightshade family (potatoes, tomatoes, aubergines, tobacco and peppers) contain toxic alkaloids. Lectins in pulses are highly toxic but are broken down by fast boiling for at least 10 minutes.

Sometimes the production of plant toxins is stimulated by damage or stress inflicted on the plant by insects, fungi or frost, for example. A number of human deaths have occurred from solanine in potatoes, produced as a result of exposing the potatoes to light. Psoralens produced by celery which has been attacked by moulds or viruses can cause skin rashes. Both natural and artificial toxins originating in poisonous plants or from pesticides consumed by an animal can be passed on to the human consumer in the meat, milk or eggs of that animal.

Under normal circumstances, natural toxins in common plant foods can be easily dealt with by the human liver, which has developed enzymes capable of detoxifying these substances. However, the overloading of enzymes in the liver's detoxification system which may occur in individuals who have been subjected to severe toxic assault, or the overconsumption of certain foods which may occur in starvation conditions where a varied selection of foods is not available, may lead to the accumulation of toxic levels of one or more plant toxins.

Selenium

Trace element
UK RNI 75 mcg
US RDA 70 mcg

FUNCTIONS
Anti-carcinogenic
DNA repair
Needed for glutathione peroxidase enzyme
Needed by the immune system
Needed for thyroid hormone activation
Prostaglandin production
Spares vitamin E

GOOD FOOD SOURCES
Brazil nuts
Cereals
Fish and shellfish
Meat
Offal

Deficiency signs and symptoms

- Age spots
- Cancerous changes
- Cataracts
- Growth impairment
- Heart disease
- Infections

- Muscle inflammation
- Pale fingernail beds
- Pancreatic insufficiency
- Reduced detoxification ability
- Reduced fertility in males

Preventing deficiency

Soil levels of selenium vary considerably in different parts of the world. Most areas of the UK, New Zealand, Finland and parts of China are very selenium-poor. A high proportion of the UK's selenium intake used to come from selenium-rich Canadian wheat. In recent years European wheat is being used instead, and the UK's average selenium intake has dropped to only 30 micrograms per day, well below the Lower Reference Nutrient Intake – the official deficiency level. Although studies have shown that levels of the enzyme glutathione peroxidase – the major indicator of selenium status – are now low in many individuals, the UK Government has refused to advocate the consumption of more selenium-rich foods or to enforce the addition of selenium to fertilizer, a practice now successfully used in Finland. One of the richest sources of selenium is brazil nuts. If either fish, meat, offal or brazil nuts are not consumed daily in low-selenium countries, it is probably wise to take a daily selenium supplement.

Comments

It used to be believed that because animals grazing in very high-selenium areas can suffer symptoms of selenium poisoning, there was a very narrow margin between selenium adequacy and selenium toxicity. This has encouraged the belief that the use of selenium supplements should be discouraged. It is now recognized that selenium toxicity is extremely rare in humans, despite the widespread availability and use of supplements.

Selenium may be effective in reducing the toxic effects of mercury (*Hansen JC: Has selenium a beneficial role in human exposure to inorganic mercury?: Medical Hypotheses 25(1):45-54, 1988.* Also *Schrauzer GN: Quecksilber-Detoxifikation durch Selen: ein Beitrag zur Losung des Amalgam-Problems (in German). Dtsch Zschr f Biologische Zahnmedizin 5:162-164, 1989*). Unfortunately selenium deficiency is common in many parts of the world. Selenium adequacy is tested for by measuring the activity of the important antioxidant enzyme glutathione peroxidase. In a 1990 UK study, it was found that 25 per cent of healthy volunteers and 50 per cent of medical patients had serum selenium values below those required for full expression of glutathione peroxidase activity (*Pearson DJ et al.: Human selenium status and glutathione peroxidase activity in north-west England. Eur J Clin Nutr 44(4):277-83, 1990.*)

Supplementation

In research studies, selenium supplements have been found to:

- Bring clinical improvements in Aids
- Enhance immune function
- Help asthma
- Help prevent liver cancer
- Improve sperm motility
- Improve thyroid function
- Increase creatinine clearance (a sign of improved kidney function)
- Raise levels of the important antioxidant enzyme glutathione peroxidase
- Reduce early childhood seizures in epileptic children
- Reduce the death rate from acute pancreatitis

- Reduce the incidence of viral hepatitis in susceptible populations
- Reduce the symptoms of osteoarthritis and rheumatoid arthritis
- Treat acne
- With vitamin E, improve muscular dystrophy

Preferred form and suggested intake

The generally preferred forms of selenium supplementation are selenium-rich yeast, and L-selenomethionine. Supplements of 50–100 mcg per day are generally regarded as safe for most individuals. Inorganic selenium selenate is most effective at increasing the activity of glutathione peroxidase.

Cautions

Some cases of selenium toxicity have arisen from the use of anti-dandruff shampoos containing the highly toxic selenium sulphide, which can be absorbed through the skin by users who wash their hair in their bath water and then lie in it. Selenium toxicity imparts a 'garlicky' odour to the breath, and there may be a loss of hair and abnormal growth of fingernails.

Serine

Amino acid

Serine can be made in the human body from glycine, with the aid of vitamin B_3, B_6 and folic acid. In the form of phosphatidylserine, it is highly concentrated in all cell membranes. Serine is used to make many important substances such as ethanolamine, choline and phospholipids, and therefore plays a key role in cell membrane stability. (*Also see Phosphatidylserine.*)

Serine can be metabolized to pyruvate and used to make energy. It is required for the proper metabolism of methionine, and is also a neurotransmitter. It is involved in DNA synthesis and is a source of methyl groups for DNA. Combined with carbohydrates it forms glycoproteins.

Apart from meat and other animal products, gluten, soya products, peanuts and gelatin are good sources of serine.

Serotonin

A neurotransmitter derived from the amino acid tryptophan, which plays a role in sleep, consciousness and mood. Higher tryptophan levels in the brain result in higher serotonin levels. A meal high in carbohydrate aids the transport of tryptophan into the brain by stimulating the release of insulin, which hinders the brain's uptake of the other large neutral amino acids which compete with tryptophan.

Shark cartilage

The shark is one of the few species that rarely contracts cancer, even when exposed to cancer-causing chemicals. Sharks have no bone – their skeleton consists of cartilage which functions without nerves or a blood supply. This cartilage actually inhibits the development of blood vessels, and this property is thought to be of potential value in the dietary treatment of human cancers. Since tumours need a network of blood vessels in order to flourish, it is reasoned that the consumption of shark cartilage would cause the tumours – especially those tumours which are heavily vascularized (have a lot of blood vessels) – to perish. This process would not affect normal tissue, which does not have such fragile blood vessels as tumours. In tumours on the other hand, the blood vessels are constantly breaking down and being replaced.

A number of animal studies have been carried out which appear to confirm this hypothesis, and some human case reports also seem to offer hope. However, a small survey of shark cartilage users in the US found that only about half of those with cancer who took it regularly as a supplement experienced beneficial effects.

Shark cartilage may also help arthritis sufferers. There have been many reports that it helps to reduce joint inflammation and pain. It is speculated that this may be because it is in some way helping to regenerate joint cartilage.

Availability: Shark cartilage can be purchased in capsules and is available from health food shops.

Shark liver oil
(see Alkylglycerols)

Shiitake mushroom

Like the Reishi mushroom (*which see*) the Shiitake is also known as one of the 'power mushrooms' because of its longstanding record of health benefits. It is also eaten as a delicacy. Shiitake's main ingredient is the complex polysaccharide lentinan, which is being researched (in Japan in particular) as a potential immune system supporter, anticancer agent, and treatment for viral hepatitis. Shiitake is also a good natural source of vitamin D.

Shoyu sauce

One of the Japanese names for soya sauce. The other name is tamari. Shoyu sauce is thinner, while tamari is more full-bodied. When buying either sauce for macrobiotic cookery, ensure that no sugar, monosodium glutamate or preservatives have been added.

Silica (see Silicon)

Silicon

Trace element

Found in nature as silica (e.g. in quartz and sand) it is not known whether silicon is an essential element in the human body, but it is found mainly in the skin, tendons, bones and artery walls. In body fluids, silicon is found mainly in the form of silicic acid. Work with animals has shown that silicon is needed for connective tissue metabolism and bone development. In the diet, silicon is found mainly in association with fibre, particularly in the husks of grains. Oats, barley, millet and soya beans are especially rich sources of silicon.

Silymarin

Herb

Silymarin is the name given to a flavonoid-rich extract from the medicinal herb milk thistle used primarily for its wide range of benefits on the liver. Widely researched, silymarin has been shown to have considerable liver protective effects, for instance in test animals it is capable of preventing liver

necrosis (death of liver tissue) caused by carbon tetrachloride, and death from consumption of the poisonous death cap mushroom. Silymarin can reduce toxic fatty degeneration in the liver (for instance as caused by alcoholism), and rapidly improves chronic hepatitis, with reduction of the related digestive problems. Good results have been reported in the treatment of cirrhosis of the liver, with bilirubin levels soon returning to normal. Silymarin stabilizes the membranes of liver cells, preventing the entry of toxic compounds and thus preventing damage to these cells. Other reported benefits include inhibition of iron-induced liver toxicity, and damage to the liver caused by the painkiller paracetamol (acetaminophen).

Availability: Widely available in health food shops.

Singlet oxygen

A highly reactive form of oxygen similar to a free radical (*which see*), and consisting of single atoms instead of molecules. Beta-carotene and lycopene are effective scavengers of singlet oxygen.

Slippery elm

Herb

The inner bark of *Ulmus fulva*, slippery elm is rich in mucilage and tannin. Sold either as lozenges or as a powder to be mixed with liquid, slippery elm is used for its soothing effect on the digestive system. It reduces the irritation which is the cause of many symptoms such as the pain of gastric ulcers and the after-effects of food poisoning.

Availability: From health food shops or through nutritional therapists.

SOD (see Superoxide dismutase)

Sodium (also see Salt)

Mineral

Sodium is required for the following functions:

- Acid-alkaline balance
- Assimilation of amino acids and glucose into body cells
- Electrolyte (*which see*)
- Energy production
- Muscle contraction
- Nerve impulse transmission
- Normal water balance and blood volume

The human sodium requirement is probably about 500 mg per day (representing about 1.3 grams of salt) although most individuals consume far more than this. Apart from the high-salt foods listed under *Salt*, other common sources of sodium include monosodium glutamate and other sodium-based food additives, baking powder, and sodium bicarbonate antacid medications. Salt itself is 40 per cent sodium and 60 per cent chloride.

Whereas potassium is mainly found inside the cells, sodium is found outside the cells, in the extracellular fluid. Large amounts are also found in bone, bile and pancreatic juice. There is no control of sodium absorption as with other minerals – the excessive dietary intakes which are so common in the Western world are readily absorbed. As the blood sodium levels rise the thirst receptors in the hypothalamus stimulate the thirst sensation, and the extra water is retained to keep the sodium diluted. At the same time the kidney will begin reabsorbing less sodium, thus allowing more sodium to be excreted in the urine. Aldosterone, a hormone secreted by the adrenal cortex, controls the rate of excretion of sodium in the urine, and vasopressin (also known as anti-diuretic hormone or ADH) produced by the pituitary, controls the rate of fluid excretion by the kidneys. Normal kidneys have no difficulty in excreting excess sodium as long as there is sufficient water to allow this.

Low-sodium diets are frequently prescribed to control the excessive retention of body water, especially in individuals with high blood pressure resulting from this excess fluid. Such diets may help to prevent an enlarged heart, and enlarged kidneys leading to nephritis. A high dietary intake of calcium and potassium can help to protect against some of the adverse effects of excess sodium consumption.

Sodium deficiency is rare in the Western world, although heavy exercise in a hot climate, causing prolonged sweating, may lead to sodium depletion. An insufficiency of the adrenal cortex gland, or prolonged vomiting or diarrhoea, kidney disease (as in renal failure), or long-term very low-sodium diets may produce a sodium deficiency, leading to weakness, lassitude, anorexia and vomiting, mental confusion, cramps and aching muscles. Addison's disease involves a loss of adrenal function and aldosterone production, thus causing sodium deficiency by impairment of the kidney's ability to reabsorb sodium. Cushing's disease, on the other hand, involves the production of excessive amounts of hormones by the adrenal cortex, thus resulting in sodium retention.

Sodium pump

All cell membranes contain a sodium 'pump' – an enzyme known as Na+/K+ATPase, which moves sodium from the inside to the outside of the cell. As sodium leaves the cell, potassium enters. It is this activity of the sodium pump which is responsible for the electrical charges in the cell membrane, which are required for the conduction of nerve impulses. The activity of the sodium pump is controlled by hormones.

Soya products

Soya beans have been consumed for 3,000 years, especially in the Far East. They are extremely rich in protein and, weight for weight, products such as soya protein isolate, soya flour and dried tofu contain more essential amino acids than meat, which makes them popular with vegans, who eat no animal produce. The soya bean is also used to make soya milk, soya oil, and the fermented products known as miso and soya sauce.

Soya milk is the liquid left after the beans have been crushed in water and strained. In many respects the nutritional value of soya milk compares very well with cow's milk, but it is lower in calories and in calcium.

Soya products are rich in phyto-oestrogens (plant oestrogens also known as isoflavones), particularly genistein, which has tumour-inhibiting effects. A high consumption of soya products has been found to prevent prostate cancer in men and to have an oestrogen-balancing effect on women. Both problems of excess oestrogen, such as breast cancer, and problems of inadequate oestrogen, such as hot flushes, are significantly reduced.

Babies. Some speculation has recently arisen about the safety of soya-based infant formula feeds for male babies because of the phyto-oestrogen content. Since at the time of writing no research has yet been carried out to determine whether the phyto-oestrogens may interfere with a male baby's sexual development, some authorities are suggesting that to err on the side of caution, soya formula feeds should only be used in case of necessity. However, the alternative of cow's milk formula feeds also poses risks due to the high rate of allergy to cow's milk. Wherever possible, breast-feeding is best.

Children. Because soya milk contains much less fat than whole cow's milk, it is not recommended for very young children unless they obtain enough calories from other sources. (This applies as a general rule to all low-fat foods since children need more fat in their diet than adults do.)

Spirulina (see Algae)

Sprouted seeds

Sprouted seeds are seeds which have been allowed to germinate and sprout. Lentils, chick peas, mung beans and alfalfa sprouts are all popular, and some sprouted seed enthusiasts believe that these foods provide more nutrients, ounce for ounce, than any other natural food known. They also believe that the high level of enzyme activity in the sprouts can stimulate the body's own enzymes into greater activity.

The simplest sprouting method is to put a few handfuls of seeds in a large glass jar, rinse them, pour off all the water and then cover the jar. The rinsing process is repeated every day until the seeds have sprouted and are an inch or so in length. After a final rinse they are then ready to eat.

St John's wort

Herb

This very valuable medicinal herb has both relaxant and anti-depressant properties, and is used to treat depressive illness. However, it is probably not effective against severe clinical depression. St John's wort does not have an immediate mood-lifting effect, but must be taken for several weeks before this effect will begin to occur. Other conditions which may respond to this herb include menopausal problems, insomnia, nervous tension, bed-wetting, and all conditions involving cramps and spasms, such as irritable bowel syndrome and period pains.

Oil in which the flowers of the St John's wort plant have been steeped can be used externally to treat neuralgic pains, wounds and mild burns.

Cautions: St John's wort causes users to develop photosensitivity of the skin. To avoid getting skin rashes, those using this herb internally or externally should not expose themselves to strong sunlight.

Starch (see Carbohydrates)

Sterols

Lipid compounds with a multiple-ring structure such as cholesterol, bile, sex hormones, adrenal hormones and vitamin D. (Cholesterol itself is the starting material for many of these substances.)

Sterols found in plants are known as phytosterols, some examples being beta-sitosterol, which can block the absorption of dietary cholesterol by competing with it, and ergosterol, which on irradiation with ultraviolet light can be converted to vitamin D_2. Phyto-oestrogens (*see Oestrogen*) are a type of phytosterol.

Stomach

The major organ of digestion (*which see*). Once food has been swallowed it passes down the oesophagus and enters the stomach, which secretes acidic gastric juices to begin protein digestion.

Sucrose (see Carbohydrates and Sugar, health effects)

Sugar, health effects
(also see Carbohydrates)

Sugar, a form of carbohydrate, occurs naturally in fruit and vegetables, where it is not in concentrated form. Concentrated sugar occurs in products such as honey, syrup and treacle, and highly concentrated sucrose crystals are sold as brown or white table sugar. In this form it is widely used in large amounts to sweeten foods such as cakes, biscuits, jam, desserts, confectionery, sweets, chocolate, candy and ice cream. It is also a main ingredient in soft drinks, colas, milk shakes and many alcoholic drinks, and is added to tea, coffee and other beverages. In the UK, the average consumption of concentrated sugar is about 2 lb per person per week. Since a large percentage of the population consumes less than the average, this means that an equally large percentage are consuming considerably more than 2 lb per week.

There is no nutritional requirement for concentrated sugar. All the energy needs of people with access to a normal diet can be met without consuming any added sugar in any form. And since large amounts of sugar can be consumed without a feeling of fullness (satiety), it is very easy for us to over-consume it and therefore to put on excess body weight, since sugar, whether white or brown, is a source of pure calories. Sugar also promotes tooth decay by being turned into acid by bacteria in the mouth.

Nutritionists connected with the sugar industry attempt to play down the role of sugar in obesity and tooth decay. They claim that there is no evidence that sugar itself is responsible for either of these problems, and that it cannot be blamed for illnesses such as heart disease which are linked with obesity. To some extent this is true since overweight and tooth decay are caused by an abuse of sugar rather than by sugar itself. But in most cases this is an unknowing abuse. Most of the public are very poorly informed about the dangers of excess sugar consumption thanks to the power and wealth of the sugar industry, which ensures that the professionals who are officially in charge of our health rarely dare to publicize them. Some of the less well-known among these dangers are as follows.

Vitamin and mineral deficiency

We can only eat a certain number of calories a day without putting on excess weight. If 20 per cent of these calories come from sugar, you are eating only 80 per cent of the amount of vitamin-rich food which a person on a low-sugar diet eats. Can you be sure that this is enough? With all the evidence now pointing to the protective effects of eating large amounts of vitamin-rich foods against cancer and heart disease, you could be putting yourself in the high-risk category if you continue to over-indulge in sugary (and fatty) foods deficient in vitamins and minerals.

In fact a high sugar consumption even robs the body of some nutrients. Chromium and some of the B vitamins are used up and lost every time you consume sugar. Chromium deficiency is now strongly linked with heart problems and with maturity-onset diabetes. Numerous other health problems including premenstrual syndrome, chronic fatigue and acne are also linked with vitamin and mineral deficiency.

In many individuals, excess sugar consumption can also cause the body to produce too much insulin. Such people show an increased tendency to atherosclerosis. Experimental high-sugar diets have been shown to increase the level of blood fats and the stickiness of blood, thus increasing the risk of cholesterol deposits and clots. Blood clots are the cause of heart attacks and strokes.

Fluid retention

The consumption of sugar stimulates the body to produce insulin, particularly if sugary foods are consumed on their own rather than as part of a meal. Some individuals are sugar-sensitive, and produce much more insulin than others. By suppressing the formation of ketoacids, high insulin levels can interfere with the body's excretion of sodium, leading to sodium retention. High insulin levels also promote low blood potassium levels. An excess of sodium and a lack of potassium encourage fluid retention.

Gall-bladder disease

Research studies have shown that individuals with gallstones frequently have a higher sugar consumption than those who do not.

Kidney disease

A high sugar consumption can cause enlarged kidneys and kidney damage, as evidenced by increased amounts of a substance known as N-acetyl-beta-glucosaminidase. This may lead to kidney stones or to kidney insufficiency.

Crohn's disease, ulcerative colitis and colon cancer

There is now much research which suggests that those with a high sugar consumption have a much higher risk of developing Crohn's disease or ulcerative colitis, both being severe inflammatory bowel conditions. There is also some evidence of a higher risk of colon cancer. The mechanism for this may be the increase in gut dysbiosis (*which see*) which occurs when sugar is not adequately digested.

Miscellaneous

Research suggests that a high sugar consumption is also linked with a greater risk of short- or long-sightedness, gout, peptic ulcers, liver enlargement due to fat accumulation, adrenal gland enlargement, and acne. The excess insulin levels stimulated by excess sugar can interfere with the body's production of beneficial prostaglandins, which are required for a host of important functions relating to blood pressure control, fluid and electrolyte balance, and control of blood stickiness and capillary permeability.

Sulphate (see Bioavailability and Detoxification)

Sulphur

Mineral

Sulphur is an essential nutrient for humans. It is a constituent of all proteins, especially hair, nails and skin. Most of the sulphur found in the human body occurs in the amino acids cysteine, cystine, methionine and taurine. Sulphur is needed to stabilize the shape of proteins, for insulin production, and to form part of vitamin B_1, biotin, lipoic acid, glutathione and coenzyme A. In its inorganic sulphate form, sulphur is an electrolyte. Sulphate is also involved in the production of mucopolysaccharides needed for collagen integrity, and helps to prepare some waste substances for excretion in the kidneys by making them more water-soluble.

Foods rich in sulphur include meat, fish, eggs, nuts, garlic, pulses, radishes and watercress.

Superoxide (see Free radicals)

Superoxide dismutase (see Antioxidants)

T

Tamari sauce
(see Shoyu sauce)

Tannins

Polyphenols found in many plants, such as tea, which may act as deterrents against insect attack. Tannins have an astringent effect on the mouth and digestive system, and precipitate proteins. They are anti-nutrients, binding to minerals such as iron and zinc in the gut to form unabsorbable complexes.

Tartrazine

Coal tar dye found in fish batter and chips, fish fingers, cakes, biscuits, confectionery, soft drinks, party foods, and fed to chickens and cows to colour butter and eggs. Linked with asthma, rashes, migraine, hyperactivity. A 1983 study on 88 children reported in the *Lancet* showed that two of the top 10 causes of intractable migraine in children were the coal-tar dyes tartrazine (E102) and benzoic acid preservative (E210). After cow's milk, tartrazine was the second most common single cause of migraine. A study on hyperactive children has found that tartrazine consumption increases the excretion of zinc in the urine, lowers body zinc levels and worsens behavioural symptoms in these children.

Taurine

Amino acid

Taurine is one of the sulphur amino acids. Unlike the others it is not incorporated into muscle proteins but it is the second most abundant free amino acid in the brain. Within the brain taurine is concentrated in the taste and smell centre, the memory centre and the pineal gland, and it has neurotransmitter functions. It is present in cell membranes, helping to stabilize them electrically and facilitating the passage of sodium, potassium and calcium ions in and out of cells. This role may account for taurine's usefulness in the treatment of epilepsy, seizures and convulsions. Taurine is also an inhibitory neurotransmitter (*which see*).

Taurine is the most abundant amino acid in the heart, and has been successfully used in supplement form to combat congestive heart failure, by regulating calcium and potassium in heart muscle cells (and therefore in nerve impulses in the heart), by acting as a heart stimulant and by encouraging the excretion of sodium and water. Taurine is needed for the formation of taurocholic acid, which helps to break down fats in the small intestine. It is also needed in large amounts by the eyes.

One of taurine's most important roles is in detoxification (*which see*). It is needed for conjugating toxic substances, and as an antioxidant, especially for the hypochlorite ion, formed by the oxidation of chloride ions and itself a powerful oxidizing agent. Because the hypochlorite ion requires adequate amounts of the amino acid taurine to control and scavenge it, taurine-deficient individuals may become very sensitive to aldehydes, chlorine, bleach and other similar chemicals, and free amino acids in their body may become toxic aldehydes. For this reason infant formula feeds should always be enriched with taurine at least to the levels found in human breast milk.

Except for young babies, the human body is able to make taurine from the amino acid cysteine although it is not known whether this is always enough for our requirements. Taurine is found in breast milk, meat, fish and organ meats. The food additive monosodium glutamate can reduce taurine levels. Adequate zinc, vitamin A and vitamin B_6, and adequate methionine intake and metabolism are required to maintain normal taurine levels in the body. Poor kidney function may result in taurine depletion. High levels of the amino acid beta-alanine, which may occur if vitamin B_6 is deficient, can result in excess losses of taurine through the urine.

In one research study, taurine supplementation was found to reduce dementia in elderly people.

Availability: Taurine supplements are available through health food shops and nutritional therapists.

Tea tree oil

The essential oil of *Melaleuca alternifolia*, related to clove, eucalyptus and myrtle. All the essential oils from this family have antiseptic properties. Aromatherapists attribute powerful immune stimulant properties to tea tree oil and recommend its use in the bath at the first sign of a cold or the flu. Vaginal douches with a few drops of tea tree oil in warm water are used to treat thrush.

Tempeh

A fermented soya product which originated in the Far East and has a firm texture, suitable for slicing and dicing. Tempeh is often used as a meat substitute by vegetarians, and in macrobiotic cookery.

Testosterone

The major male sex hormone (androgen) produced by the male testes. Small amounts are also produced by the ovaries in women, and are subsequently converted to oestrogen. Testosterone is required for sperm production, for the development of male characteristics, and promotes sex drive in both sexes. In men, testosterone can be converted into another form known as dihydrotestosterone. Increased amounts of dihydrotestosterone have been associated with abnormal prostate gland enlargement, a problem common in middle-aged and elderly men.

Tetracycline

A broad spectrum antibiotic – one which is capable of destroying a wide variety of micro-organisms. When prescribed for lengthy periods for problems such as acne, or to prevent infections in susceptible individuals, there is a very real danger of serious depletion of the beneficial intestinal flora and the development of dysbiosis (*which see*). Although antibiotics are popularly believed to be harmless drugs, this is not always the case.

Tetracycline, for instance, can cause damage to the liver and kidneys.

Theobromine (see Methylxanthines)

Theophylline
(see Methylxanthines)

Therapeutic diets

These are the diets used by the professional nutritional therapist to help individuals suffering from nutrition-responsive health problems.

Anti-Candida diet
The anti-Candida diet is intended to discourage the growth of the *Candida albicans* yeast (*which see*). Since most candidiasis sufferers have food allergies, the diet is a modified version of the hypoallergenic diet. In addition it does not permit the ingestion of any sweetened foods or any foods or drinks which are very high in natural sugars, such as bananas, fruit juice and dried fruit. This is because sugar encourages the growth of yeasts.

It used to be believed that mushrooms (which are a member of the fungus family), and yeast occurring in stock cubes, yeast extract, baked products, fermented products such as soy sauce and vinegar, or even products containing small quantities of these, such as mayonnaise, could encourage the growth of the candida yeast. It is now known that the consumption of killed yeast cannot encourage *Candida albicans*, and that the aggravation of candidiasis

symptoms which was noted by early workers in this field was almost certainly due to yeast allergy – the candidiasis sufferer having been sensitized to yeast by having a yeast infestation in his or her intestines.

An anti-Candida diet will also encourage the consumption of onions, leeks, extra virgin olive oil, unsweetened soya yoghurt and garlic, all of which help to inhibit the growth of the yeast.

Anti-herpes diet
Because a high intake of the amino acid arginine appears to encourage the herpes simplex virus, while a high intake of the amino acid lysine has the opposite effect, this diet avoids foods rich in arginine and encourages the consumption of foods which favour lysine.

Foods to eat liberally: meat, fish (except shellfish), dairy products, fruit, all vegetables except those mentioned below, butter beans, mung beans

Foods to eat less liberally: maize products and sweetcorn, millet, wheatflour, rye, oats, barley, potatoes

Foods to avoid: All nuts and seeds (their oils are OK), all beans, peas and lentils (except those mentioned above), buckwheat, rice, pumpkin, chocolate.

Blood sugar control diet
There are two types of blood sugar problem: a tendency to excessively high blood sugar (hyperglycaemia, or diabetes) and a tendency to excessively low blood sugar (hypoglycaemia). Both types are aggravated by the consumption of foods with a high glycaemic index, that is to say foods which are converted very rapidly into blood sugar. Most of these foods can be identified by their sweetness, such as sugar, honey, bananas, fruit juice, carrot juice and dried fruit. Refined starches such as white flour and white rice are also more readily converted to sugar than their whole grain counterparts.

The blood sugar control diet excludes such foods and encourages the use of foods high in soluble fibre such as pulses and oatmeal, which help to slow down the absorption of sugars into the bloodstream. It is interesting that orthodox nutritional advice for diabetics has undergone considerable change and is now identical to the advice which nutritional therapists have always given. (*Also see Glycaemic index.*)

Calorie-controlled diets

These are diets which combine the principles of healthy eating with strict rationing of high-calorie foods to promote weight loss.

Cleansing diets (alkalinizing diets)

There are many variations of cleansing diets, which stem from naturopathic tradition. Often based on raw food, they may not be suitable for people suffering from weakness, or a 'yin' condition of the body, since raw food increases any excess of yin. The main purpose of these diets is to remove excess tissue acidity, a toxic condition caused by the long-term consumption of too much protein, to correct the sodium/-potassium balance, to promote cell respiration and oxygenation, and to help decongest the liver after long-term excess fat consumption and help it to discharge toxic waste matter.

Protein, when metabolized by the body, leaves an acidic residue. This residue may build up in the tissues, causing difficulties in cell oxygenation and, by promoting free radical damage to tissues and joints, may in the long term encourage the development of degenerative diseases such as arthritis and cancers. Research carried out by Professor Louis-Claude Vincent has shown that sufferers of such diseases often have high tissue acidity levels, as shown by measuring urine pH.

Fruits and vegetables, on the other hand, leave an alkaline residue after being metabolized, so cleansing diets mainly concentrate on these, often to the exclusion of all other foods for a short while. For the first 10 days to two weeks, cleansing diets are often all raw food. After this some steamed vegetables may be added, and some brown rice and pulses. Some nuts (not peanuts) and a very small amount of olive oil may be allowed, but no other fat. The diet is deliberately low in calories, since it is designed to break up fatty deposits in the liver. Body fats (and lean body tissue) are broken down to release stored energy when calorie intake from food is inadequate for energy needs. To minimize the loss of lean tissue, care must be taken not to reduce the calorie intake too much.

Elimination diet

This is a diet which eliminates suspect foods to which an individual may be allergic or intolerant, before reintroducing them to determine the reaction.

Exclusion diet

A diet which excludes certain foods, usually because the individual has been found to be allergic or intolerant to them.

Fasting and mono diets

Fasting is a technique used much more frequently by the more traditional naturopath rather than the modern nutritional therapist. It is based on the theory that if an individual stops eating, the body will have the opportunity to break down and eliminate its diseased parts. Whether or not this is true, it is certainly true that the digestive system will have the opportunity to rest and repair its absorptive ability where impaired (if this is possible and provided dysbiosis is thoroughly treated first).

The most effective type of fast is thought to be the water fast, in which only water is consumed. Also used are juice fasts, in which carrot or apple juice, for instance, may also be consumed, especially after severe diarrhoea, when the body needs to replenish electrolytes and may be unable to tolerate food anyway. 'Mono diets', consisting of eating only one food, such as apples or grapes, are also a type of fast.

Water or juice fasts generally last from four days to two weeks. Mono diets may last up to six weeks. Lengthy fasting must only be prescribed and supervised by a knowledgeable practitioner and never self-administered in the hope that it 'might help'. People who are severely underweight or suffering from any form of weakness are not advised to fast.

Feingold diet

This diet was developed by the late Dr Ben Feingold MD, an American allergist who spent many years researching the possibility that chemical food additives may be linked to hyperactivity and behavioural disorders. The Feingold diet excludes most synthetic ingredients such as food colourings and flavouring, and also some natural fruits because of their salicylate content (*which see*) to which some children are sensitive.

Although this diet is often successful in treating hyperactivity, its successes may not necessarily be always due to the exclusion of synthetic substances. When such substances are avoided, this often results in the much greater use of fresh foods prepared at home. These may be a great deal more nutritious than the commercial foods normally consumed by the children in question, which could lead to health benefits not related to the avoidance of artificial additives. Clinical trials testing additives against placebo in hyperactive children have led to variable results, which is one reason why this whole area remains controversial. However, some studies have shown that additives are by far the most common inducers of behavioural problems and migraine in the children tested.

Few foods diet

The 'few foods diet' is a recognized medical technique for identifying food allergens and problem foods, and consists of hospitalizing a patient, starting him or her off on just a few foods, and then gradually adding more foods, observing which foods seem to set off symptoms when added to the diet. One well-known version of the few foods diet is the 'lamb and pears' diet, in which the patient is allowed to eat nothing but lamb and pears for a number of days. Other versions are the 'mackerel and courgettes' diet or the 'cod and cabbage' diet. In each case the 'few foods' chosen are those considered least likely to provoke an allergic reaction.

It is not advisable to continue with a few foods diet for more than a few days, and such a diet is only given under the strictest supervision. Although useful for identifying definite allergic reactions which occur within 24 hours, it may not pick up on the more insidious types of allergic response.

Gerson diet

This diet is famous for its use against cancer, and many so-called anti-cancer diets are variations of it. Dr Max Gerson was a physician practising from the 1930s to the 1950s who invented what was to be a revolutionary but controversial new form of cancer treatment based primarily on the consumption of organically grown fresh, wholefoods and large quantities of fruit and vegetable juices, particularly leafy green vegetables. In his book *A Cancer Therapy: Results of Fifty Cases*, Gerson wrote that cancer is 'a very slow, progressing, imperceptible symptom caused by poisoning of the liver and simultaneously an impairment of the whole intestinal tract.' His treatment therefore aimed to assist liver oxidizing enzymes (now known as cytochrome P450 mixed-function oxidases) and provide extra nourishment in easily-absorbed form (by means of the juices) as well as to enhance the elimination of toxic substances (by means of coffee enemas).

Half a century on, modern science is only now catching up with Max Gerson, as scientists are finding that green vegetables like broccoli and brussels sprouts really do contain powerful substances (indoles) which assist the function of cytochrome P450 oxidase enzymes in the liver. Research also reveals that most cancer patients have some degree of food malabsorption.

Hay diet

The Hay diet has traditionally been promoted as being effective for weight loss and digestive problems because it does not 'mix' starch and protein, thus preventing the body from having to produce starch-digesting and protein-digesting enzymes at the same time. There is no physiological rationale why this enzyme manipulation should help with weight loss. Since a proportion of people do find the Hay diet more effective than a conventional weight-loss diet, this may be because one or more meals a day are low in carbohydrate.

Another explanation may be that many people on the Hay diet avoid carbohydrate meals completely, and eat fruit-only meals, or protein with salad or vegetables. They are unknowingly avoiding some of the most common food allergens and promoters of dysbiosis (which see), such as sucrose, gluten, wheat or other grains. They may attribute their weight loss or health improvement while following this diet to the non-mixing of starch and protein, whereas the truth may be that their symptoms were due to food allergy and dysbiosis and their excess body weight to allergic fluid retention, and it was the avoidance of the problem foods which helped them.

Doubtless weak digestive organs may benefit from not having to produce all types of enzymes for all meals, but our

understanding of the factors involved in digestive disorders have advanced considerably since the development of the Hay diet, and more finely tuned options are now available. In its full form this difficult and complex diet is not a reliable or long-term solution to a weak digestion, and most nutritional therapists do not often prescribe it.

High methionine diet

The amino acid methionine (which see) is vital for the supply of sulphur compounds needed for many functions in the body, particularly in liver function and detoxification and in cell membranes. Extra dietary methionine can therefore be particularly helpful for individuals suffering from chemical sensitivities. Methionine is also involved in the control of blood histamine and so can help to prevent allergic reactions as well as to control a type of depressive illness which is related to high histamine levels. Some individuals need extra dietary methionine for these reasons. Certain foods such as brazil nuts, rice and sesame seeds are particularly rich in methionine and can be used to form the basis of a methionine-rich diet.

Hypoallergenic diet

This is often used as a basic diagnostic diet for the first two weeks of a nutritional therapy regime. It excludes the four foods which are most commonly associated with allergic symptoms (wheat and gluten, dairy produce, eggs and yeast) together with a number of dietary items which may cause actual or potential stress to the digestive system, detoxification system or endocrine system, including tea, coffee and chocolate, sugar, salt, artificial food additives, alcohol, saturated and hydrogenated fat and red meat. The diet is usually given in the form of a checklist of foods to eat and foods to avoid, with suggested recipes and advice on food preparation. In some cases individual guidance for meal planning is also given. This diet must be given under supervision since patients who are faddy eaters have been known to adapt it to taste, and to try to exist on a very small number of foods, quite inadequate for their needs.

′ People who have attempted food elimination without proper professional advice often fail to improve because they are unaware of hidden ingredients in food.

Low carbohydrate diet

This is a technique used only as a last resort by nutritional therapists, for patients with a very resistant weight problem that will not respond to a healthy reduced-calorie, high exercise programme. They must be clinically obese, not merely anxious to lose weight for cosmetic reasons. This diet is based on the premise that if you deprive the body of carbohydrate it will have to convert protein and fat into glucose, to obtain the raw energy material it needs. In the process of this conversion there appears to be some calorie wastage.

Although we are not certain that it is this calorie wastage which accounts for the success of this diet, the diet does usually succeed when other diets have failed. However it can lead to acidosis, dehydration, loss of lean tissue, and impairment of kidney function due to a build-up of waste products from the breakdown of body tissues if used for prolonged periods. Nutritional therapists take great care when administering this diet, and ensure that the patient understands it is a once-only diet, and after the target weight has been reached a healthy lifestyle with strict rationing of high-calorie foods must be permanently maintained so that excessive weight gain never recurs.

Maintenance diet

A maintenance diet is a diet prescribed for long-term use after a nutritional therapy treatment programme. It aims to keep the individual as healthy as possible, and to prevent their original problem from returning, but with the minimum of inconvenience.

The basic principles of the maintenance diet are that 90 per cent of the diet should consist of a variety of fruit, vegetables, pulses, whole grains or cereals, nuts and seeds daily, and that the remaining 10 per cent can be selected at will, provided that any appropriate calorie restrictions are observed and allergenic foods avoided. The nutritional therapist will also generally recommend that even if the individual is not allergic to wheat, eggs, yeast and dairy produce, consumption of these foods should be controlled. This is because out of all the foods which form part of the human diet, these seem to be the most highly allergenic, therefore as a species we are probably not well adapted to them and may be well advised to take care with their consumption. It is possible that the breeding to which modern wheat and yeast have been subjected (to make lesser quantities go further in manufactured products) and the antibiotics and/or hormones, food colourings, etc. fed to laying hens and dairy cattle, traces of which may remain in eggs and milk, may play some part in this poor adaptation. Some children who are severely allergic to ordinary dairy milk suffer no reaction to organic milk (milk from cows fed only traditional food and not routinely treated with drugs). Likewise, many individuals who are allergic to modern wheat products can tolerate ancient wheat (also known as 'spelt') without problems.

A maintenance diet also requires a restricted intake of tea, coffee, food additives, sugar (including honey), saturated fat and red meat.

The maintenance diet is also suitable for those without health problems who wish to follow healthy eating practices.

Oligoantigenic diet

This is similar to an elimination diet, but excludes more foods. This term is often used in clinical trials which investigate the effects of dietary restrictions on symptoms and behaviour.

Rare food diet

This is a type of elimination diet which only allows the consumption of foods which the patient has rarely eaten and to which he or she cannot therefore have become sensitized.

Raw food diet

Although some naturopaths advocate eating mainly raw food for both preventive and curative purposes, it is important to be aware that a high-raw diet does not suit everyone's constitution and may even be inappropriate. In particular the condition of individuals with chronic muscular weakness, severe fatigue and other debilitated conditions may rapidly deteriorate on such a diet. Cooking food breaks down and softens the tough, indigestible walls of plant cells, making the starch available for enzymes to work on in our intestines.

Oriental medicine does not advise individuals suffering from any of the conditions mentioned above, or with fluid retention or 'cold' conditions of the body to eat more than a small amount of raw food. On the other hand, raw food diets may be extremely beneficial for individuals who suffer from hot, inflammatory conditions.

Rotation diet

Nutritional therapists use rotation diets for patients with multiple allergies who would not otherwise be able to eat a varied diet. There are many different types of allergic response to foods, and one of these is a type which only occurs if a specific food is eaten more than once in any four-day period. Why four days, and not three or five, for instance,

we do not know. Some believe that it takes four days to clear all remains of a food completely out of the system, and that eating it more than once in that period can overload the body's ability to detoxify some of the natural chemicals found in that particular food. It is believed that the rotation diet achieves a gradual regaining of tolerance to foods by reducing an excessive demand for specific liver detoxifying enzymes that are required to metabolize specific natural food toxins. If this demand is not met, and the problem foods continue to be eaten, there may be a rise in circulating toxins or intermediate toxic metabolites, which promotes not only symptoms but biological damage. If the load is reduced, there is an opportunity not only for the enzyme systems in question to regenerate, but also for the biological damage to be repaired.

Each rotation diet must be individually devised according to the patient's own tolerances. The diet will not include foods to which the patient is severely allergic or which always cause an allergic reaction when eaten. Each food in a rotation diet may be eaten only once in any four-day period. Once the patient begins to feel better, this can be modified, and then foods to which the patient has never suffered an allergic reaction need no longer be strictly 'rotated', although they should nevertheless not be eaten too regularly.

Specific carbohydrate diet

Devised by digestion researcher Elaine Gottschall, this diet is designed to combat dysbiosis (*which see*) by avoiding those foods which require digestion by enzymes secreted by the gut wall. The production of these enzymes becomes impaired when the gut wall is damaged by bacterial endotoxins and acids. As a result, starches and disaccharide sugars in particular can be poorly digested. Undigested carbohydrates are fermented by undesirable gut bacteria, allowing them to thrive and thus worsening the dysbiosis. The end result can be problems such as an excessively permeable gut (*see Leaky gut syndrome*), inflammatory bowel disease and food intolerance or allergy. Users of the specific carbohydrate diet have reported being cured of such diverse conditions as Crohn's disease, irritable bowel syndrome, ulcerative colitis and coeliac disease (with restoration of the coeliac's tolerance to gluten). Bowel toxins can even promote hallucinations and other mental effects, as many coeliac sufferers have reported. By helping to heal the bowel in such patients, the specific carbohydrate diet has reversed some cases of schizophrenia.

Stone Age diet

This is a type of elimination diet for allergy sufferers which avoids all foods which have entered the human diet relatively recently in evolutionary terms and which man may therefore be less well adapted to: wheat, rice and other cereals, bread, biscuits, cake, sugar, dairy products, food additives, coffee, tea and alcohol. These foods are much more likely to cause allergy/sensitivity problems. Stone Age man lived a mainly hunter-gatherer existence on fresh meat, fish, vegetables, fruit and nuts.

Yin/Yang balanced diets

These diets are given to individuals whose symptoms suggest an imbalance in yin and yang energies – the energies in the Oriental macrobiotic system of medicine which, according to this system, are thought to be at the root of all illness.

Conditions of excess yang are those associated with excessive body heat, inflammations and eruptions. Acne sufferers are often a good example of this. Conditions of excess yang are thought to be much less common than conditions of excess yin in the Western world. Yin conditions are those associated with coldness and lack of energy, chest ailments, and fluid retention. They are thought to be linked with the excess consumption of ice-cream, chemicals, drugs and dietary fat and sugar, all of which are considered to be excessively 'yin'.

A diet aiming to reduce excess yang will avoid high-protein foods, and concentrate mainly on brown rice, salad and fresh fruit, vegetables and pulses. A diet aiming to reduce excess yin will avoid raw, cold foods and fruit juices, and concentrate mainly on brown rice, porridge oats, cooked vegetables, miso (*which see*), pulses and a little cooked fruit and fish.

A large variety of diets for the treatment of specific illnesses have been promoted in books and magazines. Unfortunately this 'one diet for all' approach will never have more than a hit-or-miss effect. For best results, diets should always be tailored to the individual's needs.

Therapeutic trial

If a clinician believes, for instance, that a patient has a nutritional deficiency such as zinc, the clinician may give zinc supplements in the form of a 'therapeutic trial'. This means that the results of the trial will determine whether or not the diagnosis was accurate. This is a common technique used in medicine and is particularly justified in the case of nutritional treatments, since these treatments are usually non-toxic and will often be a much cheaper, more accurate diagnostic tool than most of the testing procedures currently available.

Thiamine (see Vitamin B$_1$)

Thioctic acid (see Lipoic acid)

Threonine

Amino acid

The human body cannot make threonine and must obtain it from the diet. This amino acid may play a role in immune system function and a severe deficiency causes neurological symptoms in experimental animals.

Vegetarian sources: Weight for weight, soya protein concentrate, soya flour, tofu, peanuts and almonds are as rich in threonine as animal proteins.

Thyroid hormone

The thyroid gland secretes three different hormones. One, calcitonin, is involved in blood calcium regulation. The other two, thyroxine (T4) and tri-iodothyronine (T3) are known together as thyroid hormone and are involved in growth and energy metabolism. T3 is the more active form of thyroid hormone. T4 is converted to T3 by a selenium-dependent process. Iodine, vitamin A and the amino acid tyrosine (*which see*) are required for the synthesis of thyroid hormone. It is thought that thyroid hormone plays a part in the conversion of beta-carotene to vitamin A since hypothyroidism, the thyroid deficiency disease, result in high levels of beta-carotene in the blood (hypercarotenaemia). (*Also see Hormones.*)

Thyroxine
(see Thyroid hormone)

Tin

Trace element

Although very small amounts of tin are thought to be required by the human body, its role is not well understood.

Inorganic tin is not well absorbed by the digestive system and is not thought to accumulate in the body.

Tissue salts

Homoeopathic minerals used in accordance with the principles developed by German homoeopathic physician Wilhelm Schüssler (1822–98). Schüssler reasoned that since the remains of the human body when it is burned to ashes primarily consist of 12 mineral salts, these minerals must play a vital role in the body's integrity and function. In addition, the different organs and parts of the body in turn reveal different combinations of minerals. Schüssler's method consisted of administering the appropriate minerals to correct deficiencies which he identified in his patients using a complex diagnostic system, but he did so using homoeopathic doses.

The 12 tissue salts

Calcium phosphate
Calcium sulphate
Calcium fluoride
Potassium phosphate
Potassium sulphate
Potassium chloride

Sodium phosphate
Sodium sulphate
Sodium chloride
Iron phosphate
Magnesium phosphate
Silicon dioxide
(*Also see Celloid minerals.*)

Tocopherol (see Vitamin E)

Tocotrienols

Substances similar to vitamin E and found in association with vitamin E in certain foods. Rich sources of tocotrienols are palm oil and barley oil. Tocotrienols are thought to have cholesterol-lowering properties, which may account for the fact that although palm oil is a highly saturated fat, it has the ability to lower cholesterol levels.

Tofu

Soya milk curd pressed into blocks. Tofu is rich in protein and highly versatile for use in cookery. Plain tofu is usually crumbled or diced and may be fried. Silken tofu is a smoother variety which can be liquidized and used to make mayonnaise, 'cheesecake' or sauces.

Toxic overload

An excessive body burden of toxic substances. (*See Detoxification*)

Trace elements

Essential minerals required in very small amounts.

Trans fats (see Fats)

Triglycerides (see Fats)

Tryptophan

Amino acid

Tryptophan cannot be made by the human body and must be obtained from the diet. It is best known for its role in the production of serotonin, a brain neurotransmitter involved in sleep promotion. The concentration of serotonin in the brain has been shown to be directly proportional to the concentration of tryptophan. Carbohydrate ingestion encourages the uptake of tryptophan into the brain. Tryptophan can also be converted to vitamin B_3 within the body, and it is the precursor of the antioxidant and 'anti-jet lag' substance melatonin produced by the gut and the pineal gland.

Tryptophan metabolism is highly dependent on vitamin B_6. Due to the tryptophan-lowering effects of oestrogen, it has been estimated that women on the contraceptive pill need a minimum of 20 mg vitamin B_6 per day (10 times the RDA) to metabolize tryptophan normally.

One of the most important uses of tryptophan supplements by natural medicine and orthodox medical practitioners is as an anti-depressant. Suicidal patients often show a significant decrease in serotonin levels. It is often said that supplements of tyrosine in the morning and tryptophan at night can probably mimic the effects of most pharmaceutical anti-depressants.

Suggested dosage to aid sleep: 500 mg 30 minutes before bed-time. At the time of writing a doctor's prescription may be required to obtain tryptophan supplements since these were withdrawn from general sale in the UK and US in 1990 after supplies which were produced using genetically engineered bacteria led to cases of eosinophilia myalgia syndrome (*see Genetic engineering*).

Vegetarian sources: Weight for weight, soya protein concentrate, soya flour, tofu, almonds, peanuts, pumpkin seeds, sesame seeds, tahini, almonds and sunflower seeds are as rich in tryptophan as animal proteins.

Tyramine

A substance found in chocolate, mature cheeses, red wine, smoked fish products, dried meats, broad beans, sauerkraut, fermented pickles and other fermented products, brewer's yeast and monosodium glutamate, which produces migraine and other food intolerance reactions in susceptible individuals by releasing histamine from mast cells. Tyramine also raises blood pressure by causing the release of catecholamines (*which see*). The foods listed above, as well as the amino acid tyrosine from which tyramine is derived, must be avoided in patients taking MAO inhibitor drugs. Monoamine oxidase (MAO) is an enzyme involved in the breakdown of tyramine and catecholamines (*which see*). In the absence of adequate MAO, tyramine could rise to excessively high levels, causing dangerously high blood pressure.

Tyrosine

Amino acid

Tyrosine is made in the body from the amino acid phenylalanine and is the raw material of the three catecholamines: adrenaline, noradrenaline and dopamine. These are involved in alertness, concentration and coping with stress. Tyrosine is also used to make thyroid hormone, which is needed for growth and energy metabolism.

Some researchers have used tyrosine supplements in parkinsonism, and claim to have obtained better clinical results with fewer side-effects than conventional treatments.

Low levels of catecholamines can lead to mental apathy, low blood pressure and depression. If these low levels are due to a tyrosine deficiency, tyrosine supplementation can increase them, thus improving all these symptoms. *Suggested dose*: 1 gram on rising in the morning.

Tyrosine supplements should not be taken by people on MAO inhibitor drugs or individuals with schizophrenia or malignant melanoma.

Vegetarian sources: Weight for weight, soya protein concentrate, soya flour, tofu, peanuts, almonds, pumpkin seeds, peanuts and peanut butter are as rich in tyrosine as animal proteins.

Availability of supplements: Tyrosine supplements are widely available in health food shops.

U

Vitamin U (Cabagin)

Vitamin-like substance

Vitamin U is listed in the Merck Index as methylmethioninesulfonium chloride, a therapeutic agent for the treatment of gastric disorders. It was originally called vitamin U because of its usefulness against ulceration of the digestive system. Vitamin U is extracted from cabbages (hence its alternative name, cabagin) and has a strong cabbage-like odour.

The traditional use of raw cabbage juice as the treatment of choice for peptic ulcers would seem to support the use of vitamin U supplements (or cabbage juice) as a healing aid for damaged and eroded intestinal mucosa, and this has been extensively confirmed by scientific research, particularly in Russia and other countries of the former Soviet Union.

Availability: From nutritional therapists.

Ubiquinone
(see Coenzyme Q10)

Umeboshi

A Japanese mountain plum which has been pickled in salt with the purple-red herb shiso. It has a tart taste and is widely used in macrobiotic cookery to enhance grain, sushi, vegetable and salad dishes.

Availability: from specialist macrobiotic suppliers.

Uña de gato (Cat's claw)

Herb

A South American herb classified as a 'master healer' – regarded as sacred in the Amazon.

Uña de gato is traditionally believed to have almost unlimited curative properties and has been shown to be especially helpful to the immune system. This herb is often specifically used to combat viruses.

Availability: from herbalists.

Urea cycle

The body processes which form the waste product urea from ammonia. Ammonia is a toxic waste product of protein breakdown. It is converted to urea by the liver, and the urea is then excreted in the urine. Adequate amounts of magnesium are needed for this conversion process. The amino acids ornithine, citrulline and arginine also play an important part.

Uric acid

The end product of purine metabolism (from nucleic acids, *which see*). In susceptible people, uric acid (urate) crystals can form in the joints, causing gout. Vitamin C supplements can assist with uric acid excretion.

Uva-ursi

Herb

Also known as bearberry, uva-ursi contains the active ingredient arbutin which, when metabolized to hydroquinone in the kidney, has an antiseptic effect on the urinary tract provided that the urine is alkaline. This requires that patients taking uva-ursi should refrain from consuming acidic fruits and their juices. Uva-ursi is used for problems such as cystitis, urinary infections and prostatitis. Tests have demonstrated its effectiveness against Klebsiella, Enterobacter and Streptococcus bacteria, and a study in which 915 patients with urinary problems were given a preparation including uva-ursi, hops and peppermint resulted in improvement in about 70 per cent of cases.

Uva-ursi should not be taken on a long-term basis due to its high tannin content, which irritates the stomach. It should be avoided in pregnancy.

Availability: From specialist centres and herbalists.

V

Valerian

Herb

Often used for its relaxant properties, valerian has been clinically demonstrated to promote sleep and to combat nervous problems such as anxiety, nervous indigestion, palpitations and spasms. Many people use valerian, or combination products which include valerian, as natural alternatives to pharmaceutical sleeping pills and tranquillizers. There have been no reported side-effects to valerian.

Availability: Widely available in health food shops.

Valine

Amino acid

Valine is one of the branched chain amino acids (*which see*). It cannot be made by the human body, and is particularly involved in stress, energy and muscle metabolism.

Supplements of this amino acid may help to reverse hepatic coma, in which patients with cirrhosis of the liver are suffering from increased amounts of ammonia and tryptophan or tyrosine in the brain. Valine competes with tryptophan and tyrosine for entry into the brain, and, because it can be converted to glucose, also acts as a fuel in brain metabolism.

Branched chain amino acids (BCAAs) decrease the rate of breakdown and utilization of other amino acids.

Vegetarian sources: Weight for weight, soya protein concentrate, soya flour, tofu, pumpkin seeds and peanuts are as rich in valine as animal proteins.

Availability of supplements: Usually available only in combined BCAA products.

Vanadium

Trace element

Although vanadium is an essential trace element, little is known about its functions in humans. It appears to be involved in bone mineralization. It also has insulin-like effects, which have led to its experimental use in diabetes. In relatively small amounts vanadium can block oxidative phosphorylation, which is an important process in energy production from glucose. It can also inhibit the activity of the sodium pump, which maintains the correct balance of sodium and potassium inside and outside cells. Because of this effect vanadium has been implicated in manic-depressive illness: manic depressives who are fed a low-vanadium diet, or given vitamin C mega-doses (which lower vanadium levels) have shown improvement as their vanadium body levels fall.

Vanadium is the principal dietary antagonist of chromium. Research has shown that chromium levels are very low in a large proportion of individuals. Whenever high-sugar foods are consumed, chromium is lost in the urine but may not be sufficiently replaced if the diet is generally chromium-poor and if low chromium/high vanadium foods such as fish, seaweed, skimmed milk and intensively farmed chicken are regularly consumed. Chromium deficiency is known to cause problems such as short sight, chronic hypoglycaemia (with resultant mood problems) and elevated blood cholesterol.

Foods rich in vanadium include parsley, lobster, radishes, lettuce, bonemeal and gelatin. Vanadium is not normally available as a dietary supplement.

Vegans

Vegans are vegetarians who consume no animal produce at all. There are about 170,000 adult vegans in Britain. Reasons for veganism include concern for animal rights and for people in the third world, whose grain harvests may be fed to beef cattle for export instead of to starving humans. Some individuals are vegan for health reasons and some for religious reasons. (*Also see Section III, page 293*)

Vegetarians

Those who avoid the consumption of meat and usually also fish but may eat other animal products such as dairy produce and eggs. The vegetarian diet is generally considered to be healthy, and in many cases healthier than a meat- and animal fat-rich diet, although dairy produce can contribute substantial amounts of saturated animal fat. (*Also see Section III, page 292*)

Vervain

Herb

Vervain has traditionally been used as a nerve tonic and to encourage milk flow in nursing mothers. It is thought to be especially useful in the treatment of depression and to stimulate the immune system in feverish illnesses. Vervain also has a stimulating effect on the liver and helps to clear uric acid out of the system.

Availability: Widely available in health food shops.

Villi

Tiny finger-like projections on the wall of the small intestine. Villi serve to increase the absorptive surface area of the intestine. The greater the surface area, the better the capacity for absorption of nutrients from food.

VLDLs (see Lipoproteins)

W

Wakame

A type of salty seaweed often eaten in Japan and used in macrobiotic cookery. Wakame is similar to kombu (*which see*). It is packaged in flat, wide strips and after soaking and cooking can be added to a variety of dishes.

Availability: Health food shops or macrobiotic suppliers.

Water

Water is essential for life. It is required to maintain the health of cells and tissues, for the excretion of soluble waste matter (in sweat and urine), and for the cooling of the skin by evaporation of sweat. The body's water intake comes from liquid drunk from the natural water content of food, and (about ¼ litre per day) as a by-product of carbohydrate, fat and protein metabolism.

'Water intoxication' is a condition which can occur after heavy sweating or dehydration if a lot of liquid is consumed without replacing the lost sodium. Symptoms include weakness and apathy and may progress to convulsions and coma.

Opinions vary on how much water or fluid should be consumed on a daily basis for optimum health. There is a traditional belief in some quarters that the larger the quantities of water consumed, the better this is for health. There is no real evidence for this and some philosophies (such as macrobiotics) believe that excessive fluid consumption can place an excessive strain on the kidneys, which can show up as swellings under the eyes.

What is certainly agreed by most natural medicine practitioners is that water should wherever possible be consumed in preference to other forms of fluid, especially alcoholic and caffeinated beverages.

Wheat grass

Another name for sprouted wheat (*see Sprouted seeds*). Wheat grass is very rich in nutrients and enzymes.

Wild yam

Herb

Wild yam has the capacity to relax smooth muscle and to treat cramps (e.g. period pains) and the pains of irritable bowel syndrome. Wild yam is also added to herbal formulas for the treatment of the liver since it helps to counteract liver and gall-bladder spasms caused by other herbs.

Mexican wild yam contains diosgenin, a substance which can act as the raw material for the industrial production of the female hormone progesterone.

Availability: From specialist centres and herbalists.

X

Xenobiotics

Substances that are foreign to the body, such as drugs, pollutants and artificial food additives.

Y

Yang (see Macrobiotics)

Yeast

A substance consisting of minute fungi, used in brewing for its ability to ferment sugar and produce alcohol, or used in baking for its ability to leaven bread. Brewer's yeast is a rich source of B vitamins, chromium, phosphorus and nucleic acids and is often consumed for its nutritional value. Yeast should not be consumed live.

Some authorities in the natural medicine movement believe that modern varieties of commercial yeast, bred to be very virulent, should not be consumed even if killed. The DNA strands are said to be able to recombine in the warm, moist conditions of the gut, to form potentially harmful colonies in the gut or even in other parts of the body if the integrity of the gut wall has been impaired.

Yin (see Macrobiotics)

Yoghurt

A food produced by the bacterial fermentation of milk, and containing friendly, symbiotic bacteria such as Acidophilus and Bifidus. Yoghurt is more easily digested than other milk products, is highly nutritious, and is widely promoted as a health food. It is one of the traditional staple foods of the Hunza tribe from Kashmir, which has a reputation for being remarkably disease-free.

Z

Zinc

Trace element
UK RNI 9.5 mg
US RDA 15 mg

FUNCTIONS

Acid/alkaline balance
Alcohol detoxification
Carbon dioxide transport
Collagen synthesis
Energy metabolism
Growth
Haemoglobin
Hormones
Immunity
Insulin storage
Male fertility
Nucleic acid synthesis
Numerous enzymes
Prostaglandin function
Protein digesting enzymes
Protein synthesis
Superoxide dismutase (antioxidant enzyme)
Vitamin A metabolism and distribution

GOOD FOOD SOURCES

Eggs
Leafy green vegetables
Meat
Nuts
Seafood
Seeds
Whole grains

Deficiency symptoms

- Abnormal hair loss
- Acne
- Anorexia
- Depression
- Impaired taste and smell
- Infertility in men
- Mental illness
- Nervousness
- Nystagmus
- Poor growth in children
- Poor hair growth
- Sensitivity to light (photophobia)
- Skin rashes
- Slow wound healing
- White spots on fingernails

Preventing deficiency

The times when zinc is in most demand include pregnancy, when breast-feeding, if suffering a wound, burn or infection, and as we grow. The zinc intake should be particularly high at these times, if necessary by adding a zinc supplement to the diet.

Doctors in the UK who regularly test patients for their mineral status find that mild zinc deficiency is extremely common, and often accounts for problems such as infertility in men, acne in teenagers, and low birthweights. Zinc is not added to artificial fertilizer, therefore if natural soil levels become depleted crops may contain very little zinc. In general zinc bioavailability is better from animal foods than from plant foods. Zinc absorption can be seriously reduced by the consumption of phytic acid (found in raw whole grains and bran) or tea or coffee in the same meal.

Other causes of zinc deficiency include the contraceptive pill, and high-dosage iron and folic acid supplements prescribed by doctors for pregnant women. These can seriously lower zinc levels or inhibit zinc absorption (*Am J Clin Nutr 43:258-62, 1986*). In contrast to iron, zinc is not stored and is easily lost from the body. Zinc deficiency may be common in pregnancy (*Hambidge et al.: Zinc nutritional status during pregnancy: a longitudinal study. Am J Clin Nutr 37(3)429-42, 1983*).

For babies, the bioavailability (*which see*) of zinc from human milk is better than that from cow's milk formula. This is thought to be because of the high citric acid and picolinic acid content of human milk.

Supplementation

In research studies, zinc supplements have been found to:

- Improve abnormally low testosterone levels in men
- Improve acne
- Improve appetite in anorexia
- Improve birthweight and growth in at-risk babies
- Improve sperm count and motility in infertile men
- Improve the healing rate of gastric ulcers
- Improve the management of sickle cell anaemia
- Improve thyroid function
- Improve tinnitus
- Improve white blood cell function
- Improve wound healing, including the healing rate of gastric ulcers
- Inhibit herpes simplex virus replication
- Inhibit histamine release in inflammatory reactions
- Reduce disease activity in rheumatoid arthritis
- Reduce enlarged prostate glands
- Reduce symptoms of the common cold and shorten recovery time
- Reduce the rate of visual loss in macular degeneration
- Treat mouth ulcers

Preferred form and suggested intake
Zinc sulphate is an inexpensive form of zinc but may not be well tolerated. Highly bioavailable zinc supplements include zinc citrate, zinc gluconate, zinc picolinate and zinc monomethionine. 15 mg per day of elemental zinc in any of these forms should suffice for most purposes and is known to be safe in the short term. In the long term it is probably wise to balance this intake with a multimineral supplement containing copper.

Cautions
High-dose zinc supplements can in time deplete copper levels in the body. If used for more than three months, copper levels should be monitored.

Nutritional Causes of Illness

The Research

Although we are reluctant to believe that nutritional deficiencies are a problem of any importance in the affluent Western world where we are surrounded by plenty, there is an enormous amount of research indicating that deficiencies are involved in the development of many common chronic illnesses. Equally there is a large body of research in which dietary supplementation has been used to reverse these disease processes by efficiently correcting these deficiencies.

Doctors would be the first to admit that conventional treatments for chronic illness usually allow the disease to progress while helping the sufferer cope temporarily with pain and other symptoms. Indeed, if modern medicine was effective against chronic illness, then chronic illness would, by definition, not exist.

If you have one of the illnesses listed below, you are advised to consult your doctor before embarking on any self-help programmes. A nutritional therapist (*see Appendix V*) may also be able to help you.

Note for doctors

The collection of human research studies presented here is intended to demonstrate the great wealth of research which has found a role for nutritional factors in disease causation and treatment. There may be studies which contradict those presented here, but contradiction is not the same as refutation. Rather, the methodological factors should be analysed which have resulted in the different outcomes. For instance was the same dosage of nutritional supplement used, with the same formula and for the same time period? Was the nutritional status of the test subjects measured first to determine those suffering from deficiencies who would therefore be more likely to respond to the regimes given? Were co-factors taken into account?

It should be borne in mind that to look only for simple cause-and-effect relationships may limit our understanding of chronic illness. In the experience of those who specialize in nutritional medicine and therapy, the more chronic the illness, the more multifactorial its aetiology as over the course of time nutritional and environmental problems promote a downward spiral of multiple functions. Nutritional therapy is about reversing this spiral. It obtains its best results using a multifaceted approach to treatment. However impressive some of the trial results discussed below may be, they are best used only as clues to a better understanding of the disease processes involved, not as definitive statements of cause and effect. A treatment based on individual need, on a case by case basis, is likely to produce the best success (*Nutritional therapy in the treatment of common, minor health problems. Society for the Promotion of Nutritional Therapy, PO Box 47, Heathfield, East Sussex TN21 8ZX, United Kingdom. June 1993*). See Appendix V, *Helpful addresses* for details of how to find a nutritional therapist.

Acne

Some causative factors

- Contraceptive pill
- Deficiencies of vitamin A, vitamin B_6, vitamin E, essential fatty acids and/or zinc
- Fatty diet
- Female hormone imbalance (premenstrual acne)
- Food intolerances (e.g. chocolate, cocoa, cheese, sugar)
- Sluggish, fatty liver

Compared with controls, advanced cases of acne had significantly lower zinc levels.
Int J Dermatol 21(8):481–4, 1982.

Skin zinc levels were found to be low in a group of patients with acne, psoriasis and other skin diseases, suggesting that many of these patients have a zinc deficiency.
Acta Derm Venereol 70(4):304–8, 1990.

Promising nutritional research

Premenstrual acne improved in 72 per cent of 106 women given vitamin B_6 supplements.
Arch Dermatol 110:130–1, 1974.

Zinc intake is of borderline sufficiency in the French population. Zinc supplementation has been shown to be beneficial against several conditions, including acne, reduced immunity and infertility.
Rev Prat 15(2):146–51, 1993.

Success or failure of zinc treatment of acne depends on whether a zinc deficiency is present.
Z Hautkr 62(14):1064, 1069–71, 1075, 1987 (in German).

Zinc therapy results in significant improvement for many acne cases.
Acta Derm Venereol (Stockh) 60(4):337–40, 1980.
Acta Derm Venereol (Stockh) 69(6):541–3, 1989.

In a trial on 76 acne patients the efficacy of a vitamin B_3 gel was found to be comparable to the efficacy of an antibiotic gel (clindamycin).
Int J Dermatol 1995 34(6):434–7, 1995.

Studies have found low glutathione peroxidase levels in patients with acne and other skin disorders, indicating selenium deficiency. Clinical trials with selenium or selenium plus vitamin E supplements have given positive results.
Acta Derm Venereol (Stockh) 62(3):211–4, 1982.
Ann Clin Res 18(1):8–12, 1986.
Acta Derm Venereol (Stockh) 64(1):9–14, 1984.

Acne rosacea

Some causative factors

- B vitamin deficiency
- Gastric acid and/or pancreatic enzyme insufficiency
- Intolerance to tea, coffee and alcohol

Promising nutritional research

Of 30 acne rosacea patients, those with a hydrochloric acid deficiency improved after treatment with hydrochloric acid and B vitamins.
South Med J 38:235–41, 1945.

Aids

Some causative factors

- (*See Section I, Iatrogenic*)
- Anti-viral drugs
- Coenzyme Q10 deficiency
- Drug abuse, especially nitrite 'poppers'
- Nutritional deficiencies, especially selenium, magnesium and vitamin A

The theory that HIV is a new infectious virus causing Aids does not explain inconsistencies such as its inability to be transmitted to animals under experimental conditions. All the evidence suggests that American/European Aids is a disease caused by recreational and anti-HIV drugs.
Pharmac Ther 55:201–7, 1992.

In 95 HIV-positive patients, higher rates of death and opportunistic infection corresponded with lower levels of serum selenium. Selenium levels were predictive of the patients' prognosis irrespective of their CD4 cell count.
J Acquir Immune Defic Syndr Hum Retrovirol 10(3):392, 1995.

Compared with normals, those diagnosed as HIV positive have evidence of selenium deficiency as determined by reduced glutathione peroxidase activity.
J Parent and Ent Nutr 10:405–7, 1986.
Biol Trace Elem Res 15:167–77, 1988.

Severe selenium deficiency causes a heart muscle disease (congestive cardiomyopathy). Selenium deficiency is known to be common among Aids patients. Eight Aids patients examined at autopsy were all found to have abnormalities related to those found in cardiomyopathy.
J Parent Ent Nutr 13(6):644–7, 1989.

Low zinc status has been demonstrated in Aids sufferers and may cause failure in the production of thymus hormone.
JAMA 259(6):839–40, 1988.

A survey of vitamin supplement use and circulating concentrations of 22 nutrients and glutathione in 64 HIV-positive men and women, revealed lower mean circulating concentrations of several nutrients compared with controls. The authors conclude that the low magnesium levels may be particularly relevant to symptoms such as fatigue and that the abnormal nutrient levels may contribute to the development of the disease.
J Acquir Immune Defic Syndr Hum Retrovirol 12(1):75–83, 1996.

Mortality from Aids was compared with diet in 281 HIV-positive individuals between 1984 and 1992. Those with the highest intake (from food and supplements) of vitamin B_1 had a relative risk (RR) of dying during that period, of only 60 per cent compared with those on the lowest intakes. For vitamin B_2 the RR was 59 per cent, for B_3 57 per cent, and for beta-carotene 60 per cent. Those consuming vitamin B_6 at levels more than twice the RDA had only 60 per cent of the risk of death compared with those on low intakes. Zinc supplementation was associated with a higher risk of mortality at all levels.
Am J Epidemiol 143(12):1244–56, 1996.

Progression to full-blown Aids was compared with diet in 281 HIV-positive individuals between 1984 and 1990. Those with the highest intake (from food and supplements) of vitamin C had a relative risk (RR) of progressing to Aids during that period, of only 55 per cent compared with those on the lowest intakes. For vitamin B_1 the RR was 60 per cent, and for B_3 52 per cent. A moderate (but not high) vitamin A intake was also protective, with a RR of 55 per cent. High zinc intakes were associated with an increased risk of progression to Aids.
Am J Epidemiol 138(11):937–51, 1993.

HIV-positive women are four times more likely to transmit the infection to their children if they are deficient in vitamin A.
Nutr Rev 52(8 Pt 1):281–2, 1994.

Compared with controls, 21 HIV-positive patients were found to have higher concentrations of reduced homocysteine (which could contribute to free radical damage), normal total homocysteine, but lower concentrations of the amino acid methionine in plasma. There was a significant correlation between low methionine concentrations and a low CD4+ cell count.
Am J Clin Nutr 63(2):242–8, 1996.

Promising nutritional research

A group of Aids patients with cryptosporidium infection were given liquid allicin (garlic extract) mixed with water daily. This resulted in less diarrhoea and stabilized or increased body weight. Several patients showed negative tests for cryptosporidium parasites on follow-up.
Treat Rev 22:11, 1996.

Ten HIV-positive patients with severely low natural killer cell activity, abnormal helper-to-suppressor T-cell ratios (both these parameters are indicators of advanced Aids, probably with short life expectancy) and opportunistic infections such as cryptosporidial diarrhoea were given five grams daily for six weeks and then 10 grams daily for six weeks of an aged garlic extract. Three patients died before the trial ended, but seven of the 10 experienced a return to normal natural killer cell activity by the end of the 12 weeks. Chronic diarrhoea and candidiasis also improved.
Int Conf AIDS (Canada) 5:466 (ISBN 0-662–56670–X), 1989.

Coenzyme Q10 levels were found to be severely depressed in Aids patients. Supplementation with 200 mg CoQ10 per day produced encouraging clinical results.
Biomed and Clin Aspects of CoQ10 6:409–16, 1991.

Supplementation with selenium and antioxidant vitamins brings symptomatic improvements in Aids sufferers and may slow the course of the disease.
Chem Biol Interact 91(2–3):199–205, 1994.

Decreased vitamin B_{12} levels occur in up to 20 per cent of Aids patients, and may result in dementia symptoms mistakenly diagnosed as Aids dementia. These symptoms resolved in two months in one patient diagnosed with Aids dementia who was treated with vitamin B_{12}.
J Intern Med 233(6):495–7, 1993.

Aids patients suffer from reduced zinc bioavailability. Since zinc deficiency is associated with immune abnormalities and an increased susceptibility to infectious diseases, zinc supplements were administered for 30 days to AZT-treated stage III and stage IV Aids patients. Body weight increased or stabilized, the CD4+ cell count increased and the frequency of opportunistic infections was reduced in the following 24 months.
Int J Immunopharmacol 17(9):719–27, 1995.

Allergy and food intolerance/sensitivity

Some causative factors

- Genetic predisposition
- Gut dysbiosis
- Nutritional deficiencies
- Toxic overload

The zinc and copper status of 43 allergic children suffering from asthma or eczema was compared with healthy children. The hair zinc level was lower in allergic children and the serum and hair copper levels were higher. The investigators conclude that allergic children seem to be particularly at risk of zinc deficiency.
Acta Paediatr Scand 76(4):612–7, 1987.

The effects of magnesium deficiency on the immune system in humans may be affected by the genetic control of blood cell magnesium concentration. Abnormal activation of complement (an immune factor), excess antibody production, and susceptibility to allergy and to chronic fungal and viral infections have been reported.
Magnesium 7(5–6):290–9, 1988.

Many so-called food allergies may be caused by abnormalities of the intestinal bacteria, causing toxic chemical compounds to enter the blood. If these compounds only result from the digestion of one particular food, the patient may believe he has a food allergy.
Lancet 338(8765):495, 1991.

Promising nutritional research

The flavonoids quercetin and fisetin were found to have anti-histamine properties in a study examining the effects of flavonoids on histamine release.
Biochem Pharmacol 33(21):3333–8, 1984.

Alzheimer's disease and senile dementia

Some causative factors

- Aluminium toxicity
- B vitamin deficiency
- Poor circulation in the brain

Recent studies have investigated the possibility that supplementation with choline or lecithin may be beneficial in Alzheimer's and other psychiatric diseases where there may be a deficiency of the neurotransmitter acetylcholine, since acetylcholine is made from these nutrients.
Am J Clin Nutr 36(4):709–20, 1982.

Compared with controls, 17 Alzheimer's disease patients had significantly lower plasma vitamin B_1 levels. The authors conclude that currently used testing methods may be inadequate for such patients and point out that vitamin B_1 deficiency can in itself impair cognitive function (thought processes).
Arch Neurol 52(11):1081–6, 1995.

Vitamin B_1-dependent enzymes were found to be very low in the brain of patients with Alzheimer's disease, indicating a vitamin B_1 deficiency.
Arch Neurol 45(8):836–40, 1988.

The neurological status of 11 patients with low vitamin B_{12} levels but without definite signs of deficiency in their blood picture was examined. The patients displayed a variety of problems, including depression, dementia, neuropathy and seizure disorder. Testing procedures

and a trial of B_{12} therapy led to the conclusion that electrophysiological evidence of neurological impairment is often present even in patients who do not have obvious clinical neurological abnormalities.
Arch Neurol 47(9):1008–12, 1990.

High homocysteine levels are indicative of a vitamin B_{12} and/or folate deficiency. In a study on 70 men aged 54–81, scores for mental performance were compared with levels of homocysteine and serum levels of vitamins B_6, B_{12} and folate. Lower levels of B_{12} and folate and higher levels of homocysteine were associated with poorer mental performance. Higher concentrations of vitamin B_6 were related to better memory performance.
Am J Clin Nutr 63(3):306–14, 1996.

Vitamin B_{12} levels were found to be significantly lower in the cerebrospinal fluid of patients with dementia due to Alzheimer's disease compared with those with dementia due to blood clots.
Acta Psychiatr Scand 82(4):327–9, 1990.

Promising nutritional research

The effects of *Ginkgo biloba* extract on mental performance were assessed in 72 outpatients with cerebral insufficiency. After 24 weeks there was a significant improvement in short-term memory and learning rate.
Fortschr Med 110(5):73–6, 1992 (in German).

216 patients with Alzheimer's disease or dementia due to small blood clots were given either *Ginkgo biloba* extract or placebo. After 24 weeks there was a significant improvement in the *Ginkgo biloba* group compared with controls.
Pharmacopsychiatry 29(2):47–56, 1996.

In an analysis of 40 clinical trials using *Ginkgo biloba* against cerebral insufficiency, it was found that Ginkgo was an effective agent, as effective as the pharmaceutical agent co-dergocrine, used for the same indication.
Br J Clin Pharmacol 34(4):352–8, 1992.

Patients with cerebral circulatory disease leading to intellectual deterioration, confusion and impaired memory and concentration experienced a significant improvement after treatment with 3–4 grams a day of the amino acid taurine by mouth for several weeks.
Clin Ter 71(5):427–36, 1974.

Patients with Alzheimer's disease who were supplemented with coenzyme Q10, iron and vitamin B_6 experienced a delay in the progression of the disease amounting to two years.
Lancet 340(8820):671, 1992.

Amyotrophic lateral sclerosis (see Motor neurone disease)

Anaemia (see Section I)

Angina (see Heart disease)

Anorexia

Some causative factors

Anorexia

- Zinc deficiency

Anorexia nervosa

- Psychological (control) issues
- Peer influences
- Zinc deficiency

Zinc status was found to be low in approximately half of 24 patients with anorexia nervosa, probably due to low zinc intake, purging and vomiting. Since reduced food consumption is a major manifestation of zinc deficiency, this acquired deficiency could add to and prolong the anorexic behaviour.
J Clin Psychiatry 50(12):456–9, 1989.

Zinc deficiency is common in anorexia nervosa and bulimia nervosa and may act to sustain abnormal eating behaviour.
J Am Coll Nutr 11(6):694–700, 1992.

Promising nutritional research

Zinc levels were found to be very low in anorexia nervosa sufferers. Zinc supplementation resulted in a decrease in depression and anxiety.
J Adolesc Health Care 8(5):400–6, 1987.

Food intake rose significantly in mildly zinc-deficient children supplemented with zinc for one year.
Am J Dis Child 138(3):270–3, 1984.

In a study using zinc supplementation on 20 women with anorexia nervosa, over 8–56 months follow-up no patients suffered any further weight loss and 17 increased their body weight by 15–24 per cent. No patients developed bulimia.
Acta Psychiatr Scand Suppl 361:14–17, 1990.

Anxiety and panic attacks

Some causative factors

- B vitamin deficiency
- Caffeine sensitivity
- Magnesium deficiency
- Selenium deficiency
- Sugar sensitivity (causing hypoglycaemia)

In a group of patients suffering from panic attacks, investigation of their caffeine consumption revealed that a higher consumption was associated with higher anxiety levels.
Arch Gen Psychiatry 41(11):1067–71, 1984.

The effects of caffeine administration compared with placebo were assessed in 12 patients with general anxiety disorder. It was found that these patients are abnormally sensitive to caffeine.
Arch Gen Psychiatry 49(11):867–9, 1992.

Selenium levels in the food chain are very low in some parts of the world, including the UK. To ascertain whether selenium deficiency caused mood problems, 50 test subjects were given either supplements or placebo. Supplementation was associated with a general elevation of mood and decrease in anxiety. The lower the previous level of selenium intake, the more the reports of anxiety, depression and fatigue decreased following five weeks of selenium therapy.
Biol Psychiatry 29(11):1092–8, 1991.

20 patients with neurosis symptoms consistent with the early signs and symptoms of beriberi were found to have abnormal red cell transketolase activity (a marker of vitamin B_1 deficiency). In some (not all), this was probably due to heavy consumption of sweets and sugary foods and drinks. All patients were clinically improved by the administration of vitamin B_1, but improvement was slow.
Am J Clin Nutr 33(2):205–11, 1980.

The brain has receptor sites for benzodiazepine-type tranquillizers, suggesting that the body may naturally contain similar substances. In animal trials vitamin B_3 (in its nicotinamide form) has been shown to have anti-anxiety, anti-aggressive, anti-convulsive, and muscle relaxant properties, and to increase the body's production of the sleep-promoting substance serotonin. This suggests that it has benzodiazepine-like properties, which may shed new light on the mental problems which are associated with vitamin B_3 deficiency states.

Nature 278(5704):563–5, 1979.

Promising nutritional research

21 patients with panic disorder (some of whom also had agoraphobia) were given 12 g per day of inositol for four weeks in a randomized, double-blind placebo-controlled trial. Compared with placebo, inositol significantly decreased the frequency and severity of panic attacks and the severity of agoraphobia. There were no significant side-effects.

Am J Psychiatry 152(7):1084–6, 1995.

Asthma

Some causative factors

- Allergy
- Magnesium deficiency
- Pollution
- Selenium deficiency
- Vitamin B_6 deficiency

49 patients with asthma were found to have significantly lower selenium levels in their plasma and whole blood compared with controls.

Clin Sci 77(5):495–500, 1989.

A low forced expiratory volume (FEV) is associated with a greater severity of asthma. Dietary magnesium levels were measured in 2633 adults in England. A 100 mg/day higher magnesium intake was associated with a 27.7 mL higher FEV and a reduction in the risk of hyper-reactivity and wheeze. The investigators conclude that a low magnesium intake may be a factor in the development of asthma.

Lancet 344(8919):357–62, 1994.

In a study on 77,866 women comparing dietary factors with airway function it was found that women with the highest vitamin E intake from food had only half the risk of asthma compared with those on the lowest intake.

Am J Respir Crit Care Med 151(5):1401–8, 1995.

Promising nutritional research

In 15 adult asthma patients, plasma and red cell vitamin B_6 levels were much lower than in a group of 16 controls. Vitamin B_6 supplementation brought a dramatic decrease in asthma attacks.

Am J Clin Nutr 41(4):684–8, 1985.

In a double-blind study on 76 asthmatic children, 100 mg vitamin B_6 supplementation daily brought significant improvement and a reduction in the use of conventional medications. A dose of 50 mg per day was not effective.
Ann Allergy 35(2):93–7, 1975.

92 per cent of a group of asthma sufferers improved when given a vegan low-allergen diet.
J Asthma 22:45–55, 1985.

Patients admitted to a clean-air environment and placed on a therapeutic fast were able to significantly reduce their anti-asthma medications. On follow-up, after following a rotation diet and using Miller vaccines, 68 per cent reported being 'definitely better' and 25 per cent described themselves as 'well' or 'almost well'.
J Nutr Med 3:231–48, 1992.

322 children under one year of age with respiratory allergy were given a hypoallergenic diet for six weeks consisting of meat base formula, beef, carrots, broccoli and apricots. 91 per cent showed a significant improvement. Skin tests did not correlate with results of feeding the children with foods they reacted to. The most common problem foods were milk, egg, chocolate, soya, pulses and grains.
Ann Allergy 44(5):273, 1980.

In 19 severe asthmatics who failed to respond to conventional treatments and were given intravenous magnesium sulphate infusions in a hospital emergency department, there was a significant improvement in breathing ability compared with the placebo group.
JAMA 262(9):1210–3, 1989.

In 12 asthmatics given 500 mg vitamin C supplements daily, there was a considerable reduction in asthma symptoms after exercise, compared with placebo.
Ann Allergy 49(3):146–51, 1982.

The scientific literature points to low levels of selenium in asthmatics compared with the normal population. 24 asthmatics were given either selenium supplements or placebo for 14 weeks. The supplemented group experienced a significant increase in glutathione peroxidase levels (a marker of selenium sufficiency) and significant clinical improvement.
Allergy 48(1):30–6, 1993.

Four of five asthmatic children sensitive to sulphite food additives failed to develop bronchospasm when challenged with metabisulphite, when they were pretreated with vitamin B_{12}.
J Allergy Clin Immunol 90(1):103–9, 1992.

12 asthmatics were treated with omega-3 fatty acids for one year in a double-blind trial. A positive effect on forced expiratory volume was observed after nine months.
Int Arch Allergy Appl Immunol 95(2–3):156–7, 1991.

Autism

Some causative factors

- Magnesium deficiency
- Vitamin B_6 deficiency
- Vitamin C deficiency

Promising nutritional research

16 autistic children receiving vitamin B_6 supplements for autism were either continued on vitamin B_6 or given placebo, on a double-blind basis. The placebo group significantly deteriorated after withdrawal of the vitamin B_6.
Am J Psychiatry 135(4):1978.

A group of 44 autistic children were treated with large doses of vitamin B_6 and magnesium. There was a clinical improvement in 15 children.
J Autism Dev Disord 11(2):219–30, 1981.

In a trial administering vitamin B_6 with magnesium to 44 autistic children, 15 showed a moderate clinical improvement and worsened when the supplements were discontinued.
Acta Vitaminol Enzymol 4(1–2):27–44, 1982.

In a double-blind clinical trial on 60 autistic children given supplements of vitamin B_6 and magnesium, there was a behaviour improvement and significant improvements in biological parameters.
Biol Psychiatry 20(5):467–78, 1985.

Questionnaires on the treatment of 4,000 autistic children revealed that among the biomedical treatments, the use of high-dosage vitamin B_6 with magnesium was found to be six times more effective than the two commonly used drugs fenfluramine and thioridazine hydrochloride.
J Child Neurol three Suppl:S68–72, 1988.

In a 30-week double-blind trial, supplementation of autistic schoolchildren with eight grams per 70 kg body weight per day of vitamin C resulted in a reduction in the severity of symptoms.
Prog Neuropsychopharmacol Biol Psychiatry 17(5):765–74, 1993.

Bed-wetting (children)

Some causative factors

- Food allergy
- Nutritional deficiencies

Promising nutritional research

21 children successfully treated for migraine with an exclusion diet also suffered from bed-wetting. 12 of this group ceased bed-wetting while on the diet. The reintroduction of problem foods caused a relapse of the bed-wetting.
Clin Pediatr 31(5):302–7, 1992.

Birth defects

Some causative factors

- Alcohol consumption
- Heavy metal toxicity
- Nutritional deficiencies (zinc, selenium, folic acid, essential fatty acids)
- Obesity

Epidemiological and *in vitro* studies suggest a correlation between low selenium levels and a higher incidence of birth defects such as spina bifida.
Z Kinderchir 44 Suppl 1:48–50, 1989 (in German).

Zinc deficiency is widespread and in pregnancy is associated with premature birth, inefficient labour and increased risk to the foetus. Growth impairment and lowered immunity occur in zinc-deficient children.
J Am Coll Nutr 15(2):113–20, 1996.

Low zinc levels frequently found in pregnant women constitute a real risk of deficiency and consequent miscarriage, toxaemia, anaemia, extended pregnancy, difficult delivery, birth defects and learning disorders. Reviewing the scientific literature, the authors conclude that zinc and multi-nutrient supplementation is imperative in pregnancy.
Rev Fr Gynecol Obstet 85(1):13–27, 1990 (in French).

The use of multivitamins was compared between 731 mothers of babies born with a facial cleft or cleft lip or palate, and 734 mothers with non-malformed babies. It was found that the use of multivitamins before and during pregnancy reduced the risk of offspring with this type of deformity by 25 to 50 per cent.
Lancet 346(8972):393–6, 1995.

Zinc deficiency during pregnancy has been shown to be related to many congenital abnormalities of the nervous system in children, who may later develop reduced learning ability, apathy and mental retardation.
Biol Psychiatry 17(3):513–32, 1982.

Mothers of 538 babies or foetuses with neural tube type birth defects (incomplete development of the brain or spinal cord) were compared with mothers of 539 non-malformed controls. It was found that the risk of occurrence of this type of birth defect was almost twice as great in obese mothers as in those of normal body weight.
JAMA 275(14):1093–6, 1996.

In a study of 513 pregnancies, the nutrient intakes of mothers of babies with dangerously low birthweights were found to be well below the nutrient intakes of mothers whose babies were in the safe range of birthweights. The mother's diet around the time of conception was more important than during pregnancy. The study also found that premature babies, and those of abnormally low birthweight were frequently born with deficiencies of the essential fatty acids required for brain development (arachidonic acid and DHA).
Nutr Health 9(2):81–97, 1993.

Promising nutritional research

The risk of recurrent neural-tube defects (spina bifida and similar deformities) is decreased in women who take folic acid or multivitamins before and after the period of conception.
N Engl J Med 327(26):1832–5, 1992.
JAMA 269(10):1292–3, 1993.
Can Med Assoc J 149(9):1239–43, 1993.
Lancet 338(8760): 131–7, 1991.

Daily zinc supplementation in women with relatively low plasma zinc concentrations in early pregnancy is associated with greater infant birth weights and head circumferences.
JAMA 274(6):463–8, 1995.

In 56 pregnant women at risk of delivering a small baby and supplemented with 22.5 mg zinc daily, the incidence of growth retardation was significantly reduced and health indices were better compared with controls.
Eur J Clin Nutr 45(3):139–44, 1991.

Blood disorders (also see Section I, Anaemia)

Some causative factors

- Vitamin B_6 deficiency
- Vitamin C deficiency
- Vitamin E deficiency

Sickled red blood cells are more susceptible to peroxidation than normal red cells. Vitamin E deficiency promotes red cell susceptibility to peroxidation and could lead to cell abnormalities, capillary obstruction and tissue damage. The investigators propose that sickle-cell patients would benefit from vitamin E supplementation.
Ann NY Acad Sci 393:323–35, 1982.

Promising nutritional research

Plasma levels of vitamin B_6 were found to be very low in 16 sickle cell anaemia sufferers compared with normals. Supplementation with 100 mg vitamin B_6 per day resulted in an increase in number of red cells and haemoglobin.
Am J Clin Nutr 40(2):235–9, 1984.

Three years after beginning a wholefood diet free of added salt, with homoeopathic remedies, multivitamins, calcium pantothenate and vitamin E, a 40-year-old woman with von Willebrand's disease was free of all symptoms and abnormal bleeding.
Nutritional Therapy Today 2(2):4, 1992. Society for the Promotion of Nutritional Therapy, PO Box 47, Heathfield, East Sussex TN21 8AE, UK.

11 patients with idiopathic thrombocytopenic purpura were treated with two grams of vitamin C daily. Seven patients responded well and suffered no relapses.
Brit J Haematol 70:341–4, 1988.

Breast lumps

Some causative factors

- Essential fatty acid deficiency
- Tea, coffee, cola and chocolate consumption

Women with premenstrual syndrome and/or breast disease were found to have consistently lower levels of omega-6 essential fatty acid metabolites in cell membranes than normal women, suggesting a reduced conversion of linoleic acid to GLA.
J Nutr Med 2:259–64, 1991.

Promising nutritional research

Women suffering from painful fibrocystic breast disease were counselled to abstain from or reduce caffeine consumption. Of those who succeeded, 61 per cent reported a decrease in or loss of breast pain.
Nurse Pract 14(2):36–7, 40, 1989.

Bronchitis (chronic)

Some causative factors

- Pollution
- Smoking
- Vitamin C deficiency
- Zinc deficiency

Dietary factors were analysed in a group of sufferers from respiratory symptoms. It was found that a low intake of vitamin C and zinc and a high intake of sodium correlated with a higher incidence of bronchitis and wheezing.
Am J Epidemiol 132(1):67–76, 1990.

Promising nutritional research

2,510 patients with bronchitis, bronchial asthma and emphysema were treated for four weeks with the amino acid N-acetylcysteine in addition to the patients' usual medications. All selected parameters improved, especially for bronchitis.
Fortschr Med 110(18):346–50, 1992 (in German).

Cancer, general

Some causative factors

- Deficiencies of selenium and/or vitamins A, C and E, folic acid, carotenoids
- Fruit and vegetable deficiency
- Use of the contraceptive pill

Many studies now demonstrate the protective effects of fruits and vegetables against cancer.
Am J Clin Nutr 53(1) Suppl:226S–37S, 1991.

Crude extracts from cruciferous vegetables (broccoli, cauliflower, cabbage, brussels sprouts) have been shown to have anti-mutagenic properties. An increase in an enzyme induced by brussels sprouts has been shown to result in an 87 per cent reduction in the binding of powerful carcinogenic chemicals to DNA.
Am J Clin Nutr 59(suppl):1166S–70S, 1994.

In an area of high tomato consumption in Northern Italy, researchers found that the rate of cancers of the digestive system was particularly low.
Int J Cancer 59(2):181–4, 1994.

People who later develop cancer tend to have a lower selenium status than others.
Lancet 322:130–3, 1983.

Higher dietary intakes of selenium are associated with lower rates of cancer.
Int J Biochem 20(2):123–32, 1988.

In a population study on 10,000 men, the risk of death from cancer was 3.8 times higher in individuals consuming the lowest amounts of selenium compared with those consuming the highest.
Nutr Cancer 10(4):221–9, 1987.

In a study on 39,268 Finnish men and women it was found that men with the highest levels of selenium had only 11 per cent of the risk of contracting lung cancer compared with those with the lowest levels.
J Natl Cancer Inst 82:(10)864–8, 1990.

Antioxidant levels were measured in the serum of 25,802 individuals in Washington County. Those with the lowest levels of selenium were found to have twice the risk of developing bladder cancer compared with those with the highest levels.
Cancer Res 49(21):6144–8, 1989.

In a Finnish study, cancer risk was found to be 11 times higher in those with a low selenium and vitamin E status compared with those with a high status of these nutrients.
Br Med J 290:417–20, 1985.

In a study on 15,093 women in Finland, those with the lowest vitamin E levels had a 1.6 times greater risk of contracting cancer than those with the highest intakes.
Int J Epidemiol 17(2):281–86, 1988.

In a study on 21,172 Finnish men, it was found that those with the highest serum levels of vitamin E had only 64 per cent of the risk of contracting cancers compared with those with the lowest levels.
Am J Epidemiol 127(1):28–41, 1988.
Cancer Detection and Prevention: 9(1–2):67–77, 1986.

Levels of nutrients in stored serum samples were compared for those who developed lung cancer and those who did not. Those with the lowest vitamin E levels had 2.4 times the risk of developing lung cancer compared with those with the highest levels. For low beta-carotene levels the risk was also considerably higher.
N Engl J Med 315(20):1250–4, 1986.

The major antioxidants were measured in the plasma of 2,974 men. Low levels were associated with a significantly higher risk of developing cancers compared with high levels.
Am J Clin Nutr 53(1) Suppl:265S–9S, 1991.

Serum samples collected from 28,000 volunteers were used to assess the link between dietary habits and the development of cancers in subsequent years. Low levels of beta-carotene, lycopene and vitamin E were associated with much higher rates of lung cancer, pancreatic cancer and bladder cancer.
Am J Clin Nutr 53(1) Suppl:260S–4S, 1991.

In a 19-year study analysing the diets of 1,954 middle-aged men, it was found that those consuming the lowest amounts of dietary beta-carotene were seven times more likely to develop lung cancer. This risk was increased to 8-fold in those who were also smokers.
Lancet 2(8257):1186–90, 1981.

In an analysis of 257 cases of cervical dysplasia and 133 controls it was found that those with lower levels of vitamins A and C, folic acid and vitamin B_2 had an increased risk of cervical dysplasia (precancerous condition of the cervix).
Cancer Epidemiol Biomarkers Prev 2(6):525–30, 1993.

Many mechanisms involved in resistance to cancer are dependent on vitamin C.
Cancer Res 39(3):663–81, 1979.

From a screening of 726 subjects it was found that low red cell folate levels were associated with a higher risk of cervical dysplasia.
JAMA 267(4):528–33, 1992.

Dietary zinc deficiency is strongly linked with an increased risk of cancer of the throat.
J Am Coll Nutr 8(2):99–107, 1989.

Zinc deficiency causes the increased activation of several types of carcinogens by liver cells.
Adv Exp Med Biol 206:517–27, 1986.

A reduced intake of trace elements and vitamins may lead to a decrease in fatty acid metabolism to cancer-preventive prostaglandins PGE1 and PGI2. Adequate amounts of selenium, beta-carotene, vitamin A and vitamin E are needed to prevent the peroxidation of fatty acids which are needed to make these prostaglandins.
Nutrition 5(2):106–10, 1989.

The diets of 35,156 Iowa women aged 55 to 69 were analysed in relation to the incidence of non-Hodgkin lymphoma in this group. A high dietary intake of animal fat, saturated fat or red meat were associated with a significantly increased risk of contracting the disease. Compared with a low intake of hamburgers in particular, a high intake more than doubled the risk of non-Hodgkin lymphoma. A high intake of vegetables reduced the risk by 36 per cent.
JAMA 275(17):1315–21, 1996.

The histories of 377 women with cervical cancers were compared with 2,887 matched controls, including smoking, anogenital warts, prior use of oral contraceptives, herpes and other factors. It was found that the longer the use of the contraceptive pill, the greater the risk of cervical cancer. The risk was highest in recent and current users, especially for women under 35. The researchers conclude that women who have used oral contraceptives should be considered at increased risk of developing cervical cancer.
The World Health Organization Collaborative Study of Neoplasia and Steroid Contraceptives. Am J Epidemiol 144(3):281–9, 1996.

In a study on 1,154 post-menopausal women it was found that, compared with those who had never used hormones, those who had taken oestrogen-type hormone therapy had a four-fold greater risk of developing endometrial cancer.
Lancet 349:458–61, 1997.

Promising nutritional research

Selenium supplementation (via fortified table salt) of the general population in a town in China suffering from a high incidence of primary liver cancer resulted in a significantly reduced rate of the disease after five years.
Biol Trace Elem Res 29(3):289–94, 1991.

Vitamin and mineral supplementation, particularly with vitamin E, selenium and beta-carotene, reduced the incidence of cancer in the Linxian region of China, known for its high rate of gastric and oesophageal cancer and its low intake of several micronutrients.
J Natl Cancer Inst 85:1483–92, 1993.

People who regularly use Vitamin E supplements are found to have only half the normal risk of developing cancers of the mouth and throat.
Am J Epidemiol 135(10):1083–92, 1992.

In a randomized study on 65 patients with bladder cancer, those given large doses of vitamin and mineral supplements had a markedly reduced rate of recurrence of the disease at 10 months compared with those on RDA-level doses.
J Urol 151(1):21–6, 1994.

Compared with controls, patients with inoperable brain tumours treated with the antioxidant substance melatonin survived significantly longer.
Cancer 73(3):699–701, 1994.

The status of vitamin B_6 and other B vitamins was investigated in patients with cancers of the female reproductive system. It was found that (1) The more the carcinoma had progressed, the more pronounced was the impairment of vitamin B_6, B_1 and B_2 activation tests, indicating deficiencies of these nutrients. (2) Soon after the start of radiotherapy, a biochemical deficiency of vitamins B_1 and B_6 was provoked. (3) A similar reduction of vitamin B_1 and B_6 enzyme activities was observed after the administration of cytostatic drugs. (4) Vitamin A, C and E status was also impaired. (5) The 5-year survival rate was about 10–15 per cent better in the groups which were administered vitamin B_6 than the groups which were not. (6) Daily administration of 300 mg vitamin B_6 supplements was required to prevent impairment of vitamin B_6 status.
Strahlenschutz Forsch Prax 26:63–9, 1985.

The mean survival time of 100 terminal cancer patients treated with large daily doses of vitamin C was more than 4.2 times that of the controls.
Proc Natl Acad Sci US Oct 73(10):3685–9, 1976.

A review of cancer and vitamin C studies found that: (1) Survival and tumour control by X-irradiation may be improved by vitamin C supplementation. (2) X-ray therapy of cervical cancer in one study decreased vitamin C levels to 0.01–0.03 mg per cent, suggesting that supplements are required during X-ray therapy. (3) 500–1,000 mg per day vitamin C administered to advanced cancer patients has been found in several papers to benefit the general state of health. (4) 10 g vitamin C per day may increase the survival time of terminal cancer patients four-fold or more, and significantly reduce pain and increase strength. (5) Up to 30 g vitamin C per day may be especially effective in cancer of the uterus. In one study, about 10 per cent of the patients seemed to have a greatly extended life expectancy. (6) Three g/day vitamin C may reduce the number and size of residual rectal polyps in familial polyposis. (7) Vitamin C in high doses augments the activity of white blood cells by 100–300 per cent. (8) Vitamin C stimulates interferon production. (9) 1 gram of vitamin C per day significantly raises the serum levels of IgA, IgM and C–3 complement in humans.
Int J Vit Nutr Res, Suppl 24: Vitamins in Medicine: Recent Therapeutic Aspects. A Hanck (ed), pp 87–104, 1983.

A review of cancer and vitamin E studies found that: (1) Vitamin E enhances the growth inhibitory effect of several anti-tumour drugs. (2) Vitamin E reduces the toxic effects of some anti-tumour agents. (3) Vitamin E can kill newly transformed cancer cells directly or indirectly by stimulating the immune system, and can reverse malignancy in certain tumours. (4) Vitamin E at high doses may have anti-tumour activity against some tumours. (5) Vitamin E has been shown to stimulate immunity at a dose of 5–20 iu per kilo of body weight daily. (6) High doses of vitamin E may reduce the level of prostaglandin E2, which has been implicated in suppressing the immune system. (7) Vitamin E blocks the action of certain cancer-promoting chemicals. (8) Vitamins A and E in combination are more effective than the vitamins individually.
In Prasad KN (ed): Vitamins, nutrition and cancer. Publ Karger (Basel, New York) pp 76–104, 1984.

A review of cancer and zinc studies found that: (1) Zinc inhibits the development of cancer, and low serum zinc is associated with several forms of cancer. (2) Zinc deficiency has been found in 20 to 30 per cent of patients with head and neck epidermoid cancers. (3) Zinc treatment significantly increases lymphocyte responses. (4) A parabolic correlation between leucocyte zinc content and neutrophil phagocytic capacity has been observed.
J Orth Psych 11:28–41, 1982.

In 47 young women with cervical dysplasia (precancerous condition of the cervix), treated with folic acid or placebo, the biopsy scores after three months were significantly better in the treated group.
Am J Clin Nutr 35(1):73–82, 1982.

In human subjects at increased risk of colon cancer, calcium supplementation significantly reduces cancer-associated cell proliferation.
J Cell Biochem Suppl 22:65–73, 1995.

65 patients with bladder cancer and given BCG immunotherapy were randomized to receive multiple dietary supplements (vitamins A, B$_6$, C and E plus zinc) in the RDA range or the megadose range. The recurrence of tumours measured at 10 months was found to be 91 per cent in the RDA group and only 41 per cent in the megadose group.
J Urol 151(1):21–6, 1994.

The administration of bovine cartilage preparations for several years brought a 90 per cent response rate in 31 cases of different cancers including glioblastoma multiforme and cancers of the pancreas and lung, ovary, cervix, thyroid, prostate and rectum.
J Biol Response Mod 4(6):551–84, 1985.

In six patients with primary liver cell cancer, supplemented with evening primrose oil and vitamin C, clinical improvement and reduction in tumour size occurred in three cases – one to a remarkable degree.
Prostaglandins Leukot Med 15(1):15–33, 1984.

In a study on 429 non-smoking women with lung cancer compared with controls, women with the highest intake of dietary saturated fat were six times more likely to develop lung cancer than those with the lowest intakes. A high consumption of peas and beans was associated with a reduction in lung cancer risk, while a high intake of citrus fruit and juice doubled the risk of contracting lung cancer compared with a low intake.
J Natl Cancer Inst 85(23):1906–16, 1993.

Cancer, breast

Some causative factors

- Coenzyme Q deficiency
- Contraceptive pill
- Diet high in sugar and fat and low in fibre
- Environmental pollution, particularly pesticide use
- Essential fatty acid deficiency
- High consumption of animal meat and fat
- Hormone replacement therapy
- Silicone breast implants
- Vegetable deficiency
- Vitamin E deficiency

The dietary intake of fruit, vegetables and related nutrients was assessed in 297 premenopausal women diagnosed with breast cancer, and compared with controls. The women with the highest consumption of vegetables had less than half the rate of breast cancer compared with those eating the least vegetables.
J Natl Cancer Inst 88(6):340–8, 1996.

Of 5,004 Guernsey women whose plasma samples were stored for a prospective study, 39 later developed breast cancer. Their levels of vitamin A, beta-carotene and vitamin E were measured in the stored samples and compared with those of 39 women from the same group who had not developed breast cancer. It was found that those with the lowest vitamin E levels were five times more likely to develop breast cancer than those with the highest levels.
Br J Cancer 49(3):321–4, 1984.

Organochlorine pesticide levels were measured in serum from the stored blood specimens of 14,290 women. Mean levels of DDE and PCB pesticides were higher for breast cancer patients than for others. The investigators conclude that environmental contamination with organochlorine residues may be an important factor in the development of breast cancer.
J Natl Cancer Inst 85:648–52, 1993.

Evidence has accumulated for over three decades associating avoidable exposure to environmental and occupational cancer-causing chemicals to the escalating rate of breast cancer in the Western world.
Int J Hlth Serv 24(1):145–50, 1994.

A study of dietary factors in 133 breast cancer cases and 289 controls concluded that a low intake of fat and a high intake of dietary fibre and fermented milk products may provide substantial protection against breast cancer.
Int J Cancer 47(5):649–53, 1991.

Evidence on the risks of breast cancer imposed by silicone implants has been withheld from the public by industry and plastic surgeons. Implanted women should be given a medical alert.
Int J Occup Med Toxicol 4(3):315–42, 1995.

Fatty acids in breast tissue were analysed in breast cancer patients and controls. Post-menopausal women with breast cancer were found to have significantly lower levels of DHA (produced from fish oils). It is concluded that oily fish consumption may be protective against breast cancer in older women.
Nutr Cancer 24(2):151–60, 1995.

A study using data from 66 countries to identify the most important predictors of breast cancer found that death due to breast cancer was most strongly associated with the consumption of large amounts of meat and animal products.
Cancer Detect Prev 20(3):234–44, 1996.

The risk of breast cancer in post-menopausal women using hormone replacement therapy (HRT) was evaluated by asking study participants to complete questionnaires regularly updating information on their menopausal status, use of HRT, and any diagnosis of breast cancer. During 725,550 person-years of follow-up, 1,935 cases of newly diagnosed breast cancer were documented. The risk of contracting the disease was found to be significantly higher among women currently using oestrogen-based HRT alone or oestrogen plus progestin, compared with those who had never used hormones. The risk was particularly

increased in women who had taken the hormone treatments for more than five years, and were more than 60 years old.
N Engl J Med 332(24):1589–93, 1995.

Promising nutritional research

Of 32 patients with high risk breast cancer treated with high-dose antioxidants, fatty acids and coenzyme Q10, six showed partial tumour regression. Of these six, two were given additional coenzyme Q10 and experienced complete disappearance of their tumours.
Biochem Biophys Res Commun: 199(3):1504–8, 1994.

Of 32 patients with breast cancer spread to the lymph nodes, and given large daily doses of vitamins C and E, beta-carotene, selenium, essential fatty acids and coenzyme Q10, six showed apparent partial remission, none developed signs of further distant secondary cancers over an 18-month period, and although the expected death rate was four, none died during this period.
Mol Aspects Med 15s:s231–s240, 1994.

Three breast cancer patients with advanced disease underwent conventional treatments supplemented by a daily oral dose of 390 mg coenzyme Q10. Numerous secondary cancers (metastases) in the liver of one patient disappeared, and no signs of metastases were found elsewhere. The other two patients also became and remained free of all cancer signs.
Biochem Biophys Res Commun 212(1):172–7, 1995.

Of 17 patients with mammary dysplasia (pre-cancerous condition of the breast), administered 600 iu vitamin E per day, 88 per cent showed a clinical response, and abnormal progesterone/oestradiol ratios were normalized.
Cancer Res 41(9 Pt 2):3811–3, 1981.

14 patients who were not responding to tamoxifen were given 20 mg per day of the antioxidant substance melatonin. A partial response was observed in four patients. Mean serum levels of insulin-like growth factor were significantly reduced.
Br J Cancer 71(4):854–6, 1995.

Studies have shown that a higher intake of dietary fibre and complex carbohydrates is associated with a lower risk of breast cancer. This may be because (1) A high-fibre diet can reduce circulating oestrogen levels. (2) Many plant foods contain plant oestrogens, which compete within the body for binding sites with oestradiol. (3) A high-fibre diet is associated with lesser obesity, a condition which encourages higher levels of the biologically active varieties of oestrogen which promote breast cancer. (4) A high-fibre diet usually has a lower content of fat and a higher content of antioxidant vitamins, which may be protective against breast cancer. (5) Fibre-rich diets improve insulin sensitivity, which may also reduce circulating oestrogen levels.
Br J Cancer 73(5):557–9, 1996.

12 healthy premenopausal women given a very low-fat, high-fibre diet for two months experienced significant reductions in serum oestrone and oestradiol (highly active forms of

oestrogen) levels without affecting ovulation, suggesting that this type of diet may be protective against breast cancer.

Cancer 76(12):2491–6, 1995.

Cancer, colon

Some causative factors

- Calcium deficiency
- Dietary fibre deficiency
- Excess fat consumption
- Excess sugar consumption
- Folic acid deficiency
- Vitamin E deficiency

A study on 35,215 Iowa women showed that a high intake of vitamin E may decrease the risk of colon cancer.

Cancer Res 53(18):4230–7, 1993.

In a study comparing the sugar consumption of 953 cases of colon cancer with 2,845 controls, researchers found that compared with subjects who reported adding no sugar to their beverages, the relative risk of contracting colon cancer was 1.4 times higher for those adding one spoonful, 1.6 times higher for those adding two spoonfuls, and twice as high for those adding three or more.

Int J Cancer 55:386–9, 1993.

The diets of 50 patients with colon cancer were compared with 50 matched controls. Those with colon cancer consumed significantly more sugar and fat and less dietary fibre.

BMJ 291(6507):1467–70, 1985.

A study analysing the diet and blood of 682 subjects found that men with the highest intake of folic acid had only 50 per cent of the risk of developing colorectal polyps (a risk factor for cancer of the colon) compared with those having the lowest intake.

Cancer Epidemiol Biomarkers Prev 4(7):709–14, 1995.

1,904 vegetarians were followed-up for 11 years in Germany. Among the men, their expected death rates were 44 per cent less than for the general population, and for the women 53 per cent less. Rates of death from colon cancer were also greatly reduced. Health-conscious behaviour was thought to play an important part in addition to vegetarianism.

Am J Clin Nutr 59(5 Suppl):1143S–52S, 1994.

Cancer, melanoma

Promising nutritional research

The survival rate of 153 melanoma patients treated with the Gerson therapy, which restricts the intake of protein, sodium and fat and increases potassium and vitamin/mineral intake by the regular administration of freshly pressed fruit and vegetable juices, were compared with patients in the mainstream literature. For stage I and II melanoma, no Gerson patients suffered progress of the disease after admission, compared with an average survival rate of 79 per cent for conventionally treated patients. For stage III melanoma 71 per cent of the Gerson patients survived for five years, compared with only 27 per cent to 42 per cent of conventionally treated patients.
Alternative Therapies 1(4):29–37, 1995.

Cancer, prostate

Some causative factors

- Cadmium toxicity
- Zinc deficiency
- Selenium deficiency

In a study on 47,894 subjects it was found that higher intakes of foods rich in the carotenoid lycopene (mainly tomato products) were associated with lower rates of prostate cancer.
J Natl Cancer Inst 87(23):1767–76, 1995.

Isoflavonoid (plant oestrogen) levels in blood samples were compared in Japanese and Finnish men. Levels were 7–110 times higher in the Japanese men. Since isoflavonoids, which are found in soya products, inhibit the growth of several types of hormone-dependent cancer cells, the authors conclude that a life-long high intake of soya products may explain why prostate cancer is rare in Japanese men.
Lancet 342:1209–10, 1993.

While cadmium stimulates prostate growth, selenium inhibits this effect of cadmium.
Biochem Biophys Res Commun 127(3):871–7, 1985.

Carpal tunnel syndrome

Some causative factors

- Vitamin B_2 deficiency
- Vitamin B_6 deficiency

Promising nutritional research

Measurements of red blood cell enzymes in a carpal tunnel syndrome sufferer revealed severe deficiencies of both vitamin B_6 and vitamin B_2. Combined supplementation of these nutrients brought the total disappearance of the carpal tunnel syndrome.
Proc Natl Acad Sci 81(22):7076–8, 1984.

Cataracts

Some causative factors

• Deficiency of foods high in antioxidant nutrients, especially vitamin E and beta-carotene.

In a survey on the use of vitamin supplements, it was found that those who were free of cataracts used significantly more vitamins C and E supplements. Vitamin supplementation appeared to reduce the risk of cataracts by 50 per cent.
Ann N Y Acad Sci 570:372–82, 1989.

There is now much evidence to suggest that individuals with higher intakes of antioxidant nutrients have a reduced risk of developing cataracts.
Z Ernahrungswiss 28(1):56–75, 1989.

Individuals with a low serum concentration of antioxidant vitamins had almost twice the risk of developing cataracts compared with those with the highest levels.
BMJ 305(6866):1392–4, 1992.

The consumption of a diet rich in fruit and vegetables may be the most cost-effective way to delay the development of cataracts, since compromised functioning of the lens and retina with ageing is made worse by reduced reserves of antioxidant nutrients and reduced antioxidant enzyme function.
Am J Clin Nutr 62(6 Suppl):1439S–47S, 1995.

It has been estimated that in the United States more than half the operations carried out to remove cataracts, as well as the associated healthcare costs, could be saved if the onset of cataracts could be delayed by 10 years. The authors point out that according to the scientific literature this could be achieved by dietary measures.
J Am Coll Nutr 12(2):138–46, 1993.

Cholesterol, high

Some causative factors

- Deficiencies of vitamins C, B_6, B_{12} or folic acid
- Dietary fibre deficiency
- Essential fatty acid deficiency
- Excessive dietary saturated fat

According to 30 years of research studies, dietary cholesterol consumption has little effect on blood cholesterol levels in humans. In comparison a 1 per cent decrease in saturated fat consumption decreases plasma cholesterol.
Can J Cardiol 11 Suppl G:123G–6G, 1995.

Promising nutritional research

When 16 male volunteers with normal cholesterol levels were given a diet supplemented with nuts, the men's total and LDL ('bad') cholesterol levels dropped by 7 per cent and 10 per cent respectively after supplementation with almonds, and by 5 per cent and 9 per cent respectively after supplementation with walnuts.
Am J Clin Nutr 59(5):995, 1994.

In a meta-analysis of 16 randomized trials examining the effects of garlic on serum lipids and lipoproteins, total cholesterol in garlic-treated subjects was 12 per cent lower than in controls after one month of therapy, with the effect persisting for six months.
J R Coll Physicians Lond 28(1):39–45, 1994.

54 volunteers were found to have serum cholesterol levels reduced by 5–10 per cent after one week of supplementation with yoghurt. The intake of other foods did not significantly change.
Am J Clin Nutr 32(1):19–24, 1979.

Of 158 subjects with high cholesterol given 1,500 and 2,000 mg per day of vitamin B_3 as niacin, there was an improvement in total cholesterol, LDL-cholesterol, HDL cholesterol, and total-to-HDL cholesterol ratio compared with baseline and controls. Older subjects improved more than younger ones.
J Am Geriatr Soc 40(1):12–18, 1992.

Chronic fatigue syndrome and myalgic encephalomyelitis

Some causative factors

- Candidiasis
- Food intolerances
- Nutritional deficiencies, especially magnesium, B vitamins, carnitine
- Toxic overload

There is evidence that Candida albicans infection of the mucous membranes depresses T cell and natural killer cell function. Similar abnormalities of immune system function occur in chronic fatigue syndrome. The author proposes that chronic intestinal candidiasis may lead to immune depression which results in chronic fatigue.
Med Hypotheses 44(6):507–15, 1995.

Abnormalities in immune function are found in chronic fatigue syndrome (CFS) which may be related to essential fatty acid metabolism. As many as 90 per cent of CFS patients treated with essential fatty acids have shown significant improvement within three months.
Med Hypotheses 43(1):31–42, 1994.

Promising nutritional research

The energy score improved in chronic fatigue patients treated with intramuscular magnesium injections, and red cell magnesium levels returned to normal.
Lancet 337(8744):757–60, 1991.

Supplementation with the amino acid N-acetyl-cysteine can delay fatigue and increase muscle output by 15 per cent.
J Clin Investig 1994 94(6):2468–74, 1994.

Colic

- May be caused by food allergy

In a randomized, double-blind, placebo-controlled trial, 38 bottle-fed colicky babies were fed either casein hydrolysate or cow's milk formula, and the mothers of 77 breast-fed colicky infants were given either a low-allergen, additive free diet or a control diet. The babies on the active treatment had a significantly greater rate of improvement than those on the control diet, with distress reduced by 39 per cent, compared with only 16 per cent among controls.
J Allergy Clin Immunol 96(6 Pt 1):886–92, 1995.

Colitis

Some causative factors

- Food allergy/sensitivity
- Gut dysbiosis

Promising nutritional research

18 ulcerative colitis patients were randomized to a diet free of foods that appeared to provoke symptoms, or to a control group. At the end of the trial the diet group had significantly fewer

symptoms than the controls. No foods consistently provoked symptoms in all patients.
S Afr Med J 85(11):1176–9, 1995.

Marine fish oil supplements may reduce the inflammation associated with ulcerative colitis.
Nutr Rev 52(2):47–9, 1993.

10 patients with ulcerative colitis were given a high dose of EPA capsules for eight weeks. Seven patients had moderate to marked improvement and four out of the five patients on steroids were able to reduce their dosage.
J Clin Gastroenterol 12(2):157–61, 1990.

In a 4-month placebo-controlled trial, 29 ulcerative colitis patients in remission from the disease were given either psyllium husk supplements or placebo. The psyllium group experienced a significantly higher rate of improvement than the placebo group.
Scand J Gastroenterol 26(7):747–50, 1991.

In a placebo controlled study on 43 stable ulcerative colitis patients randomized to receive either fish oil, evening primrose oil or placebo for six months in addition to their usual treatment, it was found that evening primrose oil significantly improved stool consistency at six months, but there was no improvement in other symptoms in any of the groups.
Aliment Pharmacol Ther 7(2):159–66, 1993.

Common cold

Promising nutritional research

86 per cent of zinc-treated subjects became cold-free after seven days compared with only 46 per cent of placebo-treated subjects.
Anti-microbic agents and chemotherapy 25(1):20–4, 1984

100 volunteers who had developed a cold within the last 24 hours were randomized to receive either zinc gluconate lozenges or placebo for as long as their symptoms lasted. Those in the zinc group had significantly shorter colds (average 4.4 days) than the control group (7.6 days). They also had significantly fewer days with coughing, hoarseness, nasal congestion, nasal drainage and sore throat.
Ann Intern Med 125(2):81–8, 1996.

Treatment of colds with zinc reduced the mean daily clinical score and the mean daily nasal secretion.
J Anti-microb Chemother 20(6):893–901, 1987.

140 pre-school age children with a history of frequent respiratory illnesses were supplemented with vitamin A (450 mcg per day) or a placebo. The children given the vitamin A suffered 19 per cent fewer episodes than the placebo group.
Aust Paediatr J 22(2):95–9, 1986.

There are a large number of placebo-controlled double-blind studies which consistently and persuasively support the conclusion that vitamin C supplementation alleviates the symptoms of the common cold.
J Amer Coll Nutr 14(2):116–23, 1995.

Congestive heart failure

Some causative factors

- Carnitine deficiency
- Coenzyme Q deficiency
- Vitamin E deficiency

Coenzyme Q10 deficiency is a factor in numerous diseases including heart failure.
Clin Investig 71:S51–4, 1993.

Heart failure patients with abnormally low levels of coenzyme Q10 and vitamin E have a reduced survival rate.
Clin Investig 71:S137–9, 1993.

Promising nutritional research

Patients with congestive heart failure felt less tired, their general activity tolerance increased and breathing difficulties at rest disappeared when they were given 100 mg per day of coenzyme Q10 supplements.
Drugs Exp Clin Res 11(8):581–93, 1985.

Results of congestive heart failure treatment with coenzyme Q10 have been above and beyond those obtained from treatment with traditional principles, including reduced hospitalization and a reduced incidence of serious complications.
Clin Investig 71:S116–23, 1993.
Clin Investig 72:S129–33, 1993.
Clin Investig 71:S134–6, 1993.

2,664 patients from 173 Italian centres given 50–150 mg CoQ10 daily experienced more than 70 per cent improvement in cyanosis, oedema, palpitations and other symptoms.
Mol Aspects Med 15:s2287–s94, 1994.

Creutzfeldt-Jakob disease

Some causative factors

- Medications containing bismuth may cause a similar syndrome
- The possible potentiating role of pesticides and other xenobiotics, and nutritional deficiencies remains to be investigated
- Transmission of infective agent through contaminated growth hormone preparations and possibly through food

A patient given a bismuth preparation for 15 months developed an encephalopathy resembling Creutzfeldt-Jakob disease but recovered when the bismuth was discontinued. Bismuth preparations are commonly used in the treatment of gastritis.
Br J Psychiatry 158:278–80, 1991.

Crohn's disease

Some causative factors

- Dysbiosis leading to increased gut permeability
- Food allergy
- High sugar consumption

When the nutritional habits of 63 patients with Crohn's disease were compared with normals, sugar consumption in the Crohn's group prior to the onset of the disease was significantly higher.
Klin Wochenschr 54(8):367–71, 1976.

After comparing the diets of 30 newly-diagnosed patients with Crohn's disease with a control group, the researchers concluded that a diet high in refined sugar and low in raw fruit and vegetables precedes and may favour the development of Crohn's disease.
Br Med J 2(6193):762–4, 1979.

Promising nutritional research

In a randomized controlled trial, 20 patients with Crohn's disease were given either a diet excluding refined sugar, or a sugar-rich diet. In the worst cases, the sugar-free diet reduced the activity of the disease whereas the sugar-rich diet caused exacerbation.
Z Gastroenterol 19(1):1–12, 1981 (in German).

32 patients with Crohn's disease who had followed an unrefined diet in addition to medication for four years, were found to have spent only a total of 111 days in hospital during this period, compared with 533 days for a control group treated with medication alone. Only one patient in the diet group required surgery, compared with five in the medication-only group.
Br Med J 2(6193):764–6, 1979.

78 Crohn's disease patients currently in remission were given either nine fish oil capsules (with a protective coating to prevent dispersal in the stomach) per day or placebo. In the fish oil group 28 per cent suffered relapses during the following year, compared with 69 per cent from the control group. After one year 59 per cent of the fish oil group remained in remission, compared with 26 per cent from the control group.
N Engl J Med 334(24):1557–60, 1996.

The ability of dietary modification to maintain remission from Crohn's disease was compared with corticosteroid drug treatment. 136 patients were withdrawn from all treatments except for an elemental diet. 84 per cent achieved remission from the disease and were then randomly assigned to receive a diet free of foods which caused a return of symptoms, or were given corticosteroid treatment. The corticosteroid group remained in remission for an average of 3.8 months, and the diet group 7.5 months. The relapse rates at two years were 79 per cent for the corticosteroid group and 62 per cent for the diet group. Patients were mostly sensitive to cereals, dairy products and yeast.
Lancet 342(8880):1131–4, 1993.

Cystitis

Some causative factors

- Bacterial infections
- Candidiasis
- Food allergy or intolerance

Promising nutritional research

Bacterial infections of the urinary tract were reduced by nearly 50 per cent in women who drank 300 ml of cranberry juice daily for six months. Cranberry is effective in inhibiting the adhesion of bacteria to the bladder and urinary tract walls.
Nutr Rev 52(5):168–70, 1994.

Delinquency

Some causative factors

- Food or environmental allergy
- Lead or cadmium toxicity
- Nutritional deficiencies, especially zinc, B vitamins and essential fatty acids

Promising nutritional research

Hair mineral analysis of violent prison inmates found that lead and cadmium levels were significantly higher than non-violent inmates.
Psychol Rep 66(3 Pt 1):839–44, 1990.

In a double-blind study examining the effects of a reduction in the consumption of refined, sugary foods on 3,000 incarcerated juvenile delinquents, there was a 21 per cent reduction in antisocial behaviour, a 100 per cent reduction in suicides, 25 per cent reduction in assaults, and a 75 per cent reduction in the use of restraints compared with controls.
Int J Biosocial Res 5(2):99–106, 1983.

Depression

Some causative factors

- B vitamin deficiency, especially folate
- Hypoglycaemia
- Selenium deficiency
- Zinc deficiency

Depressive patients may have disturbances in folic acid metabolism related to vitamin B_6, B_{12}, magnesium or zinc deficiency, with improvement in depression on treatment of these deficiencies.
J Nutr Med 4:441–7, 1994.

Serum folate levels were estimated in depressed patients and found to be significantly lower than in normal controls. The lower the folate the more severe the depression.
Acta Psychiatr Scand 80(1):78–82, 1989.

Folate deficiency is common in psychiatric disorders, especially depression, and may predispose to or aggravate psychiatric disturbances.
J Psychiatr Res 20(2):91–101, 1986.

Of 11 healthy men given a selenium-rich or selenium-poor experimental diet for 99 days, those with an initially low selenium status experienced relatively more depressed moods.
Biol Psychiatry 39(2):121–8, 1996.

Promising nutritional research

In a double-blind trial, administration of the amino acid dl-phenylalanine (DLPA) was compared with the anti-depressant drug imipramine in 40 depressed patients. Both products were found to be equally effective.
Arch Psychiatr Nervenkr 227(1):49–58, 1979.

75–200 mg per day of the amino acid dl-phenylalanine was (DLPA) administered to depressed patients for 20 days. 12 patients were discharged with a complete or good response and only four patients did not respond. The investigators conclude that DLPA may have substantial anti-depressant properties.
J Neural Transm 41(2–3):123–34, 1977.

The amino acid tyrosine is precursor to noradrenaline, needed for mood balance. Trials using tyrosine supplementation against depression have shown encouraging results.
J Psychiatr Res 17(2):175–80, 1982.

12 patients with dopamine-dependent depression were treated with the amino acid L-tyrosine. On the first day of treatment a return to normal mood was observed.
C R Acad Sci III 306(3):9308, 1988 (in French).

In contraceptive pill users with depression, anxiety and other symptoms, vitamin B_6 supplementation restores normal tryptophan metabolism and relieves the related symptoms.
Acta Vitaminol Enzymol 4(1–2):45–54, 1982.

33 per cent of 123 patients with acute clinical depression or schizophrenia were found to be folate deficient. After treatment with methylfolate or placebo for six months in addition to their standard psychiatric drugs, those given methylfolate had experienced a significantly improved clinical and social recovery.
Br J Psychiatry 159:271–2, 1991.

Compared with placebo, 12 grams of inositol were administered daily to 13 patients with clinical depression, resulting in significant improvement.
Am J Psychiatry 152(5):792–4, 1995.

A systematic review and meta-analysis of studies testing the use of the herb St John's wort (*Hypericum perforatum*) against mild to moderately severe depression found that Hypericum extracts were significantly superior to placebo and equally as effective as standard anti-depressant drugs. Side-effects occurred in 19.8 per cent of Hypericum patients, as compared with 52.8 per cent of patients on standard anti-depressants.
BMJ 313(7052):253–8, 1996.

The usefulness of s-adenosyl methionine as an anti-depressant has been confirmed in several clinical trials. Compared with standard anti-depressant medications it has few side-effects.
Neurosci Biobehav Rev 12(2):139–41, 1988.

Diabetes

Some causative factors

- Excessive sugar consumption
- Nutritional deficiencies, especially chromium, vanadium, magnesium, vitamins C and E

Sugar consumption causes increased chromium losses through urine.
Metabolism 35(6):515–8, 1986.

Magnesium deficiency results in impaired insulin secretion and reduces tissue sensitivity to insulin. These are problems associated with diabetes. Sub-clinical magnesium deficiency is common in diabetics. It causes insulin resistance (reversible on magnesium supplementation) and promotes diabetic complications.
Therapie 49(1):1–7, 1994 (in French).
Ugeskr Laeger 153(30):2108–10, 1991 (in Danish).

A study on the tea and coffee drinking habits of 600 newly diagnosed diabetic children and 536 controls revealed that the risk of diabetes is increased in children who consume at least two cups of coffee daily and in those who consume one or more cups of tea daily.
Eur J Clin Nutr 47(4):279–85, 1994.

944 random men aged 42–60 without diabetes were followed up. Of the 45 who subsequently developed diabetes, a low plasma vitamin E level was associated with a 3.9-fold higher risk of contracting the disease.
BMJ 311(7013):1124–7, 1995.

Promising nutritional research

In a study carried out on elderly non-insulin-dependent diabetics and non-diabetics, supplementation with chromium-rich yeast improved glucose tolerance and reduced blood fat levels while chromium-poor yeast did not.
Diabetes 29:919–25, 1980.

The beneficial effects of chromium supplementation against diabetes are also reported in *Nutrition Research 5(6):609–20, 1985* and in *Clin Physiol Biochem 4(1):31–4, 1986.*

Of 15 controlled studies supplementing chromium compounds to subjects with impaired glucose tolerance, 12 resulted in improvement in the efficiency of insulin or in the blood lipid profile.
J Nutr 123(4):626–33, 1993.

Diabetics who do not respond to chromium supplementation may have inadequate levels of vitamin B_3. The use of both nutrients combined are more favourable than for each one separately.
Metabolism 36(9):896–9, 1987.

High doses of vitamin E improved insulin action in non-insulin-dependent diabetics.
Am J Clin Nutr 57:650–6, 1993.

High doses of antioxidant nutrients may lead to a regression of the late complications of diabetes.
Z Gesamte Inn Med 48(5):223–32, 1993 (in German).

Of 21 diabetic patients with an average age of 65, 17 obtained complete relief from pain of systemic distal neuropathy, five were able to discontinue hypoglycaemic medication, and half developed reduced insulin requirements after 25 days on a low-fat vegan diet consisting of unrefined foods.
J Nutr Med 4:431–9, 1994.

Low red-cell magnesium levels were found in 12 elderly diabetics. After magnesium supplementation for four weeks in a double-blind trial there was a significant net increase in insulin secretion and action, and decreased red cell membrane viscosity.
Am J Clin Nutr 55(6):1161–7, 1992.

Conditions associated with insulin resistance (a common type of diabetes) such as high blood pressure, are also associated with low cell magnesium levels. Long-term magnesium supplementation can contribute to an improvement in both pancreatic response and insulin action in non-insulin dependent diabetics.
Diabetologia 33(9):511–4, 1990.

Higher copper and lower magnesium levels (compared with controls) found in insulin-dependent diabetics may be associated with the development of insulin resistance (lack of effectiveness of insulin). The authors propose that patients may improve if dietary trace elements are supplemented.
Diabetes Res 26(1):41–5, 1994.

111 patients with mild diabetic neuropathy were given either supplements of the fatty acid gamma-linolenic acid (GLA) or placebo. After one year there were significant improvements in 13 parameters in the GLA-treated patients.
Diabetes Care 16(1):8–15, 1993.

22 patients with diabetic polyneuropathy were given either supplements of gamma-linolenic acid (GLA) or placebo for six months. The GLA-treated patients showed a significant improvement in symptom scores.
Diabet Med 7(4):319–23, 1990.

High dose vitamin C supplementation was found to have a beneficial effect on blood sugar control and blood lipids, and magnesium supplements reduced blood pressure, among a group of 56 diabetic patients.
Ann Nutr Metab 39(4):217–23, 1995.

Long-term vitamin C administration was found to have beneficial effects on glucose and lipid metabolism in a four-month randomized, double-blind study carried out on 40 elderly non-insulin dependent diabetics.
J Am Coll Nutr 14(4):387–92, 1995.

Diarrhoea (chronic)

Some causative factors

- Dysbiosis
- Food allergy or intolerance
- Infections
- Parasites

Promising nutritional research

In 111 Bangladeshi children with acute or chronic diarrhoea and increased gut permeability compared with normals, supplementation with five mg zinc per kg of body weight per day significantly reduced gut permeability.
J Pediatr Gastroenterol Nutr 15(3):289–96, 1992.

In a double-blind, randomized trial on children aged 6–35 months in India, zinc supplementation was found to significantly reduce the incidence of chronic diarrhoea and dysentery in those children with initially low zinc levels.
J Nutr 126(2):443–50, 1996.

Down's syndrome

Some causative factors

- Antioxidant deficiency
- Lack of fresh fruit and vegetables
- Mutations

Down's syndrome would disappear if it were not constantly renewed by new mutations. Mutations are alterations in the genetic apparatus of an organism, and can be induced by a number of environmental factors (mutagens), including smoking, prescribed and over-the-counter medicines, pollution, viruses, nutritional deficiencies, ionizing radiation and overheating of dietary fats and protein (particularly charring). Older women are likely to have been exposed to more mutagens than younger.
Wynn A & M: The case for preconception care of men and women, page 20. AB Academic Publishers, Bicester, 1991.

Dyslexia

Some causative factors

• Zinc and other mineral deficiencies

Grant EC et al.: Zinc deficiency in children with dyslexia: concentrations of zinc and other minerals in sweat and hair.
Br Med J: Clin Res 296(6622):607–9, 1988

Eczema

Some causative factors

• Contact allergy
• Essential fatty acid deficiency
• Food allergy
• Zinc deficiency

Promising nutritional research

Of 179 patients with eczema, 111 showed improvement after several weeks' supplementation with eight capsules a day of evening primrose oil. Medications were reduced in many cases.
J Nutr Med 2:9–15, 1991.

An analysis of nine controlled trials of evening primrose oil (Epogam) against eczema found that Epogam was significantly more effective than placebo, particularly against itching.
Br J Dermatol 121(1):75–90, 1989.

In a double-blind multicentre study on 145 eczema patients randomly assigned to fish oil or corn oil supplements there was a 30 per cent improvement in clinical score in the fish oil group and a 24 per cent improvement in the corn oil group.
Br J Dermatol 130(6):757–64, 1994.

In a double-blind 12-week study, fish oil supplementation resulted in improvements in scaling and itching.
Br J Dermatol 117(4):463–9, 1987.

Emphysema

Some causative factors

- Antioxidant nutrient deficiency
- Inhalation of cadmium fumes
- Smoking

Lung function and chest X-rays were compared in 101 men who had worked with copper-cadmium alloy, compared with a control group. The cadmium workers had significantly more lung abnormalities which put them at risk of emphysema.
Lancet 1(8587):663–7, 1988.

Experimental animals develop diseases similar to human bronchitis and emphysema from exposure to free radicals from pollutants (nitrous oxide and ozone). Vitamins C and E are protective against these free radicals, particularly in doses higher than the current Recommended Daily Amounts (RDA). The authors conclude that current RDAs are inadequate for maximum protection against air pollution levels.
Ann NY Acad Sci 669:141–55, 1992.

High vitamin C levels effectively contribute to protection from heart and lung diseases associated with smoking.
Proc Nat Acad Sci US 91(16):7688–92, 1994.

Promising nutritional research

2,510 patients with bronchitis, bronchial asthma and emphysema were treated for four weeks with the amino acid N-acetylcysteine in addition to the patients' usual medications. All selected parameters improved, especially for bronchitis.
Fortschr Med 110(18):346–50, 1992 (in German).

Inflammatory processes induced in lung tissue by smoking can, by hydrogen peroxide production, lead to the failure of an enzyme which protects against protein destruction. The inhalation of the amino acid glutathione could help to protect against this damage by inhibiting hydrogen peroxide.
Fundam Clin Pharmacol 8(6):518–24, 1994.

Endometriosis

Some causative factors

- Environmental pollution by dioxins
- Possibly nutritional deficiencies

16 monkeys were fed dioxin in their diet for four years. 71 per cent of those who had been fed the highest levels of dioxin were found to have endometriosis six to 10 years later. Three of these animals died from the disease.
Reported in Gibbons A: Dioxin tied to endometriosis. Science 262(5138):1373(1), 1993.

Epilepsy

Some causative factors

- Allergy
- Coeliac disease
- Deficiencies of selenium, magnesium or vitamins B_1, B_6, E or folic acid
- Pesticide poisoning

Vitamin B_6 deficiency, with requirements greatly above normal (a condition known as vitamin B_6 'dependency') should be considered in any baby suffering from seizures that are hard to control.
Am Fam Physician 27(3):183–7, 1983.

Compared with controls, 100 children with grand mal epilepsy had significantly lower plasma levels of vitamin E. The investigators point out that seizures can be prevented in experimental animals given vitamin E supplements.
Can J Neurol Sci 6(1):43–5, 1979.

Compared with controls, epileptic children were found to have significantly decreased plasma magnesium levels. The lower the magnesium, the more severe the epilepsy. In contrast, cerebrospinal fluid magnesium levels were high in epileptics, and this was attributed to a functional impairment of cell membranes.
J Neurol Sci 67(1):29–34, 1985.

Promising nutritional research

The clinical state of four epileptic children improved after anti-convulsant medication was discontinued and selenium supplementation substituted.
Lancet 337(8755):1443–4, 1991.

31 per cent of 72 epileptic patients taking the drug phenytoin were found to have abnormally low vitamin B_1 levels and 30 per cent abnormally low folate levels. After vitamin B_1 supplements were administered for six months, neurophysiological functions such as visuospatial analysis were improved.
Epilepsy Res 16(2):157–63, 1993.

10 of 12 epileptic children unresponsive to drugs and given 400 iu vitamin E per day in addition to medication experienced a significant reduction in seizures compared with controls.
Epilepsia 30(1):84–9, 1980.

Of 45 children with epilepsy, recurrent headaches and other symptoms, 25 ceased to have seizures and other symptoms after following a low-allergy diet. Most children reacted to several foods.
J Pediatr 114(1):51–8, 1989.

24 of 31 patients with epilepsy and cerebral calcifications were found by intestinal biopsy to have undiagnosed coeliac disease (gluten allergy), although they suffered no gastrointestinal symptoms. Five of 12 patients with coeliac disease and epilepsy were found on computerized tomography to have cerebral calcifications. A gluten-free diet may beneficially affect the course of epilepsy if provided early enough.
The Italian Working Group on Coeliac Disease and Epilepsy. Lancet 340(8817):439–43, 1992.

Fibromyalgia (fibrositis)

Some causative factors

• Magnesium deficiency

The average red blood cell magnesium levels of fibromyalgia patients is lower than controls. Magnesium deficiency symptoms are very similar to those of fibromyalgia and may be confused with the disease.
J Nutr Med 4:165–7, 1994.

Promising nutritional research

Of 15 fibromyalgia patients supplemented for eight weeks with magnesium malate, average tender point index scores were reduced from 19.6 to 6.5.
J Nutr Med 3:49–59, 1992.

Fluid retention (also see Premenstrual syndrome)

Some causative factors

- Excess capillary permeability due to flavonoid deficiency
- Excess salt consumption
- Excess sugar consumption
- Magnesium deficiency
- Vitamin B$_6$ deficiency

16 individuals were studied before and after consuming 75 grams of sugar (glucose). As levels of insulin rose the urinary excretion of sodium dropped significantly, indicating sodium retention. Sodium retention promotes fluid retention.
Clin Sci (Colch) 85(3):327–35, 1993.

Promising nutritional research

Ginkgo biloba extract (rich in flavonoids) was found to correct excess capillary permeability and reverse consequent fluid retention in all cases in a group of 15 patients.
Presse Med 15(31):1550–3, 1986 (in French).

Gallstones

Some causative factors

- Excessive refined carbohydrates (sugar and white flour). Excessive dietary saturated fat

13 test subjects with probable gallstones were given refined and unrefined carbohydrate diets for six weeks each. The refined carbohydrate diet increased bile cholesterol saturation and the investigators concluded that the avoidance of refined carbohydrate foods could reduce the risk of gallstones.
Gut 24(1):2–6, 1983.

Glaucoma

Some causative factors

- Nutritional deficiencies, especially B vitamins, vitamin C and magnesium

Promising nutritional research

Tyrosine metabolism normalized and the studied parameters improved in a group of glaucoma patients administered the antioxidant lipoic acid in combination with cofactors

pyridoxal phosphate, vitamin C and iron. The authors conclude that the scientific literature supports the supplementation of glaucoma patients with lipoic acid, vitamins B_1, B_2, B_5, B_6 (as pyridoxal) and vitamin C.
Vestn Oftalmol 107(3):19–21, 1991.

45 glaucoma patients were given either the antioxidant lipoic acid or placebo. Improvement of the biochemical parameters, visual function and of the coefficient of efficacy of liquid discharge was better in 45–58 per cent of the eyes examined, the better results being in stage II glaucoma.
Vestn Oftalmol 111(4):6–8, 1995.

Since magnesium is a natural calcium-channel blocker, 10 glaucoma patients were given magnesium supplements twice daily. After one month the visual fields tended to improve and all three measured blood flow parameters were significantly improved.
Ophthalmologica 209(1):11–13, 1995.

35 patients with primary open-angle glaucoma were treated by hyperbaric oxygenation combined with antioxidants for five years. Stabilization of visual function was obtained in 80 per cent of patients but in only 35 per cent of controls.
Vestn Oftalmol 112(1):4–6, 1996.

Headache and migraine

Some causative factors

- Brain tumour
- Caffeine consumption
- Chemical sensitivity
- Food intolerance
- Head trauma
- Liver dysfunction
- Poor posture
- Sleep disturbances
- Stress
- Tension

Patients with food-provoked headache can obtain relief by avoiding a few commonly eaten foods.
Postgrad Med 83(7):46–51, 1988.

Test subjects were given a single dose of caffeine or a placebo. Headache resulted 24–30 hours after the caffeine was consumed, confirming that headache is a specific caffeine withdrawal effect. Tiredness was also an indicator of caffeine withdrawal.
J Psychopharmacol 5(2):129–34, 1991.

Promising nutritional research

Two post-menopausal women with migraine were treated with a combination of vitamin D and calcium, resulting in a dramatic reduction in the frequency and duration of their migraine headaches.
Headache 34(10):590–2, 1994.

Patients suffering from cluster headaches, with low serum magnesium levels, experienced clinically meaningful improvements when treated with intravenous magnesium. The authors suggest that measurements of magnesium status may prove useful in determining the cause of some headaches, and in identifying those patients who would benefit from magnesium treatment.
Headache 35(10):597–600, 1995.

81 migraine patients were randomized to receive magnesium supplements or placebo daily for 12 weeks. In weeks 9–12 the attack frequency was reduced by 41.6 per cent in the magnesium group and by 15.8 per cent in the placebo group. The number of days with migraine and the use of medications to control symptoms per patient also decreased significantly in the magnesium group.
Cephalalgia 16(4):257–63, 1996.

Of 43 migraine sufferers given a trial diet free of allergens, 13 experienced a 66 per cent or greater reduction in headache frequency and six became headache free.
Ann Allergy 55(2):126–9, 1985.

Dietary treatment has been shown to be effective in most children with severe migraine.
Hum Nutr Appl Nutr 39(4):294–303, 1985.

93 per cent of 88 children with severe frequent migraine recovered on a few-foods diet in a double-blind trial. In most of the children whose migraine was triggered by factors such as blows to the head, exercise and flashing lights, these factors did not produce migraine attacks while the children were following the diet.
Lancet 2(8355):865–9, 1983.

Of seven migraine patients placed on a high-carbohydrate, low tryptophan diet, three of the four with classic migraine but none of those with common migraine reported an improvement.
Cephalalgia 7(2):87–92, 1987.

Hearing problems

Some causative factors

- Excessive fat in the diet
- Excessive viscosity (stickiness) of the blood, leading to poor circulation to the ears
- Excessive rigidity of the red blood cells
- Iron deficiency
- Magnesium deficiency
- Vitamin A deficiency
- Vitamin B_{12} deficiency (tinnitus)
- Vitamin D deficiency
- Zinc deficiency (tinnitus)

Decreased hearing ability associated with low vitamin A levels was found in a group of patients suffering from alcoholic liver disease. Animal studies have demonstrated degenerative changes in the ganglion cells on a vitamin A-deficient diet.
Arch Otorhinolaryngol 234(2):167–73, 1982.

Abnormally low vitamin D levels were found in 21 per cent of 47 patients with otosclerosis. Calcium and vitamin D supplementation in these patients resulted in significant hearing improvement in three cases.
Otolaryngol Head Neck Surg 93(3):313–21, 1985.

Red cell basic ferritin (a measure of iron sufficiency) was found to be significantly lower in 224 patients with hearing loss compared with normal controls.
ORL J Otorhinolaryngol Relat Spec 53(5):270–2, 1991.

When blood viscosity was measured in 49 patients with hearing loss it was found that hearing impairment at high frequencies was directly related to blood viscosity (stickiness). Red blood cell rigidity was also an important factor in hearing loss.
Lancet 1(8473):121–3, 1986.

Promising nutritional research

A number of papers have reported a 5–15 decibel improvement in the pure-tone threshold in patients with hearing loss supplemented with a combination of vitamins A and E.
Acta Vitaminol Enzymol Seven Suppl:85–92, 1985.

A remarkable (82 per cent) decrease in blood platelet adhesiveness (blood stickiness) was found after the administration of 400 iu vitamin E to normal volunteers for two weeks.
Blood 73(1):141–9, 1989.

400 iu vitamin E per day may be a near optimal dose of vitamin E to reduce platelet adhesiveness.
Thromb Res 49(4):393–404, 1988.

Treatment of vitamin D deficiency in patients with hearing problems should prevent progressive hearing loss, which may occasionally be partially reversible.
Am J Otol 6(1):102–7, 1985.

426 patients with idiopathic sudden hearing loss were found to have low haemoglobin and serum iron levels. They were administered either iron or vitamin supplements or medications. Hearing improvement was achieved in 53 per cent of those administered iron supplements, a result significantly better than the other groups.
ORL J Otorhinolaryngol Relat Spec 54(2):66–70, 1992.

Zinc supplements were given to tinnitus sufferers with low blood zinc levels, resulting in a significant improvement in symptoms in 52 per cent of cases, especially in cases of continuous tinnitus.
Acta Otorhinolaryngol Belg 41(3):498–505, 1987 (in French).

259 tinnitus sufferers were given either *Ginkgo biloba* extract (a medicinal herb) or almitrine-raubasine or nicergoline. *Ginkgo biloba* was found to be an effective treatment.
Meyer B: A multicentre study of tinnitus. Epidemiology and therapy (in French). Ann Otolaryngol Chir Cervicofac 103(3):185–8, 1986.

Some improvement in tinnitus and associated complaints were observed in 12 patients with low vitamin B_{12} levels following vitamin B_{12} replacement therapy.
Am J Otolaryngol 14(2):94–9, 1993.

In children with hearing losses, fluctuations in hearing ability appeared to vary according to their level of fat intake. Dietary changes led to a drop in cholesterol levels and a return to near normal hearing.
Laryngoscope 98(2):165–9, 1988.

300 young, healthy individuals with normal hearing, undergoing military training with exposure to high noise levels, were given either magnesium aspartate or placebo. Thresholds for noise-induced permanent hearing loss were significantly higher in the magnesium group. Magnesium supplementation was therefore found to be protective against damage to hearing caused by exposure to noise.
Am J Otolaryngol 15(1):26–32, 1994.

Heart disease

Some causative factors

- Consumption of trans fatty acids
- Deficiencies of magnesium, selenium, chromium, antioxidants, folic acid, vitamin C, vitamin B_6 or essential fatty acids
- High homocysteine levels

- Poor fibre intake
- Poor fruit and vegetable intake
- Poor HDL/LDL ratio in blood
- Use of contraceptive pill

A review of the literature concludes that heart disease patients suffer significantly from magnesium deficiency.
Ugeskr Laeger 150(8):477–80, 1988 (in Danish).

Many patients with variant angina have magnesium deficiency, according to the measurements of 24-hour retention rates in patients compared with controls.
Am J Cardiol 65(11):704(4), 1990.

The magnesium content of local drinking water was assessed for men who had died from heart disease and control cases in southern Sweden. Compared with the areas with the lowest levels of magnesium in drinking water, those with the highest levels had only 65 per cent of the risk of death from heart attack.
Am J Epidemiol 143(5):456–62, 1996.

Oestrogen promotes the shift of magnesium into bone and soft tissue. In individuals with a magnesium deficiency, high levels of oestrogen as found in the contraceptive pill may, as a result, encourage a calcium/magnesium imbalance which can lead to an increased risk of blood clotting and embolism.
Magnes Res 3(3):197–215, 1990.

A review of the literature shows that chromium is implicated in most of the known factors of heart disease risk. Chromium deficiency causes high circulating insulin levels. Since chromium levels have been found to be very much lower in patients with coronary heart disease than in normals, chromium deficiency may be a causative factor in heart disease.
Cardiovasc Res 18(10):591–6, 1984.

Low chromium levels in the aorta are found to correlate with coronary heart disease.
Clinical Chemistry 24:541–4, 1978.

Insufficient dietary chromium is associated with adult-onset diabetes and coronary heart disease. Chromium deficiency is very common. Well-controlled studies on dietary supplementation with chromium have demonstrated beneficial effects on glucose tolerance, blood fats and insulin binding.
Sci Total Environ 86(1–2)75–81, 1989.

Low selenium status is associated with a significantly higher risk of heart disease.
Lancet July 24:175–9, 1982.

In a study comparing selenium status in 84 heart attack patients and 84 controls, the patients had significantly lower levels.
JAMA 261(8):1161–4, 1989.

Test subjects with atherosclerosis (arteries narrowed by cholesterol deposits) had significantly lower levels of selenium than controls. The investigators postulate that risk of atherosclerosis is increased with low selenium levels, particularly if polyunsaturated fat intake is high.
Atherosclerosis 86(1):85–90, 1991.

A high intake of trans fatty acids from foods made with partially hydrogenated fats may increase the risk of coronary heart disease.
Lancet 341(8845)581–5, 1993.

Several studies have found a favourable change in plasma lipids in those consuming higher amounts of oily fish, or fish oil supplements.
Int J Clin Pharmacol Ther Toxicol 27(12):569–77, 1989.

Compared with individuals on a low dietary intake of omega three polyunsaturated fatty acids from seafood, those consuming at least one meal of oily fish per week have a 50 per cent reduced risk of heart attack.
JAMA 274(17):1363–7, 1995.

After studying homocysteine (a risk factor for heart disease) and nutrient levels in a group of 1,160 elderly survivors from the Framingham Heart Study, the researchers concluded that high homocysteine levels in the elderly can be attributed to vitamin deficiency in a substantial majority of cases.
JAMA 270(22):2693–8, 1993.

Plasma concentrations of vitamins C and E and carotene were measured in 6,000 men aged 35 to 54. A low level of all these nutrients, particularly vitamin E, was found to be associated with a higher risk of angina.
Lancet 337(8732):1–5, 1991.

The dietary intake of vitamin C in winter and summer was measured in 96 individuals aged 65 to 74 years. The average intake varied from 65 mg per day in winter to 90 mg per day in summer. It was found that an increase in dietary vitamin C of 60 mg daily (about one orange) was associated with a decrease in the potential for blood clotting which represented a 10 per cent lesser risk of heart disease.
BMJ 310(6994):1559–63, 1995.

The serum of 5,056 Canadian men and women aged 35 to 79 years with no history of coronary heart disease (CHD) were analysed for folate levels over a 15-year period, during which 165 of these individuals died from CHD. It was found that those who died had on average significantly lower serum folate levels than others.
JAMA 275(24):1893–6, 1996.

In a study on 1,605 randomly selected heart-disease free Finnish men followed up from 1984 to 1992, it was found that those with the lowest levels of vitamin C had a 3.5 times greater risk of suffering a heart attack compared with those who were not deficient.
BMJ 314:634–8, 1997.

In view of the increasing use of drug therapy in heart disease, the commonly accepted dietary principles of reducing saturated fat and increasing exercise are now thought inadequate. An increased consumption of leafy green vegetables, nut, seeds and pulses is advocated to take into account the beneficial effects of soluble fibre, vegetable protein, antioxidants, isoflavonoids, extra amounts of alpha-linolenic acid, and monounsaturated fats against factors which promote the development of heart disease.
Can J Cardiol 11 Suppl G:118G–22G, 1995.

Promising nutritional research

Selenium supplementation seems to exert an anti-atherogenic effect on blood lipids.
2nd meeting of the Int Soc for Trace Elem Res in Humans, 1989.

Higher intakes of chromium, copper and selenium have beneficial effects on risk factors associated with heart disease. Chromium supplementation has been reported to increase HDL cholesterol and to decrease triglycerides and total cholesterol. Individuals with the highest total cholesterol and triglycerides usually respond best.
Acta Pharmacol Toxicol (Copenhagen) 59 Suppl 7:317–24, 1986.

A meta-analysis of 27 studies concluded that a higher folic acid intake could, by reducing homocysteine levels, significantly protect against heart disease.
JAMA 274(13):1049–57, 1995.

In a study on 100 men with high homocysteine levels, treated with folic acid, vitamin B_6, vitamin B_{12} or a combination of the vitamins, it was found that folic acid was the most effective in reducing homocysteine levels and that the combination treatment was not more effective than folic acid alone.
J Nutr Oct 124(10):1927–33, 1994.

Supplementation with folic acid reduces both high and normal plasma homocysteine levels, especially if combined with vitamin B_{12}.
J Nutr 126(4 Suppl):1276S–80S, 1996.

Compared with a control group, 1,035 patients with coronary heart disease given 400 or 800 iu vitamin E daily for one year experienced only half the number of heart attacks.
Cambridge Heart Antioxidant Study (CHAOS). Lancet 347:781–6, 1996.

A remarkable (82 per cent) decrease in blood platelet adhesiveness (blood stickiness) was found after the administration of 400 iu vitamin E to normal volunteers for two weeks.
Blood 73(1):141–9, 1989.

400 iu vitamin E per day may be a near optimal dose of vitamin E to reduce platelet adhesiveness.
Thromb Res 49(4):393–404, 1988.

In a study on 44 men with angina, 22.7 per cent of the patients became free of exercise-induced angina after taking supplements of the amino acid L-carnitine for four weeks, compared with only 9.1 per cent on placebo.
Int J Clin Pharmacol Ther Toxicol 23(10):569–72, 1985.

Hepatitis

A low selenium intake is associated with a high regional incidence of hepatitis B virus infections in China.
Yu SY et al.: Chemoprevention trial of human hepatitis with selenium supplementation in China. Biol Trace Elem Res 20(15):15–22, 1989.

Herpes infections

Promising nutritional research

The long-term application of zinc products to genital and facial herpes eruptions greatly reduces or prevents recurrences of the infections.
Med Hypotheses 17(2):157–65, 1985.

A group of 27 herpes sufferers who took supplements of the amino acid L-lysine for six months experienced an average of 2.4 fewer herpes infections, and had greatly reduced severity and healing time compared with the placebo group.
Dermatologica 175(4):183–90, 1987.

Of 1,543 herpes sufferers assessed by questionnaire after six months on supplements of the amino acid L-lysine, 84 per cent reported that the supplements prevented recurrence or decreased the frequency of herpes infections. 79 per cent described their symptoms as severe or intolerable without lysine. 83 per cent reported that sores healed in five days or less on lysine, but took 6–15 days to heal without it.
J Anti-microb Chemother 12(5):489–96, 1983.

See Section I, Therapeutic diets: anti-herpes diet for foods which herpes sufferers should eat and avoid.

High blood pressure (hypertension)

Some causative factors

• Deficiencies of essential fatty acids, calcium and magnesium

The diets of 615 men were investigated and compared with blood pressure readings. A low intake of magnesium was most strongly correlated with increased rates of high blood pressure. The authors conclude that vegetables, fruits, whole grains and low-fat dairy items may be protective against high blood pressure.
Am J Clin Nutr 45(2):469–75, 1987.

Promising nutritional research

Data from 22 randomized clinical trials were pooled to investigate the effect of calcium supplementation on blood pressure. There was a statistically significant reduction in systolic blood pressure with calcium supplementation, in individuals with high and normal blood pressure.
Ann Intern Med 124(9):825–31, 1996.

Test subjects with high blood pressure who were given fish oil supplements experienced a drop in blood pressure after four weeks.
N Engl J Med 320(16):1037–43, 1989.

In 100 hypertensive patients treated with a meat-free diet of unrefined grains, fruits, vegetables, nuts, oils and cottage cheese, mean systolic and diastolic blood pressures had dropped by 10 mmHg after eight weeks compared with initial values and controls.
J Nutr Med 2:17–24, 1991.

6 grams of taurine per day for seven days were administered to 19 young patients with borderline high blood pressure. Systolic blood pressure decreased by nine mmHg in the taurine-treated group, compared with 2.7 mmHg in the placebo group. Plasma adrenaline levels also dropped significantly in the taurine-treated group.
Circulation 75(3):525–32, 1987.

Excess body weight is associated with higher blood pressure. Weight reductions of only 4–5 kg (8–9 lb) can lead to normalization of blood pressure. It is estimated that up to 50 per cent of adults in the United States who are on blood pressure controlling medications would need less of these if they lost only a modest amount of weight.
Am J Clin Nutr 63(3 Suppl):423S–5S, 1996.

Hyperactivity and behavioural problems

Some causative factors

- Birth trauma
- Candidiasis
- Chemical sensitivities
- Deficiencies of zinc, B vitamins, magnesium, chromium, essential fatty acids
- Food additive sensitivity, especially tartrazine

- Food allergy/intolerance
- Heavy metal toxicity, particularly lead
- Lack of stomach acid or digestive enzymes
- Sugar sensitivity

In eight pre-school children given 6 ounces of juice sweetened either with sugar or with an artificial sweetener, there was a drop in performance on structured tasks and more 'inappropriate' behaviour during free play after the sugary drink was consumed.
J Abnorm Child Psychol 14(4):565–77, 1986.

In a study on 20 hyperactive children, blood, serum and urine levels of zinc were measured after the administration of orange drinks containing the artificial colouring tartrazine, and control drinks free of this additive. Tartrazine was found to induce a reduction in the zinc content of serum and saliva, and an increase in the zinc content of urine, with a corresponding deterioration in behaviour and emotional responses.
J Nutr Med 1:51–7, 1990.

53 subjects with attention-deficit hyperactivity disorder were found to have significantly lower levels of key fatty acids in plasma and red cell lipids than 43 controls.
Am J Clin Nutr 62(4):761–8, 1995.

Behaviour, learning and health problems were compared between boys with high and low intakes of essential fatty acids. More behavioural problems were found in those with lower omega–3 intakes, and more learning and health problems were found in those with lower omega–6 intakes.
Physiol Behav 59(4–5):915–20, 1996.

Magnesium, zinc, copper, iron and calcium levels were measured in plasma, red cells, urine and hair of 50 hyperactive children. Average concentrations were low compared with healthy controls. The authors recommend nutritional supplementation for hyperactive children.
Psychiatr Pol 28(3):345–53, 1994.

Promising nutritional research

Of 76 hyperactive children treated with a low-allergen diet, 62 improved, and a normal range of behaviour was achieved in 21 of these. Other symptoms such as headaches and fits also often improved. 48 foods were incriminated. Artificial colourings and preservatives were the commonest provoking substances.
Lancet 1:540–5, 1985.

24 preschool-age hyperactive boys were given a baseline diet and then randomly assigned to either a placebo (control) diet for three weeks or an experimental diet for four weeks. The experimental diet was free from added sugar, artificial colouring and flavouring, chocolate, MSG, preservatives and caffeine, as well as any food which the family said affected their child. Parents recorded a 58 per cent improvement among the children on the experimental diet but little improvement in the placebo group.
Paediatrics 83, 1989.

In a study on 10 habitual juvenile delinquents with an average age of 11 years, all the children were found to be very low in zinc, and had high hyperactivity scores. Some also had manganese and chromium deficiencies. The children were given a diagnostic diet, low in all the foods which allergic people most commonly react to. Foods were then reintroduced one by one into the diet to see if a relapse would occur. If it did, that food was then permanently excluded. All the eight children who finished the programme responded to the diet with a dramatic reduction in their behavioural problems. Six months later, five of the children still remained free of problems. At the same time the rates of shoplifting, car theft and criminal damage in the town where the children lived dropped by 50 per cent. This was thought to be because these five children had been responsible for a large proportion of these local crime statistics.
The Shipley Project, National Society for Research into allergy, West Yorkshire, UK, 1992.

The hyperactivity ratings of 19 out of 26 children given a diet excluding wheat, corn, yeast, soy, citrus, egg, chocolate, peanuts, and artificial colours and flavours, dropped from an average of 25 (high) to an average of eight (low).
Annals of Allergy 72, 1994.

Hypoglycaemia

Some causative factors

- Chromium deficiency
- Magnesium deficiency

Promising nutritional research

Chromium supplementation may improve glucose tolerance and reduce symptoms of symptomatic hypoglycaemia.
Biol Trace Elem Res 17:229–36, 1988.

In a study supplementing eight female hypoglycaemia patients with 200 mcg chromium daily for three months in a double-blind trial, it was found that chromium supplementation alleviated the hypoglycaemic symptoms and significantly raised the minimum blood sugar levels following a glucose load. Insulin binding to red blood cells, and the number of insulin receptors also significantly improved.
Metabolism 36(4):351–5, 1987.

Magnesium status was measured in 24 subjects suffering from reactive hypoglycaemia, who were then administered either magnesium supplements or placebo. After six weeks, eight (56 per cent) of the magnesium group reported feeling better, compared with two (25 per cent) in the placebo group. After supplementation, no blood glucose levels dropped below the fasting level. The responders were found to have raised magnesium levels in their urine after supplementation while the non-responders did not.
Magnes Bull 4(2):131–4, 1982.

Hypothyroidism

Some causative factors

- Environmental pollution
- Food intolerance
- Selenium deficiency
- Smoking
- Zinc deficiency

Smoking habits were evaluated in 128 normal women and 135 women with primary hypothyroidism. Among those with overt hypothyroidism, the smokers had a greater degree of hypothyroidism, and the heavier the smoking habits, the worse this was. Both thyroid function and hormonal function were affected by smoking.
N Engl J Med 333(15):964–9, 1995.

Promising nutritional research

17 patients diagnosed as hypothyroid were able to discontinue thyroid replacement therapy after beginning a food elimination and replacement programme free of sugar and refined foods. Thyroid function returned to or remained normal.
XVI European Congress of Allergology and Clinical Immunology, Madrid, 1995.

Selenium is required to convert the T4 thyroid hormone to the active T3 form, a process which is frequently inefficient in the elderly, who often suffer from hypothyroidism. Selenium supplementation in a group of elderly patients was found to significantly improve selenium status and decrease T4 levels compared with controls.
Clin Sci (Colch) 89(6):637–42, 1995.

Selenium supplementation when administered to hypothyroid cystic fibrosis patients resulted in an increase in T3 thyroid hormone levels, indicating that conversion of T4 to T3 had improved. LDL cholesterol decreased, which was taken as another measure of improved thyroid hormone efficacy.
Biol Trace Elem Res 40(3):247–53, 1994.

In a group of 52 Down's syndrome patients suffering from hypothyroidism, nine were found to be zinc deficient. When administered zinc supplements their thyroid function improved.
Ann Genet 33(1):9–15, 1990.

T4 thyroid hormone requires conversion to the active T3 form for utilization in the body. Nine out of 13 subjects with low T3 levels were found to have mild to moderate zinc deficiency. After supplementation with zinc sulphate for 12 months, T3 and T4 levels normalized. The researchers conclude that zinc may play a part in thyroid hormone metabolism in patients with low T3 levels and may play a part in the conversion of T4 to T3.
J Am Coll Nutr 13(1):62–7, 1994.

Some causative factors

- Nutritional deficiencies
- Recreational drugs such as 'poppers' (nitrites) and heroin
- Toxic overload (especially organophosphate pesticides)

Vitamin and mineral deficiencies lead to impaired immune function. It is important to identify those patients whose illness is related to immune system deficiencies of nutritional origin.
JAMA 245(1):53–58, 1981.

81 per cent of 107 patients exposed to pesticides had depressed levels of T and B white blood cells. Their condition improved as pesticides were cleared from their body.
J Nutr Med 2:399–410, 1991.

The antioxidant substance melatonin, produced by the pineal gland and the gut, plays an important part in immune function. If the production of melatonin is experimentally inhibited, a state of immunosuppression is produced, which disappears when melatonin is restored. A role for melatonin treatment in immuno-deficiency states and cancers is proposed.
Bull Group Int Rech Sci Stomatol Odontol 1995.

Animal and human studies suggest that vitamin B_6 deficiency impairs immune responses, including antibody production and white cell differentiation and maturation. A B_6 deficiency has been associated with reduced immunity in the elderly, HIV-positive individuals, and rheumatoid arthritis.
Nutr Rev 51(8):217–25, 1993.

Promising nutritional research

Selenium affects all components of the immune system. A deficiency of selenium has been shown to lower resistance to microbial and viral infections, neutrophil function, antibody production, proliferation of T and B lymphocytes and effectiveness of T lymphocytes and natural killer cells. Supplementation with selenium has been shown to enhance all these functions.
Environ Res 42(2):277–303, 1987.

A group of elderly subjects experienced significant stimulation of several immune system parameters after six months' supplementation with selenium.
Am J Clin Nutr 53(5):1323–8, 1991.

An increase in the T4/T8 lymphocyte ratio occurred in 14 test subjects treated with coenzyme Q10 supplements.
Biochem Biophys Res Commun 175(2):786–91, 1991.

Supplementation with a modest amount of micronutrients improved several immune factors and decreased the risk of infection in a controlled trial on elderly people.
Lancet 340:1124–7, 1992.

Natural killer (NK) cells, which form part of the body's immune system, are known to spontaneously destroy tumour cells, virus-infected cells, and to play a primary role in immune system surveillance. Volunteers were given either 0.5 g/kg body weight of raw garlic daily, or 1,800 mg kyolic garlic daily. Compared with controls, the NK cell performance increased in both the garlic-treated groups, by 139 per cent in the raw garlic group and by 155.5 per cent in the kyolic garlic group.
Fed Proc 46(3):441, 1987.

Infertility

Some causative factors

- Environmental oestrogen mimicking chemicals
- Excess alcohol consumption
- Selenium deficiency
- Smoking
- Underweight or overweight
- Zinc deficiency in males

The body weights of 376 infertile women were compared with fertile controls. The investigators concluded that 6 per cent of infertility in which ovulatory dysfunction is present results from being excessively underweight, and another 6 per cent from being excessively overweight.
Fertil Steril 50(5):721–6, 1988.

The incidence of disorders of the male reproductive tract has more than doubled in the past 30–50 years and sperm counts have declined by half. Similar abnormalities occur in the sons of women exposed to large amounts of artificial oestrogen during pregnancy. Oestrogens may be involved in falling sperm counts and disorders of the male reproductive tract.
Lancet 341:1392–95, 1993.

Alcohol is a reproductive toxin. The authors discuss various mechanisms by which alcohol can cause infertility in males.
Br J Alcohol Alcohol 16(4):179–85, 1981.

Men with a low vitamin C intake have a markedly increased likelihood of genetic damage to their sperm. Cigarette smoke is high in oxidants and depletes the body of vitamin C and other antioxidants. Levels of a marker indicating genetic damage to sperm cells was found to be 50 per cent higher in smokers than in non-smokers. The concentration of vitamin E in

seminal fluid was 32 per cent lower. Male smokers may therefore experience mutations in their sperm which can lead to cancer, birth defects and genetic diseases in their offspring.
Mutat Res 351(2):199–203, 1996.

Promising nutritional research

Selenium supplementation to males attending an infertility clinic proved efficient in improving sperm motility.
Macpherson A et al.: The effect of selenium supplementation in sub-fertile males (abstract). 8th International Conference on Trace Element Metabolism in Man and Animals, 1993.

14 men with low sperm counts were supplemented with zinc sulphate for four months. While serum zinc levels did not change, semen zinc levels increased, sperm count increased, and the wives of three patients conceived.
Indian J Physiol Pharmacol 31(1):30–4, 1987.

Insomnia

Some causative factors

- B vitamin deficiency
- Magnesium deficiency
- Toxic overload

A patient with severe sleep disturbance who was treated with vitamin B_{12} experienced progressive improvement in his sleep disturbance. He was able to advance the timing of his sleep period for the first time in nearly 10 years and to follow a normal 24 hour sleep-wake regimen.
Sleep 6(3):257–64, 1983.

2 adolescent patients with persistent sleep-wake disorders experienced an immediate improvement after the administration of high doses of vitamin B_{12}. Neither had shown any other laboratory or clinical evidence of B_{12} deficiency.
Sleep 14(5):414–8, 1991.

Irritable bowel syndrome

Some causative factors

- Constipation
- Food intolerance
- Gut dysbiosis

Specific foods caused symptoms of irritable bowel syndrome in 14 out of 21 patients. Double-blind challenge confirmed this in six cases.
Lancet 2(8308):1115–7, 1982.

Promising nutritional research

14 patients with irritable bowel syndrome, one or more foods or food additives were shown to induce symptoms. The presence of yeast (*Candida albicans*) was found to promote the development of food intolerance reactions in some patients. The investigators concluded that dramatic clinical improvements can result from the use of a suitable exclusion diet.
Ann Allergy 54(6):538–40, 1985.

Kidney disease

Some causative factors

Poor kidney function
- Excessive sugar consumption
- Selenium deficiency
- Toxic overload

Kidney stones
- Chronic heavy metal poisoning
- Dietary fibre deficiency
- Excess dietary fat protein and/or sugar
- Magnesium deficiency
- Vitamin B_6 deficiency

When compared with controls, the diets of kidney stone patients were found to contain less vitamin C and more alcohol.
Br J Urol 63(6):575–80, 1989.

Compared with controls, the diet of 88 kidney stone patients was found to be lower in dietary fibre, magnesium and vitamin B_1.
Urol Res 14(2):75–82, 1986.

There is evidence that one third of the population shows increased risk factors for kidney stone disease after consuming sugar. These effects of sugar consumption are thought to be due to the increased secretion of insulin, which results in increased calcium excretion by the kidneys.
Nutr Health 5(1):9–17, 1987.

Sugar may cause harmful changes to kidney tissue. Ten kidney stone patients and 10 normal controls received 250 grams of sucrose daily for one week. In both groups sucrose ingestion

caused a rise in levels of urinary N-acetyl-ßglucosaminidase (NAG), a marker of kidney tubular cell damage. NAG was already at higher levels in the patients than the controls before the study began.
Br J Urol 58(4):353–7, 1986.

In a study investigating the effects of diet on calcium kidney stone patients, it was found that a high intake of carbohydrate and fat and a low intake of calcium was associated with a higher rate of urinary oxalate excretion, which is a risk indicator for this type of kidney stone.
Br J Urol 76(6):692–6, 1995.

8 kidney stone patients were given diets either low or high in animal protein for eight weeks. There was increased urinary supersaturation and risk of forming uric acid crystals on the high-protein diet.
Proc Eur Dial Transplant Assoc 20:411–6, 1983.

In a study investigating the differences in diet between 102 recurrent calcium kidney stone patients and 146 controls, it was found that the patient group had a significantly higher consumption of animal and vegetable protein. A link between the protein content of the diet and urinary calcium levels was confirmed but protein intake had little effect on oxalate excretion.
Br J Urol 67(3):230–6, 1991.

Coppersmiths exposed to chronic cadmium poisoning were found to have a 40 per cent incidence of kidney stones.
Br J Urol 54(6):584–9, 1982.

Lead interacts with kidney membranes and enzymes and disrupts energy production, calcium metabolism, glucose homoeostasis and several other functions. Lead damage to kidney function is irreversible.
Toxicology 73(2):127–46, 1992.

Mercury, which is a kidney toxic, was found at autopsy to have accumulated in the kidney cortex of seven individuals with amalgam tooth fillings, at levels significantly higher than in five amalgam-free individuals.
Swed Dent J 11(5):179–87, 1987.

Promising nutritional research

Eleven healthy volunteers were given increasing amounts of supplementary selenium (up to 700 mcg per day). Mean creatinine clearance increased significantly, concomitantly with a reduction of serum creatinine levels. This suggested that kidney function was positively influenced by selenium.
J Trace Elem Electrolytes Health Dis 4(3):157–61, 1990.

In 16 kidney stone sufferers supplemented with magnesium and vitamin B_6, there was a significant decline in the excretion of oxalate, leading to a significant decrease in kidney stone risk index after 120 days of treatment.
Urol Res 22(3):161–5, 1994.

Urinary oxalate excretion was significantly reduced in 12 kidney stone patients administered vitamin B_6 supplements in doses of 250–500 mg daily.
Int Urol Nephrol 20(4):353–9, 1988.

Urinary excretion levels of magnesium are abnormally low in 25 per cent of kidney stone patients. Supplementation with magnesium corrects this and effectively prevents the recurrence of stones.
Presse Med 16(1):25–7, 1987 (in French).

Dietary advice given to 392 kidney stone patients to increase dietary fibre and reduce sugar, refined carbohydrates and animal protein resulted in a significant reduction in the urinary excretion of calcium, oxalate and uric acid.
Br J Urol 54(6):578–83, 1982.

A meta-analysis of randomized, controlled studies using protein-restricted diets in humans with chronic kidney disease found that such diets significantly reduce the risk (by more than 30 per cent) of kidney failure or death, effectively slowing down the progression of kidney failure.
Ann Intern Med 124(7):627–32, 1996.

106 patients with IgA nephropathy were randomized to receive either 12 g per day of fish oil or placebo for two years. 10 per cent of the fish oil group died or developed end-stage kidney disease, compared with 10 per cent in the placebo group. Serum creatinine concentrations rose significantly more slowly in the fish oil group. The investigators conclude that in patients with IgA nephropathy treatment with fish oil retards the rate of loss of kidney function.
N Engl J Med 331(18):1194–9, 1994.

Learning difficulties

Some causative factors

- Essential fatty acid deficiency
- Food intolerance
- Heavy metal toxicity
- Vitamin and mineral deficiencies

There is a steady accumulation of evidence that iron deficiency limits physical performance, reduces work productivity and impairs cognitive (thinking) processes. In children it leads to lower mental developmental test scores, failure to respond to test stimuli, short attention span, unhappiness, and increased fearfulness and tension.
Bull NY Acad Med 65(10):1050–66, 1989.

An analysis of the literature confirms that exposure to lead in small amounts impairs children's IQ.
JAMA 263(5):673–8, 1990.

Young adults who had had higher lead levels in milk teeth shed at ages six or seven were still more likely to have a reading disability, lower vocabulary, poorer co-ordination and longer reaction times than those with lower levels.
N Engl J Med 322(2):83–8, 1990.

Zinc, calcium, lead and cadmium status was assessed from hair samples in 146 children aged 5–16, and measures of cognitive function were collected. Higher zinc levels appeared to protect against the harmful effects of cadmium on verbal IQ and reading performance. Higher calcium levels seemed to protect against harmful lead effects on performance IQ.
Nutrition and Behaviour 3:145–61, 1986.

Behaviour, learning and health problems were compared between boys with high and low intakes of essential fatty acids. More behavioural problems were found in those with lower omega–3 intakes, and more learning and health problems were found in those with lower omega–6 intakes.
Physiol Behav 59(4–5):915–20, 1996.

Promising nutritional research

Of 27 pupils with learning problems, 18 showed a rise of 1–5 and six showed a rise of 6–15 points in their IQ after beginning a food elimination and replacement programme free of sugar and refined foods. Hyperactivity was reduced and behaviour and concentration as assessed by the teachers improved.
Borok G et al.: Atopy: the incidence in chronic recurrent maladies. XVI European Congress of Allergology and Clinical Immunology, Madrid, 1995.

127 young adults took either 10 times the RDA of nine vitamins, or a placebo, in a double-blind trial. After 12 months better performance on two measures of attention was found in the women only.
Psychopharmacology 117(3):298–305, 1995.

A multivitamin/mineral preparation or placebo was administered double-blind for eight months, resulting in a significant increase in non-verbal intelligence.
Lancet: Jan 23:140–3, 1988.

Macular degeneration

Some causative factors

- Zinc deficiency
- Dietary vegetable deficiency

Dietary factors and eye health were compared in 1968 subjects aged 43 to 86. Those with the highest zinc consumption from foods had a lower risk of age-related macular degeneration.
Arch Ophthalmol 114(8):991–7, 1996.

Eye health and dietary factors were compared in 976 subjects. Despite the fact that none had any clinical nutritional deficiencies, high dietary vitamin E consumption (from food, not supplements) was associated with a protective effect against age-related macular degeneration, and vitamin C and beta-carotene were also protective.
Arch Ophthalmol 112(2):222–7, 1994.

Levels of individual carotenoids and tocopherols (vitamin E) were measured in subjects with age-related macular degeneration (ARMD) of the eyes and in controls. Individuals with the lowest levels of the carotenoid lycopene (found in tomatoes) were twice as likely to have ARMD.
Arch Ophthalmol 113 (12):1518–23, 1995.

Carotenoids and antioxidant vitamins may help to retard some of the destructive processes in the retina that lead to age-related macular degeneration.
Am J Clin Nutr 62(6 Suppl):1448S–61S, 1995.

Promising nutritional research

In a double-blind placebo-controlled study, a group of patients suffering from macular degeneration experienced significantly less visual loss after receiving zinc supplementation than a control group.
Arch Ophthalmol 106(2):192–8, 1988.

In a randomized, double-blind, placebo-controlled trial, zinc supplements or placebo were given to 151 patients with drusen (white eye deposits) or macular degeneration. The zinc group experienced significantly less visual loss than the placebo group after a follow-up of 12 to 24 months.

Arch Ophthalmol 106(2):192–8, 1988.
In a double-blind placebo-controlled trial the herb *Ginkgo biloba* or a placebo was given to 10 patients with macular degeneration. A statistically significant improvement in long-distance visual acuity was observed after treatment with *Ginkgo biloba*.
Presse Med 15(31):1556–8, 1986 (in French).

Manic-depressive illness

Some causative factors

- Vanadium excess
- Vitamin C deficiency

Promising nutritional research

In a double-blind, placebo-controlled trial, manic-depressive and depressed patients given a single dose of 3 grams of vitamin C improved significantly. In addition, both manic and depressed patients were significantly better on a reduced intake of vanadium.
Psychol Med 11(2):249–56, 1981.

In five out of six manic patients given lecithin supplements in a double-blind placebo-controlled trial, improvement was significantly greater than improvement with placebo.
Am J Psychiatry 139(9):1162–4, 1982.

75 patients on lithium therapy for manic depressive illness were given 200 mcg folic acid or a placebo. Those with the highest plasma folate concentrations were found to show the most significant reductions in symptoms.
J Affect Disord 10(1):9–13, 1986.

Therapies based on decreasing vanadium levels in the body, including the use of vitamin C supplements, have been reported to be effective in both depressive illness and mania.
Nutr Health 3(1–2):79–85, 1984.

Measles (complications from)

Some causative factors

- Vitamin A deficiency

Low vitamin A levels are associated with greater measles severity.
Nutr Rev 50(10):291–2, 1992.
Am J Dis Child 146(2):182–6, 1992.
BMJ 306(6874):366–70, 1993.

Promising nutritional research

Treatment with vitamin A reduces complications and mortality in measles. The researchers conclude that all children with severe measles should be given vitamin A supplements whether or not they are thought to have a nutritional deficiency.
N Engl J Med 323(3):160–4, 1990.

Menopausal hot flushes

Some causative factors

- Adrenal gland insufficiency
- Reduced oestrogen production

Promising nutritional research

Soy contains daidzin, a powerful plant oestrogen. 58 menopausal women suffering from at least 14 hot flushes per week were given a daily diet supplemented with soya flour or wheat flour, in a randomized, double-blind trial. There was a significant, rapid improvement in the menopausal symptom score, particularly in the soya flour group, with symptoms decreasing by 40 per cent over 12 weeks.
Maturitas 21(3):189–95, 1995.

Motor neurone disease

Some causative factors

- Calcium and magnesium deficiency

The conditions which produce calcium deficiency may also lead to a shift of calcium from bone to soft tissue. This may promote not only osteoporosis but also arteriosclerosis and

high blood pressure, due to increased levels of calcium in the blood vessel walls. Motor neurone disease and senile dementia could result from the calcium being deposited in the central nervous system.
J Nutr Sci Vitaminol 31(Suppl):S15–19, 1985.

Chronic deficiencies of calcium and magnesium stimulate the chronic release of excess parathyroid hormone. This can result in the increased intestinal absorption of toxic metals, the mobilization of calcium and magnesium from bone, and the deposition of these elements in nervous tissue.
Nippon Rinsho 54(1):123–8, 1996.

Food, water and soil were assessed for mineral content in Hohara, Japan, a location with a high incidence of motor neurone disease. Compared with control areas, Hohara inhabitants had a significantly higher manganese intake and significantly lower magnesium intake.
Sci Total Environ 149(1–2):121–35, 1994.

Multiple sclerosis

Some causative factors

- Dental mercury toxicity
- Selenium deficiency

Blood findings were compared in multiple sclerosis (MS) sufferers who had had their amalgam (silver) dental fillings removed and those who had not. MS subjects with amalgams were found to have significantly lower levels of red blood cells, haemoglobin, haematocrit, thyroxine (thyroid hormone), T-lymphocytes and T–8 suppressor cells and serum IgG. The amalgam group also had significantly higher blood urea nitrogen and hair mercury, and had suffered significantly (33 per cent) more exacerbations of their illness during the past 12 months.
Sci Total Environ 142(3):191–205, 1994.

In a comparison of the mental health of 47 multiple sclerosis (MS) sufferers with amalgam (silver) dental fillings, compared with 50 whose fillings had been removed, the amalgam group suffered significantly more depression, anger, hostility and obsessive-compulsive behaviour.
Psychol Rep 70(3 Pt 2):1139–51, 1992.

Promising nutritional research

Multiple sclerosis patients have low levels of the important antioxidant enzyme glutathione peroxidase. A group of patients given high doses of vitamins C and E and selenium for five weeks experienced a five-fold increase in the activity of this enzyme.
Biol Trace Elem Res 24(2):109–17, 1990.

Muscular dystrophy

Some causative factors

- Selenium deficiency
- Vitamin E deficiency

Promising nutritional research

High doses of selenium with vitamin E may bring improvement in this condition.
Acta Med Scand 213:237–9, 1983.

High doses of selenium and vitamin E improved grip strength and physical capacity in five patients with muscular dystrophy, especially in patients in earlier stages of the disease.
Acta Med Scand 219(4):407–14, 1986.

A boy diagnosed with myopathy and motor neuropathy was found to have a defect in the enzyme NADH dehydrogenase and dramatically improved on vitamin B_2 and carnitine therapy, with normalization of the enzyme defect.
Arch Neurol 1991 48(3):334–8, 1991.

Neurological disease

Neurological dysfunction is a known complication of coeliac disease (gluten sensitivity). 30 of 53 patients with neurological disease (ataxia, peripheral neuropathy, mononeuritis multiplex, myopathy, motor neuropathy) of unknown cause were found to have antibodies to the substance gliaden found in gluten. This suggests that gluten sensitivity may be a significant causative factor in neurological diseases of unknown cause.
Lancet 347(8998):369–71, 1996.

Osteoarthritis

Some causative factors

- Injury
- Food allergy or intolerance
- Essential fatty acid deficiency
- Toxic overload

The association between vitamin C, beta-carotene and vitamin E intake and the incidence and progression of osteoarthritis was compared with that of non-antioxidant vitamins in 640 individuals given knee evaluations. It was found that a high intake of vitamin C reduced

the rate of cartilage loss by 70 per cent in osteoarthritis sufferers. A reduction in the risk of osteoarthritis progression was also found for beta-carotene and vitamin E, to a lesser degree.
Arthritis Rheum 39(4):648–56, 1996.

Promising nutritional research

Movement ability and pain were assessed in three double-blind 4–6 week trials of glucosamine sulphate compared with placebo or with the painkiller ibuprofen in osteoarthritis sufferers. Glucosamine sulphate was significantly more effective than placebo and equally as effective as ibuprofen. While glucosamine sulphate was well tolerated, 37 per cent of patients suffered adverse drug reactions from the ibuprofen.
Int J Tissue React 14(5):243–51, 1992.

A study carried out by 252 doctors in Portugal on 1,208 arthritis sufferers found that symptoms of pain at rest, on standing and on exercise, and limited active and passive movements, improved significantly in 59 per cent and 'sufficiently' in a further 36 per cent of patients, following supplementation with glucosamine sulphate for approximately two months. The improvement lasted for 6–12 weeks after the end of treatment.
Pharmatherapeutica 3(3):157–68, 1982.

In a study on 26 osteoarthritis sufferers, supplementation with folic acid and vitamin B_{12} were found to be more effective than conventional medications in controlling tenderness of hand joints, and to be free of side-effects as well as significantly cheaper.
Flynn M A et al.: J Am Coll Nutr 13(4):351–6, 1994.

Osteoporosis

Some causative factors

- Excess caffeine consumption
- Excess phosphorus-containing food additives
- Excess protein consumption
- Excess salt consumption
- Excess sugar consumption
- Lack of exercise
- Nutritional deficiencies, especially magnesium, calcium, boron, and vitamins D and K

Magnesium deficiency may be important in the development of osteoporosis.
Voeding 21:424–34, 1960.

Serum vitamin K levels were found to be much lower in 51 elderly women with hip fractures compared with controls. A large number had undetectable levels of vitamin K. The investigators conclude that elderly patients with hip fracture have vitamin K deficiency.
J Bone Miner Res 8(10):1241–5, 1993.

Those who followed a lactovegetarian diet for at least 20 years had only 18 per cent less bone mineral by age 80 compared with 35 per cent less bone in matched meat-eaters.
Am J Clin Nutr 48(3 Suppl):837–41, 1988.

In an analysis of 560 calcium balance studies carried out on 190 women aged 34–69, it was found that to maintain calcium balance, an additional intake of 40 mg calcium is required for every six fluid ounce (177.5 ml) serving of caffeine-containing coffee consumed.
Osteoporos Int 5(2):97–102, 1995.

In a study on 13 individuals consuming a beverage containing two grams of added sugar per kilo body weight, it was found that there were significant calcium losses in urine.
J Nutr 117(7):1229–33, 1987.

The intake of 14 nutrients was measured in 159 women aged 23–75 and compared with bone mineral density. No correlation with calcium intake was found. Higher bone density was associated with higher intakes of iron, zinc and magnesium.
Bone Miner 4(3):265–77, 1988.

Recent studies in young women have shown that a diet high in phosphorus (which is often hidden in the form of food additives) and moderately low in calcium results in the over-secretion of parathyroid hormone, leading to increased calcium losses from bone.
Adv Nutr Res 9:183–207, 1994.

Promising nutritional research

The published literature does not support the value of calcium megadoses against post-menopausal osteoporosis. Magnesium supplementation may be more important. When a magnesium-emphasizing programme was given to 19 post-menopausal women on hormone replacement therapy, a significant increase in mineral bone density occurred within one year.
J Reprod Med 35(5):503–7, 1990.

The effect of magnesium-emphasized supplementation on bone density in a group of post-menopausal women on hormone-replacement therapy was 16 times greater than that of dietary advice alone.
J Nutr Med 2:165–78, 1991.

Healthy older post-menopausal women with a daily calcium intake of less than 400 mg can significantly reduce bone loss by increasing their calcium intake to 800 mg per day.
N Engl J Med 328:878–83, 1990.

Available evidence indicates that post-menopausal women should consume 1,000–1,500 mg of calcium and 400–800 iu of vitamin D daily to minimize bone loss. Vitamin D appears to enhance the effectiveness of supplemental calcium.
J Nutr 126 (4 Suppl):1165S–7S, 1996.

59 healthy post-menopausal women were given calcium supplements, calcium plus zinc, manganese and copper, or placebo, and the rate of bone loss was evaluated over two years. There was no significant difference between calcium and placebo but there was a significant difference between the calcium plus trace mineral and the placebo groups, suggesting that bone loss can be further arrested by administering trace minerals.
J Nutr 124(7):1060–4, 1994.

Vitamin K is required for mineralization of the bone matrix and if supplemented can help to increase the bone mass.
J Clin Invest 91(4):1268, 1993.
Bone 17(1):15–20, 1995.

Undercarboxylation of bone protein (a factor which promotes osteoporosis) is frequently found in post-menopausal women. Supplementation of these women with vitamin K results in an increase in these markers for bone formation, and a reduction in bone loss.
J Nutr 126(4 Suppl):1187S–91S, 1996.

The supplementation of 12 post-menopausal women with boron reduced the total plasma concentration of calcium and the urinary excretion of calcium and magnesium and elevated the serum concentrations of oestradiol and testosterone.
Environ Health Perspect 102 Suppl 7:59–63, 1994.

In a controlled trial on 31 healthy women aged 50–73 years assessing the effects of an exercise programme on bone density, it was found that the lumbar spine bone mineral content of the exercise group increased by 3.5 per cent while in the control group it decreased by 2.7 per cent.
Clin Sci 64(5):541–6, 1983.

Pancreatitis

Some causative factors

- Antioxidant nutrient deficiency
- Free radical attack

Promising nutritional research

To test the hypothesis that acute pancreatitis is a free radical disease, selenium injections were given to eight acute cases in a randomized clinical study. No patients died in this group, whereas 8/9 (89 per cent) of patients in the control group died.
Z Gesamte Inn Med 46(5):145–9, 1991 (in German).

In a 20-week double-blind trial using daily supplements of selenium (600 mcg), beta-carotene (9,000 iu), vitamin C (540 mg), vitamin E (270 iu) and methionine (2 g) on

recurrent pancreatitis, a number of biochemical markers were normalized, particularly those relating to oxidative stress.
Aliment Pharmacol Ther 6(2):229–40, 1992.

Of 330 acute pancreatitis sufferers treated with selenium, there were only eight deaths, and complications occurred only if the selenium treatment was begun too late.
Med Klin 90 Suppl 1:36–41, 1995 (in German).

Parkinson's disease

Some causative factors

- A deficiency of antioxidant nutrients
- Manganese
- Pesticide exposure
- Solvent abuse
- Toxic overload particularly heavy metals (including mercury from silver tooth fillings)

42 parkinsonian patients were compared with controls in terms of environmental factors. A lower risk of the disease was found to be associated with residence in rural areas. A higher risk of contracting the disease seemed to be associated with occupational exposure to manganese, iron and aluminium. Pesticide handling and farm work did not seem to be associated with Parkinson's disease.
Can J Neurol Sci 17(3):286–91, 1990 (in French).

Possible disease-causing factors were assessed in 130 cases of Parkinson's disease. A family history of the disease was the strongest predictor of risk, followed by head trauma then occupational use of herbicides (weed-killers).
Neurology 43(6):1173–80, 1993.

Rates of death from Parkinson's disease (PD) in Michigan were compared with exposure to heavy metals. Areas with a paper, chemical, iron or copper-related industry showed significantly higher death rates from PD than areas without these industries. The investigators suggest that there is a geographical association between PD mortality and the industrial use of heavy metals.
Mov Disord 8(1):87–92, 1993.

Data on environmental and other factors, including pesticide exposure, heavy metals, general anaesthesia and head trauma, were collected from 380 parkinsonian patients and compared with controls. Factors which appeared to increase the risk of parkinsonism included cigarette smoking, pesticide use, amalgam (silver) tooth fillings, exposure to wood preservatives, general anaesthesia, head injury, and the presence of parkinsonism in other family members.
Neurology 46(5):1275–84, 1996.

A patient who abused solvents developed Parkinson's disease and responded to the treatment usually given for parkinsonism, levodopa.
Ann Neurol 35(5):616–9, 1994.

Promising nutritional research

High doses of vitamins C and E administered to patients with early Parkinson's disease delayed the need for levodopa by an average of 2.5 years compared with control patients. This study was intended to test the endogenous toxin hypothesis of Parkinson's disease (the development of parkinsonism as a result of 'internal pollution').
Am J Clin Nutr 53(1) Suppl:380S–2S, 1991.

In 11 patients with previously untreated Parkinson's disease, treated with supplements of the amino acid L-methionine for two weeks to six months, there were improvements in movement and rigidity within about three weeks. The effects of this treatment were comparable to those obtained with the conventional treatment L-dopa.
Rev Neurol 138(4):297–303, 1982 (in French).

10 parkinsonian patients were given supplements of the amino acid L-tyrosine. For some, three years of L-tyrosine treatment was followed by better clinical results and fewer side-effects than with conventional treatments.
C R Acad Sci III 309(2):43–7, 1989 (in French).

Periodontal (gum) disease

Some causative factors

- Coenzyme Q10 deficiency
- Poor oral hygiene

Promising nutritional research

Six people with varying degrees of gum disease experienced a reduction in bleeding and inflammation after 30–100 mg CoQ10 was administered for 6–12 weeks.
Biomed and Clin Aspects of CoQ10 4:6–11, 1991.

Periods, painful

Some causative factors

- Essential fatty acid deficiency
- Magnesium deficiency

An assessment of the diets of 181 women with painful periods revealed that the problem was significantly worse among those with a low intake of dietary fish oils.
Eur J Clin Nutr 49(7):508–16, 1995.

Promising nutritional research

In a double-blind study, 21 out of 25 women with painful periods treated with magnesium supplements showed a reduction in symptoms.
Zentralbl Gynakol 111(11):755–60, 1989 (in German).

In a randomized double-blind trial on 32 women with painful periods, those treated with magnesium supplements for six cycles had less back pain and lower abdominal pain on the second and third day of the cycle, and markedly less absence from work than the control group.
Schweiz Rundsch Med Prax 79(16):491–4, 1990 (in German).

42 adolescents with painful periods were given either fish oil supplements or placebo. The fish oil group experienced a significant improvement in symptoms after two months.
Am J Obstet Gynecol 174(4):1335–8, 1996.

Pregnancy-related problems (Also see Birth defects)

Some causative factors

- Moderate and high alcohol consumption
- Nutritional deficiencies, especially zinc, magnesium, calcium, selenium, folic acid
- Smoking

On the basis of low serum, hair and white blood cell levels, it would appear that at least 5 mg per day of additional zinc is required in pregnancy, which is not covered by the diet or available from material reserves. The risk of deficiency is real, and is associated with miscarriage, toxaemia of pregnancy, treatment-resistant anaemia, abnormally prolonged pregnancy and difficult delivery. In babies it is associated with decreased immunity, learning or memory disorders or birth defects.
Rev Fe Gynecol Obstet 85(1):13–27, 1990.

High-dosage iron and folic acid supplements prescribed by doctors for pregnant women can seriously lower zinc levels or inhibit zinc absorption.
Am J Clin Nutr 43:258–62, 1986.

Serum selenium levels were measured in women who had miscarried, and compared with pregnant women and healthy volunteers. Although it is usual for selenium levels to decline in pregnancy, those who had miscarried had significantly lower selenium levels than normal. The authors recommend that research to assess the benefits of selenium supplementation should be carried out.
Br J Obstet Gynaecol 103(2):130–2, 1996.

Cigarette-smoking habits were compared in 574 women who had suffered miscarriages, and 320 control women who had carried a baby to term. Women who had miscarried tended to smoke more often than controls. Smoking mothers had an 80 per cent higher risk of miscarriage than non-smoking mothers.
N Engl J Med 297(15):793–6, 1977.

Alcohol and smoking habits were recorded in 32,019 women at their first visit to an antenatal clinic and compared with rates of miscarriage. Women consuming 1–2 alcoholic drinks daily were twice as likely as non-drinkers to miscarry in the second trimester of pregnancy (15–27 weeks), and women consuming more than three drinks daily had more than three times the risk of miscarriage.
Lancet 2(8187):173–6, 1980.

A meta-analysis was carried out on trials using calcium supplements to treat pre-eclampsia (a condition involving high blood pressure in pregnancy). The pooled analysis showed a significant reduction in systolic and diastolic blood pressure. Compared with placebo, calcium supplementation reduced the risk of pre-eclampsia by more than 60 per cent.
JAMA 275(14):1113–7, 1996.

Promising nutritional research

In 27 pregnant women with pregnancy-induced high blood pressure, supplemented with magnesium, there was a significant reduction in mean blood pressure. The babies born to the magnesium-treated group spent fewer days in the neonatal intensive care unit.
Acta Obstet Gynecol Scand 70(6):445–50, 1991.

Eclampsia, in which high blood pressure is associated with convulsions in pregnancy and can lead to death, may be treated with magnesium, the tranquillizer diazepam or the anticonvulsant drug phenytoin. Outcomes of these three treatments were compared in 1,687 randomized women. Women allocated magnesium treatment had a 52 per cent lower rate of recurrent convulsions than those allocated diazepam and a 67 per cent lower risk compared with phenytoin. Women allocated magnesium treatment were also less likely to develop complications and to be admitted to intensive care, as were their babies.
Collaborative Eclampsia Trial. Lancet 345(8969):1455–63, 1995.

Premenstrual syndrome (PMS)

Some causative factors

- Deficiencies of magnesium, calcium, B vitamins or essential fatty acids
- Poor diet

The average red blood cell magnesium levels were significantly lower in a group of PMS sufferers compared with normal women.
Am J Clin Nutr 34(11):2364–6, 1981.

While plasma magnesium levels appeared to be normal, red cell magnesium levels were significantly lower than normal in a group of 105 patients with premenstrual syndrome.
Ann Clin Biochem 23(Pt 6):667–70, 1986.

Concentrations of all metabolites of the essential fatty acid linoleic acid were significantly reduced in 43 women with well-defined premenstrual syndrome, suggesting that there was a defect in their ability to convert linoleic acid to gamma-linolenic acid (GLA).
Am J Obstet Gynecol 150(4):363–6, 1984.

Promising nutritional research

Evening primrose oil significantly alleviated premenstrual symptoms – especially premenstrual depression – in a group of 30 women with severe premenstrual syndrome.
J Reprod Med 30(3):149–53, 1985.

Results of randomized trials and open studies in 291 patients with severe breast pain show that a good response is obtained from evening primrose oil supplementation in 45 per cent of cases where the breast pain is of the premenstrual variety.
Lancet 2(8451):373–7, 1985.

Two women with a history of menstrual-related migraines supplemented with a combination of vitamin D and calcium reported a major reduction in their headaches and premenstrual symptoms within two months of beginning therapy.
Headache 34(9):544–6, 1994.

In a randomized double-blind crossover trial comparing calcium supplementation with placebo in 33 women with premenstrual syndrome, it was found that the supplements significantly reduced negative emotions, fluid retention and pain.
Psychopharmacol Bull 27(2):145–8, 1991.

In a randomized double-blind crossover trial comparing calcium supplementation with placebo in 78 women with premenstrual syndrome, it was found that after three months there was a significant reduction in negative emotions, fluid retention and pain. Period pain was also reduced. The investigators conclude that calcium supplementation is a simple, effective treatment for premenstrual syndrome.
J Gen Intern Med 4(3):183–9, 1989.

In a randomized double-blind crossover trial, the effectiveness of vitamin B_6 supplementation at 50 mg per day for three months against premenstrual syndrome was compared with placebo in 63 women. The B_6 group observed a significant beneficial effect on emotional symptoms: depression, irritability and fatigue.
J R Coll Gen Pract 39(326):364–8, 1989.

617 patients diagnosed with premenstrual syndrome were randomized to treatment with vitamin B_6 supplements or placebo in a double-blind trial. A global assessment after three cycles revealed significant improvement in the B_6 group.
J Int Med Res 13(3):174–9, 1985.

In a study on 11 premenstrual women there was laboratory evidence of significant deficiencies in vitamin B_6 and magnesium. Other deficiencies also occurred frequently. A multivitamin/mineral supplement was found to correct some of these deficiencies and, at the appropriate dosage, to improve symptoms.
J Reprod Med 32(6):435–41, 1987.

21 patients with severe premenstrual breast pain were given either a low-fat, high complex carbohydrate diet or general dietary advice. After six months there was a significant reduction in symptoms in the first group.
Lancet 2(8603):128–32, 1988.

Fluid retention symptoms decreased in a group of women with premenstrual syndrome who were placed on a low-fat diet (20 per cent of calories from fat).
Physiol Behav 40(4)483–7, 1987.

In a randomized double-blind study comparing vitamin E supplementation with placebo against premenstrual syndrome in 46 women, there was a significant improvement in emotional and physical symptoms.
J Reprod Med 32(6):400–4, 1987.

In a double-blind randomized study, the efficacy of vitamin E supplements at different doses was compared with placebo on 75 women with benign breast disease suffering from premenstrual symptoms. Vitamin E supplementation improved three of the four classes of PMS symptoms and was significantly more effective than placebo.
J Am Coll Nutr 2(2):115–22, 1983.

A multi-nutrient product 'Optivite' was administered to 31 women with premenstrual syndrome for six menstrual cycles. The symptom score before menstrual periods decreased from 31.5 to 10.3. The best responses were seen in women taking 6–12 tablets a day for three or more cycles.
J Reprod Med 28(8):527–31, 1983.

Prostate enlargement and prostatitis

Some causative factors

- Essential fatty acid deficiency
- Toxic overload
- Zinc deficiency

Promising nutritional research

In a study on 15 patients with chronic prostatitis and prostatodynia, the pollen extract Cernilton brought either complete and lasting relief of symptoms or a marked improvement

in 13. The product is believed to have anti-inflammatory and anti-hormonal properties.
Br J Urol 64(5):496–9, 1989.

In a study using the pollen extract Cernilton N on 90 patients with chronic prostatitis, 78 per cent of those without complicating factors had a favourable response including 36 per cent who were cured of their symptoms.
Br J Urol 71(4):433–8, 1993.

A decrease in zinc levels and increase in cadmium levels has been implicated in prostate abnormalities. Cadmium stimulates prostate growth. When present at high levels in laboratory studies, selenium inhibits the stimulatory effect of cadmium on prostate cells.
Biochem Biophys Res Commun 127(3):871–7, 1985.

Psoriasis

Some causative factors

- Alcohol consumption
- Fruit and vegetable deficiency
- Nutritional deficiencies
- Sluggish liver function

In a study on 100 patients with chronic psoriasis, heavy alcohol consumption was significantly more common in the most severe cases, in men.
Dermatologica 172(2):57–60, 1986.

The diets of psoriasis patients from 14 hospitals in Italy were compared with controls. Overweight was significantly associated with a higher risk of psoriasis. The consumption of higher amounts of carrots, tomatoes, fresh fruit and foods containing beta-carotene appeared to be the most protective against the disease.
Br J Dermatol 134(1):101–6, 1996.

Promising nutritional research

Psoriasis sufferers given fish oil capsules experienced a significant reduction in symptoms.
Br J Dermatol 117(5):599–606, 1987.
Lancet 1(8582):378–80, 1988.

18 patients with psoriasis received capsules of fish oil or placebo together with ultraviolet therapy for 15 weeks. The patients in the fish oil group improved significantly compared with the placebo group.
Br J Dermatol 120(6):801–7, 1989.

17 patients with psoriasis were given supplements containing a combination of fish oil, linoleic acid and gamma-linolenic acid (GLA). After four months good or moderate improvement had occurred in 10 patients.
Acta Derm Venereol 69(3):265–8, 1989.

30 patients with psoriasis vulgaris were given a low-fat diet and fish oil supplements for four months. Moderate or excellent improvement was observed in 58 per cent.
Acta Derm Venereol 69(1):23–8, 1989.

Vitamin D_3 was administered orally (for six months) or topically (for eight weeks) to 40 patients with psoriasis. Improvement was observed in 75 per cent of those who received the higher oral doses of the vitamin, and in 84 per cent of those who received the vitamin topically. [Vitamin D_3 is found in cod liver oil.]
Br J Dermatol 115(4):421–9, 1986.

Raynaud's disease

Some causative factors

- Essential fatty acid deficiency
- Possibly magnesium deficiency

Promising nutritional research

32 patients with primary or secondary Raynaud's disease were randomly given either 12 fish oil capsules or olive oil capsules daily, and followed up after six and 12 weeks, at which times they were asked to place their fingers in cold water and the time of onset of Raynaud's symptoms were noted. In the fish oil group at six weeks the average time interval before the loss of circulation began increased from 31 minutes to 46 minutes. At the 6-week and 12-week visits, five out of 11 of the primary Raynaud's patients in the fish oil group could not be induced to develop Raynaud's, compared with only one out of nine patients in the control group.
Am J Med 86(2):158–64, 1989.

Rheumatoid arthritis

Some causative factors

- Essential fatty acid deficiency
- Food allergy or intolerance

25 patients with psoriatic arthritis (arthritis with psoriasis) were compared with controls and found to have lower levels of omega–6 essential fatty acids and serum selenium, and higher levels of saturated fatty acids and plasma copper. The investigators conclude that an abnormal fatty acid pattern may play a part in the development of rheumatic diseases.
J Rheumatol 22(1):103–8, 1985.

Promising nutritional research

An experimental diet high in polyunsaturated fat with a daily supplement of EPA resulted in improvement in morning stiffness and a number of tender joints after 12 weeks.
Lancet 1(8422):184–7, 1985.

In a 24-week trial using high doses of blackcurrant seed oil (which is high in GLA) on rheumatoid arthritis sufferers, signs and symptoms of disease activity were significantly reduced.
Br J Rheumatol 33(9):847–52, 1994.

1.4 grams per day of GLA (as borage seed oil) resulted in a clinically important reduction in the signs and symptoms of disease activity.
Ann Intern Med 119(9):867–73, 1993.

94 patients with rheumatoid arthritis were given either an allergen-free or a low-allergen diet for 12 weeks. Nine patients showed a favourable response and relapsed when the diet was stopped.
Ann Rheum Dis 51(3):298–302, 1992.

In a blind, placebo-controlled study, patients with rheumatoid arthritis showed a significant improvement during periods of dietary therapy, compared with placebo.
Lancet 1(8475):236–8, 1986.

Numerous peer-reviewed studies have established the value of supplementation with fish oils in reducing tender joints and morning stiffness in patients with rheumatoid arthritis. Recent studies also suggest that some patients no longer require non-steroidal anti-inflammatory drugs while taking fish oil supplements.
Lipids 31 Suppl:S243–7, 1996.

Schizophrenia

Some causative factors

- Abnormal essential fatty acid metabolism
- Deficiencies of vitamins C, B_3 and/or B_6, folic acid or zinc
- Food allergy
- Gluten intolerance

- Heavy metal poisoning
- Histamine imbalances
- Prenatal (before birth) starvation
- Starvation

Low levels of coenzyme Q10 were found in a group of schizophrenic patients compared with normals.
Jap J Psych Neurol 43(2):143–5, 1989.

Biochemical markers of vitamin B_1, B_2 and B_6 deficiency were measured in 172 successive admissions to a hospital psychiatric unit. 53 per cent of the patients were deficient in at least one vitamin and 12 per cent in more than one. Schizophrenics tended to be deficient in vitamin B_1, and mood disorder patients to be deficient in B_2 and B_6.
Br J Psychiatry 141:271–2, 1982.

The vitamin B_1 status of 42 physically healthy non-alcoholic psychiatric patients was measured by assessing transketolase activity. 16 of the patients showed evidence of vitamin B_1 deficiency, despite, in some cases, having received vitamin B_1-containing supplements for up to six weeks before testing.
J Clin Psychiatry 40(10):427–9, 1979.

Comparisons between mentally ill subjects with and without mercury amalgam (silver) tooth fillings revealed significant differences in reports of mental health. Subjects who had amalgam fillings removed reported a subsequent reduction or disappearance of mental symptoms.
Am J Psychother 43(4):575–87, 1989.

Current evidence indicates that a disturbance in the balance of trace elements in the human body can lead to various psychiatric syndromes. The role of trace elements is important in treatment and prevention.
Br J Hosp Med 32(2):77–9, 1984.

Zinc deficiency during pregnancy may give rise to schizophrenia in genetically susceptible offspring.
Med Hypotheses 31(2):141–53, 1990.

Essential fatty acids and the prostaglandins derived from them are important regulators of nerve cell function. There is evidence that the production of prostaglandin E1 is impaired in schizophrenia. Clinical trials with E1 and its precursors GLA and DGLA have shown modest therapeutic benefits.
Prostaglandins Leukot Essent Fatty Acids 46(1):71–7, 1992.

Four lines of evidence in the literature support prenatal nutritional deficiencies as a plausible risk factor for the development of schizophrenia. For instance prenatal malnutrition affects maternal functions which are critical to the nervous system of the developing foetus.
J Nerv Ment Dis 184(2):71–85.

The risk of schizophrenia was compared in individuals exposed or not exposed to the Dutch Hunger Winter of 1944–45 in Holland. It was found that those conceived at the height of the famine were twice as likely to develop schizophrenia.
Arch Gen Psychiatry 53(1):25–31, 1996.

Promising nutritional research

Vitamin C seems to have an increased turnover in schizophrenia patients and supplementation appears to help them.
Nutrition Report 8(9):65–72, 1990.

Folic acid treatment for sub-acute degeneration of the spinal cord due to folate deficiency was associated with an improvement in the patient's mental condition, diagnosed as schizophrenia.
Ir Med J 83(2):73–4, 1990.

Folic acid supplementation may alleviate symptoms in psychiatric illness.
Lancet 336:392–5, 1990.

33 per cent of 123 patients with acute clinical depression or schizophrenia were found to be folate deficient. After treatment with methylfolate or placebo for six months in addition to their standard psychiatric drugs, those given methylfolate had experienced a significantly improved clinical and social recovery.
Br J Psychiatry 159:271–2, 1991.

Trials treating schizophrenia with essential fatty acids or prostaglandins have shown modestly promising results, particularly those where essential fatty acids were combined with nutritional supplements.
Prostaglandins Leukot Essent Fatty Acids 46(1):67–70, 1992.

In a controlled study of red cell membrane fatty acids in schizophrenia patients, both omega–3 and omega–6 fatty acids were at low levels, particularly arachidonic acid and docosahexaenoic acid. While dietary fatty acid intake was not abnormal, a higher intake of omega–3 fatty acids was associated with less severe symptoms. A significant improvement in symptoms was obtained with supplementation of 10 g per day of fish oil supplements.
Lipids 31 Suppl:S163–5, 1996.

Stroke

Some causative factors

- Flavonoid deficiency

The dietary intake of 552 men aged 50 to 69 years was followed up for 15 years. The lowest intake of dietary flavonoids – particularly quercetin – was associated with the highest risk of developing a stroke. A reduced stroke risk was also associated with higher beta carotene intakes from vegetables. About 70 per cent of the total flavonoid intake consisted of black tea. The researchers conclude that the habitual intake of flavonoids and their major source (tea) may protect against stroke.
Arch Intern Med 156(6):637–42, 1996.

Promising nutritional research

A remarkable (82 per cent) decrease in blood platelet adhesiveness (blood stickiness) was found after the administration of 400 iu vitamin E to normal volunteers for two weeks.
Blood 73(1):141–9, 1989.

400 iu vitamin E per day may be a near optimal dose of vitamin E to reduce platelet adhesiveness.
Thromb Res 49(4):393–404, 1988.

Systemic lupus erythematosus

Some causative factors

- Possible antioxidant deficiency
- Possible nutritional deficiencies
- Possible toxic overload

Promising nutritional research

Treatment with the hormone dehydroepiandrosterone (DHEA), sold as a dietary supplement, for 3–6 months in SLE patients with mild to moderate disease resulted in an improvement in indices for overall SLE activity.
Arthritis Rheum 37(9):1305–10, 1994.

In a double-blind, placebo-controlled trial, treatment for three months with the hormone DHEA on 28 women with SLE resulted in a decrease in disease activity whereas the placebo group experienced a small increase in disease activity.
Arthritis Rheum 38(12):1826–31, 1995.

Auto-immune diseases such as lupus erythematosus can result from destructive enzymes which escape from lysosomes (digestive particles found inside cells) whose membranes have been damaged by lipid peroxidation. If these enzymes attack and denature normal tissue proteins the immune system may treat the proteins as 'non-self' and initiate antibody attacks. The investigators gave large doses of vitamin E to patients with auto-immune diseases on the grounds that it is a physiological stabilizer of cellular and lysosomal

membranes. Finding that lupus and several other diseases responded to the supplements, the researchers postulate that vitamin E deficiency may be involved in the onset of auto-immune diseases by promoting damage to lysosome membranes.
Cutis 21(3):321–5, 1978.

Tinnitus (see Hearing problems)

Ulcerative colitis (see Colitis)

Ulcers

Some causative factors

• Zinc deficiency

Promising nutritional research

Chronic leg ulcers are associated with low serum zinc levels and healing is promoted by zinc supplementation.
J Parenter Enteral Nutr 9(3):364–9, 1985.

In a randomized, controlled clinical trial comparing the effectiveness of vitamin A supplements with that of De-Nol liquid, sucralfate and pirenzepine against chronic gastric ulcers, all treatments resulted in a significant reduction in ulcer size. In the second week the dynamic of ulcer healing was the most favourable in the vitamin A group.
Acta Physiol Hung 64(3–4):379–84, 1984.

In a double-blind study on 18 patients, those taking zinc sulphate supplements had a gastric ulcer healing rate three times that of patients treated with placebo.
Med J Aust 2(21):793–6, 1975.

36 of 50 patients with gastric and duodenal ulcer treated with a vitamin U preparation experienced a reduction or complete disappearance of their main clinical symptoms. Gastric secretion, motor activity and emptying of the stomach and permeability of the secretory cells of the stomach were significantly improved and there were signs of regenerative processes in the stomach.
Tsimmerman YaS et al.: TER.ARKH (USSR) 48(3):29–35, 1976.

Urticaria

Some causative factors

• Food allergy or intolerance

Promising nutritional research

64 patients with urticaria were given a diet free of items to which individuals are commonly sensitive, including food additives. Symptoms ceased or were greatly reduced within two weeks on the diet in 73 per cent of the patients. Follow-up at six months showed complete remission in 46 per cent of those on the diet.
Acta Derm Venereol 75(6):484–7, 1995.

SECTION 3

You and Your Family

Slimmers

The first thing to remember about losing weight is that your body will base its long-term weight on your habits over several months. So there's no point in starving yourself for a week and then going back to the same diet that you followed previously. You will simply go back to the same weight that you were previously! In fact, if you follow too many 'crash' diets, you can end up slowing down your metabolism permanently, so that after every diet, you end up weighing a bit *more* than you did before, without eating more. When your body thinks it is in starvation mode, it slows down its metabolism, trying to make each calorie go further and last longer. The result is an increased tendency to put on weight.

Although hormones, toxins and other substances can affect the rate at which we burn calories, the basic formula for weight loss is always the same: if calorie output (exercise) is less than calorie input (food), body weight increases. If calorie output is more than calorie input, body weight decreases. Most people think that they cannot lose weight because a weight-loss diet leaves them feeling too hungry. In fact everyone can lose weight without feeling hungry. The problem is keeping down consumption of those highly addictive high-calorie sugary, fatty foods and alcoholic drinks.

One of the biggest mistakes made by slimmers is the 'all or nothing' syndrome. If you have tried, unsuccessfully, to slim several times, you may have gone straight from your usual diet to a severely punishing regime, allowing yourself only salad meals, small amounts of other low-calorie foods, and cutting out all treats. As your body slowed down its metabolism, and you lost energy and started to feel depressed, you probably developed irresistible cravings for all the 'forbidden' foods and either succumbed to them little by little or decided that you could stop the diet since you had lost a few pounds. Every slimmer knows the depression of regaining those few pounds within 24 hours. They are just water which is always lost when the body's carbohydrate reserves are low, and regained immediately after normal eating is resumed.

Don't fall into the 'all or nothing' syndrome. Plan a diet which is low in fattening foods, but which allows you a small treat every day so that you have something to look forward to and don't feel too deprived. If you have a tendency to food addictions, don't select a treat that you are seriously addicted to! The following tips are all helpful.

Do

- Eat three meals a day, especially breakfast.
- Each meal should contain a little protein. Protein plus vegetables is an ideal meal and keeps you feeling full for longer.
- Cut out fat from your diet, but not oils. We need a little oil every day. The ideal is a few nuts or some sunflower seeds at the end of each meal, or a teaspoon of tahini (creamed sesame seeds) in soup or gravy or spread on toast.
- The smallest meal of the day should be dinner.
- Have a pan of home-made vegetable soup ready to heat up whenever you feel hungry. It fills the stomach while being low in calories. If away from home use miso soup (a nutritious Japanese broth available in packets, which you can stir into a cup of hot water).
- Adding oat bran to hot soups and stews helps you feel fuller.
- Decide on your daily 'treat'. Make sure it is something you have to buy every day. Do not be tempted to keep a supply of it at home.
- If you are addicted to chocolate, have a hot chocolate drink or some chocolate blanc-mange instead of a chocolate bar (which is almost 100 per cent sugar and fat).
- Eat low-fat varieties of cheese and spreads.
- Eat wholemeal bread and brown rice rather than white. They contain fewer calories for the same weight.
- Eat fruit and raw vegetables or hot soup if you need something between meals.
- Your drinks should be water, water and water. Your body needs it to help flush out the waste products which are released as you lose weight.
- Exercise will help you lose weight. Strength-building exercises (ask in your local gym) are the best form, since they improve your lean-to-fat ratio, which makes for a faster metabolism.

Don't

- Don't diet if your weight is normal or less than normal. What looks to you like body fat may be poorly toned lean tissue which just needs the right exercises.
- Don't eat all cold food unless you really enjoy it. It can increase depression and cravings.
- Do not eat or drink sugary things except as part of a meal, otherwise they may make you feel more hungry later.
- Don't eat fried food or food cooked in fat or in batter.
- Eating too much salt makes you retain fluid which adds to your weight.
- Don't eat creamy sauces or dips unless guaranteed low fat.
- Don't eat anything made from minced meat unless you have seen what went into the mincer. It is quite lawful to sell meat as 'lean' when it is one-third fat.
- Don't go on a total deprivation regime. It doesn't work.
- Don't go back to your old habits once you reach your target weight. If you want to keep your new figure, you will need to continue rationing the most fattening foods.

Remember

- Potatoes themselves are not fattening. It is what people cook them in and put on them that makes them fattening.
- Alcoholic drinks are fattening.
- Most foods and drinks which taste very sweet are fattening unless they are artificially sweetened.

If a low-calorie diet doesn't work

- See a nutritional therapist for help with meal balancing and detoxification, especially if you tend to have a low body temperature. Nutritional therapists can also help you identify food allergies. These sometimes cause fluid retention amounting to 8 or more pounds in weight.

Supplements

- B vitamins 50 mg/day and magnesium 100 mg/day to aid energy metabolism
- Vitamin C 1 gram/day to aid toxin release
- Carnitine 500 mg/day to assist fat metabolism.

Your Immune System: Resisting Illness

Also see Section II, Immune system impairment and *Appendix IV, An end to the common cold.*

There is a lot of talk about 'boosting' the immune system with vitamin supplements. This gives the mistaken impression that the more vitamins you take, the better you will be able to resist illness. While this is simply not true, it *is* true that a poor diet and faulty lifestyle can be definitely harmful to the immune system, resulting in lowered immunity. If you then improve your diet and use supplements to help repair damage done by nutritional deficiencies, you may well see an improvement, which is really a normalization, of your immunity. Many nutritional deficiencies have been found to have harmful effects on the immune system, especially vitamins A, B_6, C, E, selenium and zinc.

Diet advice

Follow the healthy eating guidelines in Appendix I.

Supplements

If you live in a low-selenium area such as the UK or New Zealand, and especially if you are a vegetarian, it is important to take a daily selenium supplement of up to 100 mcg.

Other suggested daily supplements are

- Vitamin C 1,000 mg
- Vitamin E 200 iu
- Zinc 10 mg
- Multivitamin providing vitamins A and B complex
- Coenzyme Q10

High levels of pesticides in the human body have been found to impair immunity. Once these levels have been reduced, immunity improves. Some of the above nutritional supplements will aid this process. Others are listed below in *Coping with pollution* on page 299.

Recreational drugs such as heroin and 'poppers' (nitrites used as aphrodisiacs) can severely damage the immune system and have been implicated as the primary cause of the immune depletion found in Aids.

Stress

There are several different types of stress.

Emotional stress

Emotional stress can take many different forms, and may be caused by
- Long-term, seemingly hopeless situations such as living with a bullying parent or partner, being disabled or having to take care of a disabled spouse or relative, or being in a job which you hate but feel that you cannot leave, or long-term unemployment.
- Shorter-term, often more intense situations which must be borne for a while, such as coping with illness, injury or bereavement, divorce, financial problems, loss of home or job, or a lawsuit.
- Stressful incidents such as being stuck in a traffic jam while late for an important appointment, having a row with your boss or someone you live with, a burglary, mugging or theft of your property, or burst water pipes. Even moving house is recognized by experts as being near the top of the list of the most stress-causing events.

Physical stress

Chronic physical stress is suffered by many people, often those in executive positions or with a heavy social calendar. They may work extremely long hours, battle against constant deadlines, and/or feel that they have to fit many activities into their leisure time, with little thought for their body's needs for rest and sleep. Some jobs, like those of ambulance drivers, firemen or police are subject to regular episodes of extreme physical and mental stress.

Nutritional stress

Certain substances which you eat or drink can mimic the effects of emotional and physical stress by causing the same hormones to be released. Caffeine, for example, found in tea and coffee, is a central nervous system stimulant which can increase feelings of stress and anxiety. Sugary foods can increase the body's production of insulin, which if too high may lead to the release of stress hormones such as adrenaline, as the body attempts to balance the blood sugar. Like stress, salt can also raise the blood pressure.

Tea, coffee and sugary or salty snacks are often consumed in large amounts by people who are under a lot of physical stress. Someone who is always short of time may miss meals and eat instead what is most easily available: salted peanuts, burgers, crisps, biscuits and chocolate.

There are no magic foods which you can eat to prevent feeling stressed, but there are several important steps you can take hopefully to prevent some of the harmful effects which stress can have on your health.
- *See Appendix I for healthy eating guidelines.*
- Plan your meals. If you know that you will be working late, take food with you to work, or ensure that when you get home there is something quick and easy to heat up. Vegetable soups and stews are ideal and can also be placed in a thermos flask.
- Plan your sleep. Your body needs sleep to regenerate and heal itself.

- Try to think more about planning your life around your body's needs rather than always putting your life first. Treat your body like a friend whom you love, not a machine to be driven without proper maintenance until it breaks down.
- If you find it impossible to relax, go to meditation classes and learn!
- Constant high levels of stress hormones have an adverse effect on the immune system.
- There is no substitute for reducing your stress levels if at all possible. Do you really need to be in your present home or work situation? Could anyone else share your responsibilities? Could you consider seeing a counsellor to help you discuss options you may not have thought of?

Supplements

B vitamins and magnesium help to keep the nervous system healthy. If you have been under a lot of strain they may have become depleted. Supplements could help to insure against this. To help prevent illness, you may wish to think about increasing your intake of antioxidants such as vitamins C, E, selenium and glutathione.

Children

Children can become fussy eaters, refusing vegetables and accepting only foods like chips, canned soup, burgers and ice cream. It is important to remember that if they are not given these foods they cannot develop a taste for them. Problems may occur because commercial foods are often highly flavoured. Canned or packet soups, for instance, contain sugar, salt, flavour-enhancing additives and artificial flavourings. Compared with such foods, home-cooking may seem bland. Then if children learn that by refusing to eat it they will get their favourite foods instead, you will have difficulty enticing them to eat anything else!

It is worth trying to get children to eat a healthy diet. A poorly balanced diet can have harmful effects on a child's behaviour, learning and athletic ability and immune system. With childhood asthma rates rising steeply, all protective measures to help prevent damage to your child's immune system will be worthwhile.

Breaking the habit

Breaking fussy eating habits is difficult, but there are some avenues you can explore. First, your child may have developed a mild zinc deficiency, which is not unusual in those consuming a diet high in sugary, fatty foods. One of the symptoms of zinc deficiency is a deterioration in the sense of taste and smell. Quite simply, bland foods taste blander, and it may be that the only foods your child can actually taste are those containing a lot of salt, sugar, flavouring and flavour enhancers. Check to see how much salt your child adds to meals – this is sometimes a good indicator of deficient taste buds. A zinc supplement designed for children may in time help wean your child off bad habits, provided that junk foods are, at least temporarily, withdrawn.

Second, you may find that making your home cooking more interesting and tasty will help. Children like colourful food – crunchy raw red and green peppers in a salad, with peanuts and carrot sticks may be found appetizing when boiled cabbage is not! And why not imitate the food companies? Putting lots of herbs, seasoning, some lemon juice and even a little honey into a vegetable soup may appeal to your child's taste buds. You can gradually reduce any excessive seasoning over a period of time.

At school

If school meals leave a lot to be desired, a packed lunch may be the answer: a thermos of hot soup, a small chopped salad with nuts, wholemeal bread sandwiches and fruit. A tight control over your child's pocket money may help to avoid peer pressure from other children leading to the over-consumption of sweets, or even to smoking habits.

Failure to thrive

Research has shown that low vitamin A levels in children are linked with growth problems related to a lack of growth hormone (*Lancet 343(8889):87–8, 1994*).

Supplements

Since it is not always possible to know what your child is consuming when away from home, it may be a good idea to give your child a daily multivitamin with minerals as an insurance policy. A child's academic performance cannot be improved by supplements if the child is not nutritionally deficient, but supplements can help to prevent a deficiency.

Vegetarians and vegans

Most vegetarians have been told 'you'll get ill if you don't eat meat'! Some have heard this so often that they begin to lack confidence in vegetarianism as a healthy lifestyle. While certain basic precautions need to be taken, you can rest assured that vegetarianism and veganism are both perfectly compatible with good health. In fact, studies have shown that these lifestyles can be healthier than an omnivorous regime. Nevertheless, vegetarians who rely heavily on dairy produce should remember that these foods can contribute substantial amounts of saturated animal fat to the diet.

Potential concerns about veganism include sufficiency of protein and vitamin B_{12}. Vegetable proteins are often low in some amino acids. These are known as the 'limiting' amino acids, for instance lysine in grains and seeds, and methionine in pulses. This has given rise to a concept that vegans, who eat only plant foods, should carefully combine their foods to ensure that each meal provides a good balance of all essential amino acids. But several human studies have shown that this is not necessary, at least in healthy volunteers eating calorie-adequate rice-based diets. Volunteers eating diets in which the protein was derived virtually only from rice, compared with those eating both rice and chicken, have shown no significant difference in nitrogen balance, indicating that their protein intake was sufficient. Rice as the sole source of their protein still provided between 1.5 and 4.5 times the WHO recommended amounts of all essential amino acids. The American Dietetic Association now confirms that, because amino acids obtained from food can combine with amino acids made in the body, it is not necessary for vegans or vegetarians to combine protein foods at each meal. The ADA also states that soy protein has been shown to be nutritionally equivalent in protein value to animal protein and can thus serve as the sole source of protein intake if desired. Nuts are also a good source of protein.

Although vitamin B_{12} is only found in animal foods, vegans survive because our requirements for this vitamin are very small. Yeast extracts used as food flavourings are often fortified with vitamin B_{12}, and vegans should ensure that they consume such foods regularly, or some other product with a guaranteed vitamin B_{12} content, such as a B_{12} supplement. Algae and seaweeds are sometimes promoted as plant sources of this vitamin, but it is now known that they contain only vitamin B_{12} *analogues* – substances which are quite similar to vitamin B_{12} but may actually block the bioavailability of the real vitamin.

Good protein foods for vegetarians and vegans

	Comments
Nuts	Low in lysine, rich in methionine
Seeds	Low in lysine, rich in methionine
Peanuts	Low in lysine and methionine
Soya	In general low in methionine.
products	Soya concentrates may be better.
Dairy produce	
(eggs, milk, yoghurt, cheese)	Well balanced
Grains	Low in lysine, some (e.g. rice) are rich in methionine
Pulses	Low in methionine and tryptophan, rich in lysine
Rice	Low in tryptophan and threonine

Fruits and most vegetables are low in protein and eaten alone do not form a balanced diet.

Supplements

Vegetarians have been found to have lower levels of some minerals such as copper, zinc and especially selenium in their blood (*Kadrabova J et al.: Selenium status, plasma zinc, copper and magnesium in vegetarians. Biol Trace Elem Res 50(1):13–24, 1995*). This may be because meat and fish provide substantial amounts of these minerals (the diets of livestock are frequently fortified), but other foods do not. Crops grown with artificial fertilizer may be lacking in minerals. These fertilizers contain little more than nitrate, which helps the plant to grow but does nothing to replenish the mineral content of the soil. As minerals such as zinc in the soil become ever more depleted by constant crop-growing, the content of these minerals found in crops is becoming less and less. So it may be a sensible precaution for vegetarians to take a daily multimineral supplement.

The Single Person

Single people may be especially at risk of eating poorly. They often say 'it's hardly worth cooking a meal just for myself.' Snacking on packet foods, or heating up ready-made meals bought from supermarkets and freezer centres is a lifestyle quite hard to resist for many people who live alone.

Obviously this can be quite an expensive lifestyle, and it is worth adding up how much money you could save if you started preparing your own food. The health benefits could also be substantial. Commercial foods often contain large amounts of food additives, particularly preservatives, colouring, flavouring, flavour enhancers (such as monosodium glutamate) and salt. You have no control over the content of these items unless you prepare your own food. Neither do you have any control over the nutritional value of commercial foods. They may contain sub-standard ingredients, such as dried potato powder, which is often made from damaged crops that could not otherwise be sold and may be subject to higher levels of pesticide residues. The ingredients may have been prepared and stored in such a way that their vitamin and mineral content is seriously reduced.

A case history (true story)

Jenny worked as a freelance secretary from her home – a London flat which received limited daylight and often needed the lights on during the daytime. She was busy and worked hard, having very little spare time to prepare food. It didn't seem worth cooking for one when she could buy ready-cooked meals from the supermarket and heat them up.

After a year or two, Jenny noticed that her hair was coming out very easily. Every time she ran her hands through it, she would lose many strands. This had never happened before. Also, Jenny occasionally felt quite nauseous. Once or twice for a few days at a time her food would go all the way through her completely undigested. This was frightening, especially as she also felt very peculiar during these times, and sometimes nearly passed out. Eventually she associated these symptoms with eating a particular brand of ready-made shepherd's pie.

Finally, Jenny noticed that her eyesight was no longer 20/20. She had difficulty focusing her eyes when at home, although bright light seemed to help. Jenny decided it was time to do something about her lifestyle. Since she didn't know whether supermarket meals were really enough for her body's needs, she stopped eating them, and instead began cooking. Having little time, she made a lot of thick soups and stews, with meat, fish or pulses and vegetables, and ate them with wholemeal bread. They would last for two or three days, which saved her from having to cook too often. She also bought a book on eye exercises, and practised them. Jenny's eyes took only two weeks to return to 20/20 vision. She wasn't sure exactly when her hair loss began to improve, but the problem did soon disappear and never returned.

Hints and tips

- Buy a big bag of pulses like marrowfat peas, kidney beans or chick peas and soak/cook them all at the same time. Once they are cold you can spread them out on a tray, freeze them, and then put them in bags ready for adding to soups and stews.
- Do the same thing with a bag of brown rice. Cooked rice will keep for several days in the fridge and need only be heated up in a lidded pan with a tablespoon of water.

- Make lots of thick, chunky soups and stews. These will last for several days and ensure that there is always something ready to heat up when you arrive home hungry and don't want to cook.
- It is always best to eat freshly cooked vegetables, but you can also save time by cooking more vegetables than you need and heating up the leftovers the next day. The quickest way to heat them up is to stir-fry them in a wok with a little olive oil.
- Frozen vegetables can be a good stand-by, but much of the goodness is lost if the defrost juices are discarded. You can avoid this by stir-frying frozen vegetables in a little olive oil rather than boiling them.
- If cooking is impossible, many take-away ethnic foods, particularly Chinese, are fresh and nutritious and may be a much better option than supermarket meals.

Having a healthy baby

Also see Section II, Infertility

It has been known for a long time that the chances of conceiving and giving birth to a healthy baby are increased by paying attention to the diet of both parents, not just around the time of conception and during pregnancy, but up to six months before. After the Dutch food shortage in the winter of 1944–5, there was a sharp rise in the number of stillborn babies in Holland. After World War II in Germany, when the population was badly malnourished, defects such as spina bifida rose from three per 1,000 births to eight.

Two specialist researchers in this area, Margaret and Arthur Wynn, have written a book which puts forward a strong case that diet and environmental factors may be responsible for a much larger proportion of birth defects, stillbirths and even miscarriages than anyone has so far realized. Sifting through 500 scientific studies, they have come up with some truly startling conclusions.

The strongest link between miscarriage and birth defects of various types, and problems such as epilepsy, diabetes and Down's syndrome in babies, seems to be something known technically as a mutation, or genetic change.

Down's syndrome is caused by mutations in parental germ cells (egg and sperm). It would disappear if it were not constantly renewed by new mutations (*Margaret and Arthur Wynn, The Case for Preconception Care of Men and Women, 1991*).

Many hundreds of substances capable of causing mutation (known as mutagens) have now been identified. They include alcohol, cannabis, tobacco and diesel engine smoke, lead, overheated cooking oil, charred meat, coal dust, radiation, diazepam tranquillizers, paracetamol (acetaminophen), and a number of other drugs, as well as viruses and other infections. Many mutagens are also capable of causing cancer through their ability to interfere with the healthy multiplication of cells.

Studies have shown that mutation is definitely promoted by nutritional deficiencies – particularly of folic acid and other B vitamins, vitamins C and E, and zinc. Several of these nutrients are also now known to have an anti-cancer effect. This is because they help to neutralize mutagens when found in adequate amounts in our bodies.

Foods or nutrients which neutralize mutagens are known as 'anti-mutagens'. 'Most of the known anti-mutagens are naturally occurring constituents of plants including familiar vegetables and fruits', say Margaret and Arthur Wynn. They report that the Japanese Institute of Genetics has measured the ability of certain plant juices to neutralize mutagens. The most effective ones appear to be burdock, mint, broccoli, green pepper, apples, shallots, pineapples, ginger, cabbage, aubergine, parsley and grapes. Unfortunately the beneficial effect seems to be lost when the plants are boiled. Unrefined olive oil and linoleic acid (from fresh nuts and seeds) have been shown in tests to be highly effective against a large number of mutagens.

Research has also shown that there are times when the egg and sperm cells are particularly vulnerable to mutation. For women this time begins three days before ovulation and ends two days after conception. For men, it begins as long as four months before conception. Abnormal sperm can cause miscarriage. In a Swedish study, when researchers examined the semen of men married to women who had had miscarriages, it was found that about half the miscarriages were attributable to the man.

Many thousands of women with a history of infertility, miscarriage or abnormal pregnancies have been helped by doctors and practitioners who believe in the importance of good nutritional status and a healthy lifestyle. Not everyone with these problems can be helped, but often a history of repeated miscarriages can be due to a problem as simple as a high coffee consumption in the woman or a slight zinc deficiency in the man. Factors such as excessive lead or pesticide levels in the body, or high levels of oestrogen-mimicking pollutants, are also likely to be detrimental.

Hints and tips

- Both prospective parents are advised to give up smoking and alcohol six months before they plan to conceive a baby. Even moderate drinking and smoking can be detrimental.
- Eat fresh fruit and vegetables every day – five portions is the general rule. Include some raw salad vegetables.
- Eat wholemeal rather than refined bread and cereals.
- Include some fresh nuts or seeds in your daily diet, for instance chopped brazil nuts or sunflower seeds in breakfast cereal, or a spoonful of tahini (creamed sesame seeds) added to soups and gravy just before serving.
- Don't eat char-grilled food.
- Wherever possible, avoid drugs and medicines unless your doctor insists on them.
- Use extra virgin olive oil in salad dressings.
- Avoid exposure to pollutants as best you can (see *Coping with pollution* on page 299).
- Avoid coffee.

After conception, the female partner should continue with all the above throughout pregnancy and breast-feeding.

Supplements

Both prospective parents may wish to take a multivitamin and mineral supplement as an insurance policy. This is *not* a substitute for a healthy diet. The product should contain at least 400 mcg of folic acid. If it does not also contain at least 10 mg zinc, take a zinc supplement separately. One gram of vitamin C daily and 200 iu vitamin E, if taken by the male partner, help to promote healthy sperm.

Coping with pollution

Also see Section II, Detoxification and *Pesticides*.

There are 60,000 chemicals in current commercial production. 3,000 of these are used as food additives, and 800 are found in drinking water. We can absorb pollutants from:

- Factory and power station discharges into air, rivers and seas
- Fish caught in polluted waters
- Food contaminated with pesticides, antibiotic drugs and industrial fall-out which has landed on the crops used to feed us and the animals we subsequently eat
- Invisible clouds of pesticide can be blown half-way across the world for us to breathe in. Pesticide is sprayed on pavements and parks, used in gardens, as wood preservatives, on footpaths, road margins and in buildings. It is washed into the water table which provides our drinking water.
- Traffic fumes

We can also bring pollution into our own homes by the products and services we use:

- Artificial air fresheners
- Artificial food additives
- Chemical-filled soap-powders and detergents
- Cosmetic aerosols and sprays, e.g. deodorants, hairspray, perfume
- Dry cleaning fumes
- Dust
- Fly spray and other insecticides
- Formaldehyde gas released by new carpets and furnishings
- Fumes from garages built underneath bedrooms or adjacent to living quarters
- Fumes from gas cookers and central heating
- Garden sprays
- Household sprays
- Mould from damp surroundings
- Strong-smelling fabric conditioners
- Strong-smelling polishes, toilet cleaners and carpet cleaners
- Tobacco smoke
- Unnecessary medications or recreational drugs
- Wood preservative

Pollution damages the body by disrupting vital processes and interfering with nutrient absorption and utilization. It also generates free radicals – destructive oxygen molecules that are capable of initiating the changes responsible for causing cancer and many other diseases. Chronic fatigue syndrome and damage to the immune system have been particularly linked with pollutant and pesticide exposure.

Our natural defences against free radicals are the antioxidant nutrients vitamins A, C and E, and beta-carotene obtained from the diet. The nutrients are destroyed in the process. The body can also manufacture antioxidant enzymes to carry out a similar task, such as glutathione peroxidase, which is dependent on an adequate supply of the amino acid glutathione and the mineral selenium, now officially recognized to be dangerously deficient in the British diet and in other countries with low soil selenium levels.

Self-help

If you believe that your health is being harmed by pollution, the first thing to do is to stop more pollutants getting into your body and then aid the release of those already present:

- Do everything you can to reduce your exposure to the items in the home pollution list
- Buy organic food
- Drink bottled or filtered water
- Follow the healthy eating guidelines in Appendix I
- Take regular saunas to sweat out toxins
- Several hours before taking a sauna, swallow a few tablespoons of organic linseed (flax) oil
- Certain foods such as radish, watercress, beetroot, broccoli, cauliflower and other cruciferous vegetables assist liver function and drainage
- Eat adequate protein. Brazil nuts, sunflower and sesame seeds are particularly good.
- To help drain your liver, use turmeric (yellow Indian spice) regularly in cookery, and drink dandelion coffee

Supplements

The following nutrients are involved in and used up by detoxification processes in the body. Taking them as supplements may help these processes to work more efficiently. (Amounts given are per day.)

- Vitamin C 2–4 grams
- Vitamin E 500–1,000 iu
- B complex vitamins 50 mg
- Selenium 100 mcg
- Zinc 15 mg
- Magnesium 200 mg
- N-acetyl cysteine (NAC) 500–1,000 mg
- Reduced glutathione 100 mg
- Taurine 500 mg
- Methionine 500–1,000 mg
- Silymarin (milk thistle) herb as per label instructions. (Stabilizes the membranes of liver cells, preventing the entry of toxic compounds.)

Your Senior Years

Is poor health really inevitable as we reach advanced age? Or can we take measures to improve our chances of living to a ripe, old age free of pain, disability, medication and failing mental and physical fitness? Current research seems to indicate that we can. The scientific literature of the 1990s is rich with studies which compare lifestyle with the risk of developing the chronic diseases associated with older age: osteoarthritis, osteoporosis, diabetes, parkinsonism, heart disease, angina and high blood pressure, Alzheimer's disease and senility.

Time after time, these studies come to the following conclusions:

- That most of these diseases are much more common in individuals with the lowest intake of fresh, wholesome foods like fruit and vegetables
- That most elderly people have nutritional deficiencies
- That most diseases of the elderly are strongly linked with nutritional deficiencies
- That when you give elderly people more nutrient-rich foods, or add dietary supplements to their diet, their health improves, which strongly suggests that a lot of diseases currently attributed to old age should really be attributed to nutritional deficiency.

Causes of nutritional deficiency include poor diet, poor chewing (due to badly-fitting dentures), poor digestion, poor absorption of nutrients through the intestines, and poor assimilation of nutrients at the cellular level. Elderly people living alone may not feel motivated to prepare good quality meals. As age progresses, a deficiency of hydrochloric acid in the stomach becomes more common. This can cause nutritional deficiency since the rest of the digestive process is dependent on the proper acidification of food in the stomach. These factors make elderly people very vulnerable to developing nutritional deficiencies, as the following research studies illustrate:

- The most efficient way to determine if an individual has a deficiency of vitamin B_{12}, folic acid or vitamin B_6 is to measure levels of substances in their body which only accumulate in the presence of these deficiencies. These so-called 'marker' substances are homocysteine, cystathione, methylmalonic acid and 2-methylcitric acid. In a 1993 study, the serum concentrations of these markers were measured in 99 healthy young people, 64 healthy elderly people and 286 elderly hospitalized patients. It was found that 63 per cent of the healthy elderly and *83 per cent* of the hospitalized elderly people were deficient in one or more of these nutrients.
  (*Am J Clin Nutr 58(4):468-76, 1993.*)

- An antioxidant cocktail consisting of beta-carotene, vitamins B_6, C and E, zinc and selenium with GLA was given to a group of elderly people, resulting in the improvement of several problems connected with ageing. The researchers concluded that elderly people often suffer from nutritional deficiencies.
  (*Swed J Biol Med 4:24-6, 1987.*)

Immunity

The immune system is dependent on a wide range of nutrients. The following studies illustrate that elderly people are particularly vulnerable to depleted immunity due to inadequate nourishment.

- 180 healthy elderly people selected at random were found to have an average zinc intake of 9 mg per day. 36 of these had immune system deficiencies. Supplementation with zinc normalized copper levels and several immune factors. The authors concluded that zinc deficiency is a significant problem among the elderly.
  (*Nutrition 9(3):218-24, 1993.*)

- 96 independently living elderly subjects were randomly assigned to receive nutritional supplements or placebo. After 12 months, those in the supplemented group had higher numbers of certain T-cells and natural killer cells, improved immune responses and higher antibody and natural killer cell activity. They had less than half the risk of infection compared with the placebo group.
  (*Lancet 340:1124-7, 1992.*)

Functional capacity

Functional capacity is the ability to lead a relatively independent life without the need for help with washing and dressing yourself, walking, standing, eating and so on.

- Researchers studying a group of elderly nuns living in the same accommodation, found that those with the highest levels of a carotenoid known as lycopene in their blood tended to have the best functional capacity. Carotenoids are substances in plants, known for their orange colour. (Beta-carotene is a well-known carotenoid.) The best source of lycopene is tomatoes, but lycopene is also found in watermelon, pink grapefruit and guava.
  (*J Gerontol A Biol Sci Med Sci 51(1):M10-6, 1996.*)

Life expectancy

- A study comparing diet with survival in elderly Greek people found that the Mediterranean diet, rich in fruit, vegetables, salads and olive oil favourably affects life expectancy among elderly people.
  (*BMJ 311:1457-60, 1995.*)

Research summaries for the following conditions which are common in the elderly can be found in Section II.

Mental function

One of the greatest fears of many people is that as they get older their memory will fail and their thought processes deteriorate. When severe this is known as senility or senile dementia. When it happens before old age it is known as Alzheimer's disease. There is now a lot of research to suggest that mental deterioration is not an inevitable consequence of ageing. B vitamin deficiency in particular seems to be associated with this problem, and the herb *Ginkgo biloba* is protective. One trial has successfully used the amino acid taurine. Supplementation with antioxidant nutrients has also been found beneficial.

Arthritis

Osteoarthritis affects most people over the age of 70 and occurs when destructive oxygen molecules called free radicals cause damage to joint cartilage. Free radicals are thought to be promoted by high levels of tissue acidity and 'internal pollution' as well as with a lack of antioxidant vitamins and minerals. High levels of vitamin C, and to a lesser extent beta-carotene and vitamin E in the diet have been found protective against arthritis.

Diabetes

Diabetes which starts late in life is known as 'adult-onset' diabetes. It is not (as commonly supposed) caused so much by a lack of insulin, but by a problem known as *insulin resistance*. That is to say, the pancreas is able to produce insulin, but the body does not respond to the insulin. The reasons for the condition are not as yet fully understood but the success of dietary supplementation in so many clinical trials suggests that nutritional deficiencies are, at least partly, involved in an impairment of the insulin quality or of the function of the body's receptor sites to which insulin attaches itself. The most common nutritional deficiencies associated with adult-onset diabetes are magnesium, zinc, chromium and vitamin E. A high sugar consumption may promote the development of diabetes.

Heart disease

Although heart disease is usually thought of as a problem of middle age, a lot of elderly people suffer from angina pain, which indicates a narrowing of the important coronary artery which supplies the heart muscle.

Hints and Tips

- The sooner you make positive dietary improvements, the better. Don't wait until the symptoms start.
- Eat tomatoes several times a week.
- If you live alone, use the tips given in *The Single Person* on page 295.
- As you get older more people offer to do things for you. Don't accept unless you have to. Remaining as active as possible helps to keep you young.
- If activity leaves you in pain, try to find some therapies to treat the underlying cause of the pain. A nutritional therapist may be able to help with arthritis, for instance. Poor posture can also lead to chronic pain, but could possibly be corrected by a combination of therapies.
- Loneliness and depression in old age can sometimes lead to self-neglect if the elderly person is subconsciously wishing to join a loved one who has passed away. If you know someone who fits this description, try to help them understand that illness may not bring early death. On the contrary, illness is liable to be chronic and to make every day seem twice as long.

Supplements

- 1 multivitamin with minerals (ensure that it contains zinc and selenium)
- 1 tablet or capsule of mixed antioxidants
- 1 capsule of an evening primrose oil/fish oil combination

Looking and Feeling Your Best

Nutrition can make a big difference to your appearance. Not only does your diet play a part in determining what kind of figure you have, it also affects your skin, hair and energy levels. Energy is as important a part of being attractive as your clothes, complexion and hairdo. An individual who looks tired and irritable is never as physically appealing as someone with an air of vitality. On the other hand someone with lively, smiling features does not need to be beautiful to be attractive.

Skin

In naturopathic philosophy, the condition of your skin is said to reflect the condition of your liver. Spotty, sallow skin indicates a liver full of toxins (waste products) and the body's attempt to excrete them. Your diet may be too fatty, which reduces your liver's efficiency, and your colon (large intestine) may be sluggish, causing soluble waste matter to be too easily reabsorbed back into the bloodstream. The liver then has to deal with this waste for a second time, in addition to the day's new waste. In the long term it can get overloaded. This affects not just your skin but also your general energy levels.

Your skin can also become spotty if your diet provides too little of the vitamins and minerals needed to keep it strong and resistant to infections. It is all very well cleaning your pores with antiseptic lotions every day, but if you have a zinc deficiency or a vitamin A deficiency, this will only partially solve the problem, if at all.

Your hair is equally as sensitive to your diet. A fatty, sugary diet low in vitamins, minerals and essential fatty acids can deprive your hair of its natural shine and promote dandruff. Forget the anti-dandruff shampoos – if you are eating the right diet you don't need them!

Eating for beauty

To improve your skin, hair and energy you don't have to go on an austere 'spring clean' like we sometimes read about in magazines, which leaves us feeling hungry and miserable. There are some simple rules which you will need to follow, but they need not leave you feeling hungry.

- Eat proper meals consisting mainly of fresh vegetables and low-fat protein foods (with the exception of oily fish, which are beneficial).
- Beware of cooking with fat, except for small amounts of olive oil.
- Become aware of how processed foods are made and what they contain. For instance, do you know that one third to one half of the weight of pastry consists of pure butter or margarine? That a pork pie is approximately 70 per cent fat and that meat described as 'lean' can quite legally contain up to one-third fat?
- Chocolate is a particularly fatty food, and a lot of people react to it with spots. Try to find other foods which you still think of as a treat but which contain less fat and sugar and more nutrients. For instance, one small square of very dark, fat-reduced chocolate, a handful of unsalted peanuts or almonds, a banana or an oatmeal biscuit.

- It is easier to avoid eating junk food if you are not hungry, so make sure that at the times when you are most likely to eat junk food, you have already eaten something else.
- In the macrobiotic system of medicine, bags under the eyes are said to be related to a strain on the kidneys caused by the consumption of too much fat and sometimes too much fluid.
- Drink water in preference to other drinks.

Supplements

(Amounts given are per day)

- 1 Multivitamin with minerals
- Magnesium 100 mg
- Vitamin C 1 gram
- For dry skin: one capsule of an evening primrose oil/fish oil combination
- For spots: zinc 15 mg and vitamin A 7,500 iu daily for 3 months

Other advice

Pay attention to your posture, and the way you walk. Take some brisk exercise every day.

Cellulite

As any plastic surgeon can confirm, it *does* exist. (Only doctors who don't know how to treat it will tell you it doesn't.) However you may not need plastic surgery to have it removed. 15 minutes' vigorous daily massage in combination with a low-fat diet of vegetables, fish and whole grains, and avoiding all dietary stressors (see page 312) may be the answer for you.

Tips for Travellers

Constipation

If you have a tendency to become constipated when away from home, take some magnesium supplements with you. An extra 200 mg magnesium daily may make all the difference. If your diet is low in fibre, you should also take a tablespoon of linseeds mixed into a large glass of water (drink immediately before they swell up) every morning or evening.

Jet Lag

Melatonin supplements are said to be extremely useful in helping to readjust your body clock by aiding sleep.

Mosquitoes

Some bugs don't like the taste of B vitamins. You may be able to avoid being bitten by taking a 50-mg B complex supplement every day.

Sunburn

To avoid sunburn, use a conventional sun-screen. If you do get burnt, one of the best treatments is to dab yourself with a dilute vitamin C solution (dissolve 1 level teaspoon vitamin C powder in a large glass of water) then apply vitamin E cream. Aloe vera lotion is also soothing and healing.

Travellers' Tummy

Bugs can cause problems if they are not killed off by the (normally strong) acid in your stomach. Not everyone has strong stomach acid so a supplement of betaine hydrochloride may be a useful preventive. (Do not be tempted to exceed the manufacturer's dosage instructions.) Garlic supplements may also be helpful in preventing infection. You should still take your travel agent's recommended precautions for whichever country you are visiting, as regards avoiding tap water, raw foods and so on.

Athletes

Athletes have very special needs, especially if they are involved in competitive or performance sports or arts and need to drive their body to its physical limits of strength and endurance. For these reasons, athletes must pay even more attention than others to the rules of healthy eating (*see Appendix I*). Fatty or sugary foods may indeed provide calories as a source of energy, but the energy itself cannot be produced without the right amounts of accompanying nutrients: B vitamins, magnesium, iron, their co-factors, and all the other substances involved in energy metabolism. These substances require a wide range of nutrients. So it is really an old wives' tale to say that 'sugar gives you energy'. If your body cannot process the sugar you will not feel very energetic at all.

Athletes also need to pay attention to their bowel movements. The accumulation of metabolic waste products in the blood and tissues as a result of constipation hinders the efficient functioning of various body systems and could impair performance. Likewise an overworked, sluggish liver due to constipation, high saturated fat consumption and stressors like food additives, medicines and alcohol does nothing at all for physical performance. It is more likely to leave you feeling as if you cannot get out of bed in the morning.

Athletes do, of course, need to eat larger quantities of food than other individuals, in order to cater for their extra energy requirements. The foods themselves do not need to be different from those required for a normal, healthy diet. The one exception is that after intensive exercise in a warm climate, or after strenuous world-class athletic events, the athlete may lose large amounts of water and electrolytes as sweat, which should be replenished. Sports drinks containing sodium, potassium, chloride and other electrolytes are available for this purpose, but a drink made from water with fresh orange juice, lemon juice and a pinch of salt would do equally well.

It is now also known that athletes lose large quantities of magnesium during exertion. (*Casoni I et al.: Changes of magnesium concentrations in endurance athletes. Int J Sports Med 11(3):234-7, 1990*. Also *Deuster P A et al.: Responses of plasma magnesium and other cations to fluid replacement during exercise. J Am Coll Nutr 12(3):286-93, 1993*.) Research has also shown that magnesium supplementation helps to build strength in strength-training programmes. (*Brilla L R et al.: Effect of magnesium supplementation on strength training in humans. J Am Coll Nutr 11(3):326-9, 1992*.)

Carbohydrate

The concept of 'carbohydrate loading' has for some time been fashionable in sports nutrition. However, studies on top-class athletes comparing the results of the standard high-carbohydrate diet and the so-called 'Zone' diet have found the latter to be superior.

So during the summer of 1991 we put nine of Marv's athletes (six top college football players and three professional basketball players) on a Zone-favourable diet for six weeks …These athletes were chosen because they had already come off intensive spring conditioning programs and wanted to continue their conditioning program to be ready for September. As any top trainer will tell you, once you're at a peak level of conditioning, any further performance gains are usually very small. But without continuing workouts you can lose much of your performance edge. That loss of performance is called 'detraining' ... So the true test of Zone benefits would be if these athletes showed any significant performance *increases* during the six-week study period.

When Marv sent me the data for analysis, the results were so startling that I had to call him for confirmation ... Every one of the performance categories we tested improved, with a statistical significance of greater than 99.95 per cent ... First of all, the vertical jump, which indicates coordinated leg strength, improved by 10 per cent ... Next came endurance ... the athletes were seven per cent faster in the last sprint than they had been at the beginning of the study period ... And their cardiovascular fitness – perhaps the most important category in terms of overall health – increased by an amazing 118 per cent.

(From *The Zone*, by Barry Sears, 1996.)

The Zone diet is based on the simple principle that if all meals and snacks are balanced with protein, carbohydrate and fat, the body's blood sugar will remain on an even keel instead of surging to high levels, as after excessive carbohydrate consumption. Even complex carbohydrates as found in pasta, bread and potatoes can result in rapid increases in blood sugar, since they have a high glycaemic index (*which see*). Rapid increases in blood sugar lead to rapid rises in insulin production, which Sears has identified as a performance inhibiting factor for athletes. The Zone diet is becoming popular among athletes in the United States, and it is likely that we shall be hearing a great deal more about it. Particularly as athletes (college swimmers) on a high-carbohydrate diet did no better than those on a diet containing only 40 per cent of calories from carbohydrate in a 1990 study carried out at Ohio State University, Sears' claim that the high-carbohydrate diet is a myth may soon become accepted.

Dietary Supplements

- Multivitamin with minerals
- Magnesium 200 mg/day
- Carnitine 500 mg/day
- Antioxidant combination product

Healthy eating on a low budget

It is often said that eating healthily is beyond the means of people on low incomes. This isn't necessarily true. In fact, healthy eating can be very affordable, for the simple reason that the foods most lacking in nutritional value are usually expensive processed foods. With processed foods you pay not just for the food, but also for the processing and (often elaborate) packaging.

Some healthy eating guidelines

- The healthiest foods are vegetables, raw salad vegetables, fruit, whole grains, pulses, fish, poultry, nuts and seeds. The secret of avoiding deficiencies is to eat a good variety of foods from these groups every day (omitting the fish and poultry if you are vegetarian).
- The more fat, sugar and white flour a food contains, the more unhealthy it becomes. Some of the worst examples are sausages, batter, ice cream, sweets, chocolate, doughnuts, croissants, crispy snacks in packets, packet soups and packet dessert mixes. Everybody needs to ration their intake of these foods.
- Cooking methods are important. Steaming, or stir-frying or braising vegetables with a tablespoon of olive oil is a good way of preserving nutrients, but boiling causes heavy vitamin losses if the water is thrown away. Deep-frying is not recommended. Deep-fried food absorbs excessive quantities of oil or fat.
- Artificial food additives are usually not tested by independent laboratories and very little is known about their effects in combination. Singly they have caused health problems in many people, particularly children.
- It is advisable to keep alcohol consumption down to no more than one glass per day.
- Try to keep all salt consumption down, and use a 'low-salt' product instead of ordinary salt.
- Since grains are very small, they can absorb more pesticide than other foods. So if you are limited in what organic produce you can afford, put grains at the top of the list.

Saving money

There are a few simple rules you need to understand if you want to save cash on food, while doing the most for your health.

- Buy foods in their 'natural' state (e.g. fresh potatoes instead of oven chips). Don't buy ready meals, pizzas, crisps, pies, etc.
- Save meat (if you eat it at all) for occasional use. Cheap meat is usually full of hidden fat. Fish and chicken are better value. Pulses (beans, lentils, dried peas and chick peas) are cheap vegetable sources of protein and can be freely used instead of animal protein.
- Shop around. Fruit and vegetables are cheaper from market stalls and greengrocers; pulses, porridge oats and brown rice may be cheaper from a wholefood shop, while eggs, cheese, butter and wholemeal bread are generally cheaper in large supermarkets.
- Don't waste food. Fish bones, vegetable peelings and chicken carcasses can be boiled to make soup stock.

Some menu suggestions

Breakfast
- Porridge made with oats, water or skimmed milk, and a few sunflower seeds. Add chopped dates to sweeten if necessary, or a little sugar;
- Or stewed apples and raisins with natural yoghurt;
- Or fresh grapefruit.

Lunch
- Pilchards, cold chicken or smoked mackerel, with salad and wholemeal bread or baked potato or potato salad;
- Or lentil and onion soup with wholemeal bread, cheese and salad. Add a little tahini (creamed sesame) to the soup before serving.

Dinner
- Grilled herring or mackerel with mashed parsnips and braised vegetables;
- Or vegetable stew of dried peas, potatoes, leeks and carrots, with wholemeal bread and butter;
- Or pasta with lentil, tomato and mushroom sauce.

Desserts
- Fresh fruit 'au naturel' or chopped and made into fruit salad or fruit jelly, served with home-made natural yoghurt;
- Or brown rice flakes made into rice pudding. (Sweeten with chopped dates);
- Or home-made flapjacks with raisins and dates.

Snacks
Fruit; bananas and oatcakes; Ryvita, oatcakes or wholemeal toast with tahini and a little sugar-free fruit spread; fresh almonds or brazil nuts; a piece of fresh coconut; home-made flapjacks; preservative-free dried fruit. If you really crave chocolate, have a cup of home-made cocoa instead (watch out for the sugar content) – or a plain chocolate-coated oatmeal biscuit.

Drinks
Instead of ordinary tea and coffee, try mint tea (especially if you can grow your own mint), rose hip tea or fennel tea, or chicory coffee (available from health shops). Home-made vegetable stock or miso dissolved in hot water make good savoury drinks. Pure fruit juice mixed with fizzy mineral water is cheaper than canned drinks.

Time-Saving Hints
- Buy a big bag of brown rice, cook all at once, and when cold, freeze it in portions. Defrost portions before use, warm over a low heat for a few minutes in a tightly lidded saucepan with a tablespoon of water, and serve.
- A bag of kidney beans or chick peas can also be cooked in advance and frozen (on a shallow tray). Large pulses like these can be cooked in 10 minutes in a pressure cooker; otherwise may take much longer. Don't forget to soak all pulses (except lentils) overnight before cooking.

The Rules of Healthy Eating: Getting the Balance Right

Your daily diet should consist of foods from the groups shown in the pyramid, in proportion to the size of the panel. You may also select other foods of your own choice in proportion to the size of the 'Free Choice' panel. The secret of avoiding deficiencies is to ensure the daily consumption of a good variety of foods from each group and not to become dependent on a small range of foods.

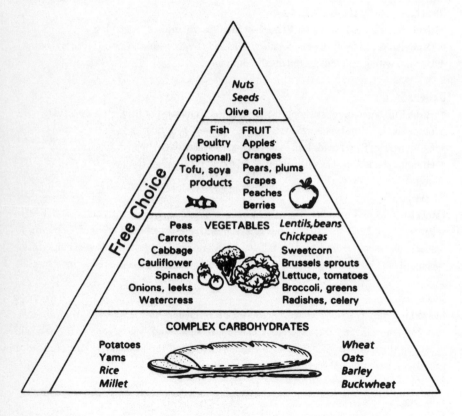

Important

If you do not eat fish or poultry regularly, and if you have cut red meat, eggs and dairy produce down to very low levels or do not eat them at all, then you should ensure that you eat a selection every day of the vegetables, complex carbohydrates and other foods listed in the pyramid in italics.

What Supplements Should I Take?

When using dietary supplements it is usually a good idea to use a multivitamin and multi-mineral preparation as a foundation. This helps to prevent imbalances caused by taking one nutrient on its own for too long. Check the labels so that the combination of products you take provides approximately the following:

Recommended Basic Formula

Vitamin A	7,500 iu [1]
Vitamin B_1, B_2, B_6	25–50 mg
Vitamin B_{12}	50 mcg
Niacin (Vitamin B_3)	50 mg
Folic acid	400 mcg
Pantothenic acid (vitamin B_5)	50 mg
Vitamin C	100 mg
Vitamin D	200 iu [2]
Vitamin E	50 iu [3]
Boron	2 mg
Chromium	50 mcg
Copper	0.5 mg (500 mcg)
Iron	5 mg
Manganese	5 mg
Selenium	50 mcg
Zinc	10 mg
Evening primrose, borage or blackcurrant seed oil [4]	250 mg
Fish oil [5]	250 mg

[1] 1 iu = 0.3 micrograms (mcg or ug) of vitamin A
[2] 1 iu = 0.025 micrograms of vitamin D
[3] 1 iu = approx 0.7 milligram (mg) of vitamin E
[4] The active nutritional ingredient in these oils is gamma linolenic acid (GLA)
[5] The active nutritional ingredients in these oils are eicosapentaenoic acid (EPA) and docosahexaenoic acid (DHA). Fish oil supplements are not the same as fish liver oils, which contain little EPA and DHA but are a good source of vitamin A.

Values given for minerals are elemental.
Children: Reduce dosages in proportion to body weight.
Pregnancy: The above dosages are considered safe in pregnancy.

Magnesium (approx 100 mg/day) will normally need to be taken separately, since adding the required amount to a multi-nutrient formula would make each tablet or capsule too bulky. Many people also take additional vitamin C, up to 1,000 or 2,000 mg a day, to help combat pollution and prevent infections. If these amounts of vitamin C look very large to you, remember that almost all other mammals produce (proportionally) much more vitamin C than this in their own bodies every day. Humans are missing the last stage in the liver enzyme process which produces vitamin C from glucose.

If you have any of the following health problems, then you may have a more deep-seated nutritional deficiency requiring additional supplementation. Many people have found the following daily regimes helpful in addition to the basic multi-nutrient formula:

Special Supplement Regimes

Amounts given as daily intake unless otherwise stated

Acne	Vitamin A 10,000 iu (except in pregnancy), zinc 15 mg
Adult-onset diabetes	Vitamin B complex 50 mg, magnesium 200 mg, chromium 100 mcg. Caution: Report any hypoglycaemia symptoms to your doctor, since this regime may reduce your requirements of insulin or other medication
Age spots (brown marks on the hands of elderly people)	Vitamin E 400 iu, selenium 100 mcg
Angina	See *High Blood Pressure*
Anaemia	In addition to iron prescribed by doctor, vitamin C 100 mg with each meal, zinc 10 mg, copper 1 mg
Anxiety and panic attacks	Vitamin B complex, 50 mg, magnesium 200 mg
Arthritis	Evening primrose oil 500 mg, fish oil 500 mg, boron 3 mg
Hyperactivity (children)	50-kilo child: zinc 7 mg, evening primrose oil 250 mg, magnesium 100 mg. Younger children: proportionally less according to body weight
Birth defects	Folic acid 200 mcg (expectant mothers)
Chronic fatigue	Pantothenic acid 500 mg, carnitine 250 mg, vitamin B complex 50 mg
Constipation	Magnesium 200 mg, fibre supplement
Dandruff or dry skin	Zinc 15 mg, evening primrose oil 500 mg, fish oil 500 mg
Depression	L-tyrosine 500 mg (morning), L-tryptophan 500 mg (evening), lecithin 1 tablespoon

Eczema and other skin disorders and rashes	Zinc 15 mg, evening primrose oil 500 mg, fish oil 500 mg
Flaking or white-spotted fingernails	Zinc 15 mg, evening primrose oil 500 mg
Frequent infections (e.g. flu or vaginal thrush)	Zinc 15 mg, vitamin C 2 x 500 mg*, cod liver oil 1 teaspoon
High blood pressure	Vitamin E 200 mg, magnesium 200 mg, evening primrose oil 500 mg, fish oil 500 mg, vitamin C 3 x 1,000 mg*
Infertility	Zinc 15 mg, vitamin C 2 x 500 mg (men and women)
Insomnia	Magnesium 200 mg, zinc 15 mg
Menopausal symptoms	Vitamin B complex 50 mg, vitamin E 200 iu, magnesium 200 mg, zinc 15 mg, Agnus castus herb as per manufacturer's instructions
Mental illness	Hallucinations, depression or manic depression can be due to unusually high needs for certain nutrients, including vitamin B_6, niacin, zinc, and sometimes chromium, vitamin C and other B vitamins. Sufferers should seek help from a knowledgeable doctor or other practitioner (*see Appendix V*)
Mood swings	Magnesium 200 mg, vitamin B complex 50 mg, chromium 100 mcg
Nausea and vomiting of pregnancy	Zinc 10 mg, iron 5 mg, magnesium 100 mg, folic acid 200 mcg
Osteoporosis	Magnesium 200 mg, boron 3 mg, comfrey as per manufacturer's recommendations, vitamin D 200 iu
Period (menstrual) pains	Vitamin B complex 50 mg, magnesium 200 mg, zinc 15 mg, evening primrose oil 500 mg, fish oil 500 mg
Poor vision in dim light	Vitamin A 7,500 iu (except in pregnancy), zinc 15 mg
Premenstrual syndrome	Vitamin B complex 50 mg, magnesium 200 mg, zinc 15 mg, evening primrose oil 500 mg, fish oil 500 mg

* Vitamin C is best taken in divided doses at two or more intervals each day.

Prostate enlargement	Zinc 15 mg, evening primrose oil 500 mg, fish oil 500 mg, Saw palmetto herb as per manufacturer's recommendations
Prematurely greying hair	Vitamin B complex 50 mg, folic acid 400 mcg, PABA 250 mg, zinc 15 mg

More serious illnesses, such as cancers, motor neurone disease, multiple sclerosis, Alzheimer's disease, rheumatoid arthritis and asthma may be aggravated by nutritional deficiencies, allergies, dysbiosis and/or an inefficient liver which has difficulty eliminating toxic waste substances. Professional help with supplementation should be sought (*see Appendix V*). Liver function can be greatly assisted by supplements of vitamin C, evening primrose oil, the amino acids glutathione and taurine, and the daily consumption of tomatoes and vegetables from the Brassica family (cabbage, cauliflower and broccoli, among others). Supplements of Acidophilus and time-released caprylic acid are helpful against dysbiosis.

The safety of dietary supplements

All persistent or worrying symptoms should be reported to a doctor before you consider self-help. Keep your doctor informed of any self-help measures you intend to take.

Dietary supplements are generally safe at the levels described above, but do not be tempted to exceed these amounts without professional advice and supervision, since it is always possible to create harmful imbalances if excessive amounts are taken for lengthy periods of time. Particular caution should be exercised with vitamins A and D.

If your symptoms do not begin to abate within six months then your problem may need a different approach, possibly requiring the assistance of a specialist practitioner. You should then revert to taking the basic multi-nutrient formula alone.

If your symptoms do begin to abate, you should continue with the regime until they have stopped or no further improvement has occurred for six months. At this point you can begin to wean yourself off the supplements until you are just taking the basic multi-nutrient formula, which should be sufficient to prevent the symptoms from returning.

Official Figures

Daily vitamin and mineral requirements for healthy people published by the United Kingdom and United States Governments.

Nutrient	UK Reference Nutrient Intake (RNI)	US Recommended Dietary Allowance (RDA)
Vitamin A (retinol)	700 mcg (2,310 iu)	1,000 mcg (3,300 iu)
Vitamin B$_1$ (thiamine)	1.0 mg	1.5 mg
Vitamin B$_2$ (riboflavin)	1.3 mg	1.7 mg
Vitamin B$_3$ (niacin/niacinamide)	17 mg	19 mg
Vitamin B$_5$ (pantothenic acid)	*3–7 mg*	*4–7 mg*
Vitamin B$_6$ (pyridoxine)	1.4 mg	2.0 mg
Vitamin B$_{12}$ (cobalamin)	1.5 mcg	2.0 mcg
Biotin	*10–200 mcg*	*30–100 mcg*
Folic acid (folate)	200 mcg	200 mcg
Vitamin C (ascorbic acid)	40 mg	60 mg
Vitamin D (calciferol)	none	5 mcg (200 iu)
Vitamin E	*More than 4 mg (5 iu)*	10 mg (7.5 iu)
Vitamin K	*1 mcg/kg body weight*	80 mcg
Calcium	700 mg	800 mg
Chloride	2,500 mg	*750 minimum*
Chromium	*25 mcg*	*50–200 mcg*
Copper	1.2 mg	*1.5–3 mg*
Iodine	140 mcg	150 mcg
Iron	8.7 mg	10 mg
Magnesium	300 mg	350 mg
Manganese	*1.4 mg*	*2–5 mg*
Molybdenum	*50–400 mcg*	*75–250 mcg*
Phosphorus	550 mg	800 mg
Potassium	3,500 mg	*2,000 mg minimum*
Selenium	75 mcg	70 mcg
Sodium	1,600 mg	*500 mg minimum*
Zinc	9.5 mg	15 mg

RNI values given are for males aged 19–50. RDA values are for males aged 25–50 years weighing approximately 174 lb (12 stone). Where no RNI or RDA exists, the safe adequate range is given in italics.

An End to the Common Cold

The debate about whether vitamin C supplements really can cure the common cold has mainly been in progress since 1970, when Linus Pauling first helped to publicize it with his book *Vitamin C and the Common Cold*. Thousands of people all over the world carried out experiments to see if drinking more orange juice would cure their colds. Clinical trials were carried out with vitamin C supplements. The scientific consensus was that vitamin C was a worthless treatment.

Research

So why did Pauling continue to assert that vitamin C is effective?

In 1986 Pauling – twice a Nobel Laureate – published another book, *How to live longer and feel better*. Part of this book is a careful analysis of the clinical trials which have been conducted into vitamin C and the common cold. Pauling points out that the general trend of these trials demonstrates that the higher the doses of vitamin C taken by the test subjects, the greater the benefit.

Most research in this area has concentrated on doses of 1,000 mg a day or less. Usually the duration of treatment was very short (2–3 days). Pauling maintains that this research only reveals that the *protocols* (regimes used) in these trials are ineffective.

The best results have been obtained from a trial in Pernambuco, Brazil, in which 133 test subjects were given 6 grams a day of vitamin C, to take starting on the first, second or third day of their cold (groups I, II and III respectively). Only 13 per cent of group I failed to recover within 15 days; 20 per cent of group II failed to recover within 15 days, and 41 per cent of group III failed to recover within 15 days. Of those who did respond to the vitamin C treatment, the average number of days' illness was 1.82 days for group I, 2.71 days for group II, and 5.10 days for group III.

Studies have also been carried out to assess vitamin C's ability to prevent the common cold. Pauling agrees that most of these have had disappointing results, but again blames the trial protocols. For instance, in a 1975 Canadian study by Anderson, Beaton and colleagues, the subjects were given only one 500-mg vitamin C tablet *per week*. Despite this there was a 25 per cent degree of protection.

Dosage

Why have vitamin C trials on the whole used such small doses?

We have to remember that in medical training, vitamin C is a drug used for the treatment of a disease, scurvy. An intake of about 10 mg a day is thought to be the minimum needed to prevent this disease. So, in short, vitamin C is thought of as a drug measured in *milligrams*. Moving too far above the anti-scurvy dose would seem as inappropriate to the uninformed doctor or trial designer, as using a whole bottle of aspirin instead of one tablet to cure a headache. And probably rather frightening too, for the same reasons.

Pauling was really ahead of his time. And the whole issue has been clouded by the mixed results obtained from clinical trials, and the lack of conviction or understanding that this is a dosage-related problem.

How does it work?

Research into the effects of large doses of vitamin C has generally shown a beneficial effect on the immune system. The number, size and mobility of white blood cells can be improved. Vitamin C also seems to have some direct anti-viral action, perhaps by promoting an increased production of interferon.

Other treatments

Vitamin A is an important protector against infection, and large amounts are needed when an infection occurs. Cod liver oil is a rich source of vitamin A. The traditional wisdom about cod liver oil preventing colds now has scientific evidence to back it up. In a recent study in New Zealand, researchers gave children small daily supplements of vitamin A. The result was a 22 per cent reduction in the number of cases of colds and flu. (The children's vitamin A intake had previously been considered adequate.)

Zinc is needed in adequate amounts for stored vitamin A to be released. Zinc itself plays (as do most nutrients) an important part in the immune system – our body's natural defences against infection.

Some herbs – particularly Echinacea – are also thought to be able to 'boost' immune function.

Self-treatment

1. *At the first sign* of a cold or the flu, take 1 level teaspoon of pure vitamin C powder dissolved in a glass of cold or lukewarm water or juice.
2. The first signs of a cold are:
   Beginning to sneeze, with a slight loss of energy and probably a slightly raw or 'scratchy' feeling in the throat, as if all is not quite right.

3. Repeat this dose every 2 hours until symptoms disappear. (They usually will if caught early enough. Often one dose of vitamin C is enough.) Also take 1 tablespoon cod liver oil and 15 mg zinc per day.

4. If the symptoms disappear rapidly, take 1 quarter teaspoon vitamin C powder or 1 gram tablet every 8 hours for the next 24 hours, then every 12 hours the day after. You may wish to continue with this as a maintenance (preventive) dose.

5. If the symptoms take longer to disappear (2 days or more), tail the vitamin C off more slowly, gradually reducing the dose and increasing the interval over about 4 days. If you do not do this, the cold or flu may return with a vengeance. Vitamin C seems to work first by suppressing the symptoms and second by fighting the infection. If you stop too soon the infection-fighting action may not yet be complete.

Important

As long as vitamin C is being absorbed from the intestines it is well tolerated and causes no discomfort. Once it is no longer being absorbed, it causes loose bowel motions, rather like a laxative. This happens at a daily intake of 1–10 grams in most healthy individuals.

If you have an infection like a cold or the flu, vitamin C users agree that the worse the infection, the more vitamin C can be absorbed. Someone with severe flu may have no loose bowel motions even at an intake of 50 grams a day.

If you do experience a laxative effect, you should reduce the dosage to comfortable levels. *See Section I, Vitamin C* for safety comments.

Useful Addresses

United Kingdom

The Breakspear Hospital
Belswains Lane
Hemel Hempstead
Herts HP3 9HP
Tel: (0144) 261333
International environmental medicine treatment unit, for laboratory diagnosis of chemical poisoning and environmental illness, and medically supervised nutritional detox programmes

Bristol Cancer Help Centre
Grove House
Cornwallis Grove
Clifton
Bristol BS8 4PG
Tel: (0117) 974 3216
A residential and day centre for cancer patients who wish to learn about holistic approaches to cancer care

British Association of Nutritional Therapists
c/o SPNT
PO Box 47
Heathfield
East Sussex TN21 8ZX
Send £2 for a register of practitioners

British Society for Allergy, Environmental and Nutritional Medicine
PO Box 28
Totton
Southampton
Hants SO40 2ZA
A society of doctors who apply the principles of nutritional medicine and treat patients accordingly

British Society for Mercury-Free Dentistry
1 Welbeck House
62 Welbeck St
London W1M 7HB
Send sae or international postal coupon for information

Community Health Foundation
188 Old Street
London EC1V 9BP
Tel: (0171) 251 4076
International centre for training in macrobiotics

Eating Disorders Association
Sackville Place
44 Magdalen St
Norwich
Norfolk NR3 1JE
Tel: (0160) 362 1414
Provides help and guidance for those with eating disorders

Society for the Promotion of Nutritional Therapy
PO Box 47
Heathfield
East Sussex TN21 8ZX
Tel: (01825) 872921
Email and Internet:
100045.255@Compuserve.com.
Educational and campaigning organization with branches throughout the UK and members in many foreign countries. Publishes quarterly journal *Nutritional Therapy Today* for members. Factsheets and other publications also available, including *Clinical Pearls News*, which provides monthly research summaries, and *Nutritional Influences on Illness*, an excellent sourcebook of clinical research.

Send £16 (UK/Europe) or £24 (rest of the world) to join the Society for one year.

United States

American Academy of Environmental Medicine
4510 W. 89th Street
Prairie Village, Kansas 66207
Tel: (913) 341 3625
Register of practitioners of environmental medicine

American Environmental Health Foundation
8345 Walnut Hill Lane
Suite 200
Dallas, Texas 75231–4262
Tel: (214) 368 4132
Organization for the recognition and appropriate treatment of environmental illness. Books and publications available.

American Preventive Medical Association
275 Millway
PO Box 732
Barnstable, Maine 02630
Tel: (508) 362 4343
Register of practitioners sympathetic to a natural approach to medicine

Citizens for Health
PO Box 1195
Tacoma, Washington 98401
Tel: (206) 922 2457
Campaigns for consumer rights in natural medicine

HealthComm International
PO Box 1729
Gig Harbor, Washington 98335
Tel: (206) 851 3943
Provides educational materials for healthcare practitioners interested in functional and nutritional medicine

ITServices
3301 Alta Arden #2
Sacramento, California 95825
Tel: (916) 483 1085
Publishers of *Clinical Pearls News*, an excellent monthly summary of the latest research

Linus Pauling Institute
440 Page Mill Road
Palo Alto, California 94306–2031
Centre for research into vitamin C

Australia

**Australian College of Nutritional &
Environmental Medicine**
13 Hilton St
Beaumaris
Victoria 3193
Tel: 9589 6088
For a referral service for all conventionally trained GPs and specialists who are interested in a wider and more natural approach to illness

Australian Natural Therapists Association
Taren Point
PO Box 2517
Sydney 2232

Canada

**International Society for Orthomolecular
Medicine**
16 Florence Avenue
Toronto M2N 1E9
Tel: (416) 733 2117
An international society for health professionals

New Zealand

Association of Natural Therapies
81 Forrest Hill Road
Milford
Auckland

Society of Naturopaths
Box 19183
Auckland 7

Index

Diesel smoke 157
Diet
   alkalinizing 183
   and kidney stones 259
   anti-cancer 184–5
   anti-candida 182
   anti-herpes 182
   blood sugar control 182–3
   calorie-controlled 183
   cleansing 183
   elimination 183
   exclusion 183
   Feingold 184
   high carbohydrate, and kidney
      stones 259
   high fat, and kidney stones 259
   high methionine 185
   hypoallergenic 185–6
   'lamb and pears' 184
   low carbohydrate 186
   low-allergen and epilepsy 241
   low-allergen, and hypothyroidism
      254
   low-allergen, and urticaria 283
   maintenance 186
   mono 183, 184
   rare food 187
   raw food 187
   rotation 187
   specific carbohydrate 187–8
   Stone Age 188
   unrefined and Crohn's disease 231
   Yin/Yang balanced 188
Dietary fat and calcium absorption 35
Dietary fat and hearing loss 246
Dietary fibre 63–4
   and breast cancer 222, 223
   and cholesterol 45
   and colon cancer 224
   and kidney stones 258
   and short chain fatty acid
      production 64
   digestion by bacteria 63, 64
   insoluble 63
   soluble 63
Dietary Reference Values 64
Dietary supplements, definition 64
Digestion 64–6
   incomplete, and allergy 8
Digestive inflammation and
      chamomile 44
Digestive juices and acne rosacea 203
Digestive relaxant, peppermint as
      151
Digestive stimulant, cardamom as 39
Dihydrotestosterone 181
Dimethioate 152
Dimethylglycine 23
Dioscorine 170
Diosgenin 196
Dioxin and endometriosis 240
Disaccharidases 65

Disaccharides 38, 39
Disodium chromoglycate and
      quercetin 80
Diuretic
   celery as 42
   dandelion as 57
   juniper berries as 112
Diuretic drugs and potassium 158
Diuretic drugs and potassium 66
Diuretics 66
Dizziness
   and anaemia 10
   and potassium deficiency 157
DLPA 154
   and depression 233–4
   and pain control 154
DL-phenylalanine see DLPA
DMG see Dimethylglycine
DNA 89, 138
   and alanine 5
   synthesis, and glutamine 94
Dolomite 36, 66
   and magnesium 126
Dong quai 66
Dopa 41
Dopamine 41, 42, 191
   and manganese 127
   and prolactin 42
   and schizophrenia 42
   and vitamin B$_1$ 16
Double-blind clinical trials 66–7
Down's syndrome 237
   and mutations 237, 297
   causative factors 237, 297
Dreams and vitamin B$_6$ 20
Dysbiosis 67
   and barberry 24
   and hydrochloric acid 3
   and sugar consumption 179
   grapefruit seed extract for 98
   poor digestion causing 187–8
Dyslexia 238
   and zinc deficiency 238

E Coli 158
E numbers 82–3
EAR 64
Echinacea 70
Eczema 238
   and evening primrose oil
      supplements 238
   and fish oil supplements 238
   and milk intolerance 132
   supplements for 315
Edetic acid see EDTA
EDTA 70
Eggs, adaptation to 186
Eicosanoids 120, 161
Eicosapentaenoic acid see EPA
Elderberry 71
Elderly, the 301–4
   and angina 303
   and arthritis 303

and B vitamin deficiencies 301
and carotenoids 302
and diabetes 303
and digestive ability 301
and functional capacity 302
and immunity 302
and mental function 302–3
and nutritional deficiencies 301–2
and self-neglect 303
and zinc deficiency 302
supplements for 304
tips for 303
Electrolytes 71
Electron transport chain 72
Eleutherococcus 92
Elimination diet 183
ELISA test 107
Embolism, oestrogen and
      magnesium deficiency 247
Emotional stress 289
Emphysema 239
   and cadmium 239
   and NAC 239
   and pollution 239
   remedy, coltsfoot as 52
Empty calorie foods 138
Encephalin and methionine 131
Endocrine system 71
Endometriosis 240
   and dioxin 240
Endorphin
   and methionine 131
   and pain control 154
Endotoxins 67, 72, 158
Enemas, coffee 185
Energy
   and carbohydrate 39
   production 72
   production, and aspartic acid 14
   production, and copper 53
   production, and cysteine 55
   production, and fluoride 81
   production, and iron 109
Energy, as term for calories 15
Entero-viaform 106
Environmental factors and
      parkinsonism 270
Environmental medicine 73
Enzyme inhibitors in raw grains 134
Enzymes 73
Eosinophilia myalgia syndrome 191
   and genetic engineering 90
EPA 70–71
   and alcohol 5
   and cod liver oil 50
   and prostaglandins 161
   supplements 77
EPA/fish oil and rheumatoid arthritis
      278
Epilepsy 240–41
   and gluten sensitivity 241
   and glycine 96

Ischaemia 111
Isoflavones 147, 176
Isoleucine 111
Isomers 9, 111
  of phenylalanine 154
Itai-itai disease 111
IU see International Units
IU metric equivalents 108

Japanese food 124
Jejunum 112
Jerusalem artichokes
  and dietary fibre 63
  and FOS 159
  and inulin 159
Jet lag and melatonin 128, 307
Jojoba 112
Juniper berries 112

Kelp 114
Ketoacidosis 114
Ketone bodies 114
  and carnitine 40
Ketosis 114
  and alanine 5
Kidney 114
  and vitamin D 114
Kidney damage
  and cadmium 34
  and lead exposure 259
  and N-acetyl-beta-
    glucosaminidase 259
  and sugar consumption 179, 258–9
Kidney function 258–60
  and fish oil supplementation 259
  and low carbohydrate diets 186
  and protein restriction 259
  and selenium 259
  and taurine sufficiency 181
Kidney stones
  and alcohol consumption 258
  and calcium deficiency 259
  and coppersmiths 259
  and dietary advice 259
  and dietary fibre consumption 258
  and high carbohydrate diet 259
  and high fat diet 259
  and magnesium consumption 258
  and protein consumption 259
  and vitamin C 34, 258
  risk of, and magnesium
    supplementation 259
  risk of, and vitamin B$_6$
    supplementation 259
Kinky hair and copper deficiency 53
Klebsiella
  and FOS 159
  and uva-ursi 193
Koji 114, 132
Kombu 115
Kombucha 115
Krebs cycle 72, 162

and acetyl CoA 3
Krebs, Dr Ernst 116
Kuzu 115
Kwashiorkor 115, 139
Kyolic garlic 115

Laboratory tests for nutrient
  deficiencies 143, 144–5
Lactase 116
Lactates 26
Lactic acid 72, 116
Lactic acid cycle see Cori cycle
Lactobacillus bacteria 158
Lactose intolerance 132
Laetrile 116–17
Lamb and pears diet 184
Lapacho 117
Lathyrism 170
Laverbread 138
Laxative
  alder buckthorn as 6, 41
  cascara as 41
  flax seeds as 80
LDL cholesterol 46
Lead 117–18
  and calcium absorption 142
  and delinquency 233
  and IQ 261
  and kidney damage 259
  and reading disability 261
  harmful effects of 117
  interaction with calcium 117–18
  removal, horsetail for 104
  sources of 117
Leaky gut syndrome 118–19
  and candidiasis 37
  and gluten 95
  and iron deficiency 119
  golden seal for 97
  tests for 119
Lean meat 286
  fat content of 75
Learning difficulties 261–2
  and essential fatty acid deficiency
    261
  and zinc 213, 214
Leber's optic atrophy 61
Lecithin 96, 119
  and Alzheimer's disease 206
  and mania 263
  as choline supplement 47
  as source of inositol 108
  calorific value of 119
Lectins 120, 170
Legumes 163
Leguminosae 83
Lemons as source of flavonoids 79
Lentinan 166, 173
Leucine 120
Leukotrienes 120, 161
  and arachidonic acid 11
Life expectancy 302

Lignins 63
Liliaceae 83
Limiting amino acids 162
Lindane 152
Linoleic acid 76
  and arachidonic acid 11
  and prostaglandins 161
Linseeds see Flax seeds
Lipase 65
Lipids 75, 121
Lipofuscin 121
  and vitamin E 69
Lipoic acid 11, 121
  and glaucoma 242–3
  and sulphur 179
Lipoproteins 121
  and cholesterol 45–6
  and choline 47
  and garlic 227
  and vitamin C 33
Lipotropic effect, choline 47
Lipotropic factors 121
Lipoxygenase enzyme and flavonoids
  79
Lips, dry, peeling, burning 17
Liquorice 121–2
Listeria infection 84
Lithium and mania 42
Liver 122
  and vitamin A 122
  as source of vitamin A 1
  cancer of, and vitamin C
    supplements 221
  damage and vitamin B$_3$ 19
  detoxification, overload from
    candidiasis 37
  eating of in pregnancy 2
  function, nutrients to help 316
  treatments and wild yam 196
Lorenzo's oil 74
Low birthweight and mother's diet
  214
Low carbohydrate diet 186
Low-allergen diet
  and hyperactivity 252, 253
  and rheumatoid arthritis 278
  vegan diet and asthma 211
Lower Reference Nutrient Intake see
  LRNI
Low-fat diet
  and breast cancer prevention
    223–4
  vegan diet and diabetes treatment
    236
Low-fibre diet and butyric acid
  deficiency 31
LRNI 64
Lucerne 6
Lung disease
  and sodium 216
  and vitamin C 216
Lupus erythematosus

and alfalfa 6
and DHEA 63
and vitamin E 69
Lutein 40, 41
Luteinizing hormone 103
Lycopene 11
and bladder cancer 217
and free radicals 40
and lung cancer 217
and macular degeneration 262
and pancreatic cancer 217
and prostate cancer 225
and singlet oxygen 86
food sources of 41
inhibition of cancer growth rate 40
Lymphatic system, food absorbed into 66
Lymphocytes and alanine 5
Lysine 122
Lysine high, arginine low diet 182
Lysine supplementation and herpes infections 250

Macrobiotics 188, 124
Macrocytic anaemia 139
Macronutrients 138
Macular degeneration 262–3
and antioxidant vitamins 262
and beta-carotene consumption 262
and carotenes 40
and ginkgo biloba supplements 262
and lycopene consumption 262
and vitamin C consumption 262
and vitamin E 69, 262
and zinc consumption 262
and zinc supplementation 262–3
Magnesium 124–6
and allergy 206
and asthma 210, 211
and athletes 308
and autism 212
and chemical sensitivity 60
and epilepsy 240
and glaucoma 243
and headaches 244
and HIV 204
and kidney stones 258
and motor neurone disease 265
and oestrogen 126
and PMS 125, 273–4, 275
and stress 125
bioavailability 125
injections and chronic fatigue 228
sulphate 73
Magnesium deficiency
and angina 247
and diabetes 235
and embolism and oestrogen 247
and fatty acid metabolism 77

and fibromyalgia 241
and heart disease 247
and hypertension 251
and insulin resistance 236
and osteoporosis 267
Magnesium supplementation
and diabetes treatment 236
and hypoglycaemia 253
and kidney stone risk 259
and migraine 244
and noise-induced hearing loss 246
and osteoporosis 268
and oxalate excretion 259
and period pains 272
and pre-eclampsia 273
Maintenance diet 186
Malathion 152
Malic acid and metabolism 3
Mammary dysplasia and vitamin E 223
Manchurian mushroom 115
Manganese 126–7
and motor neurone disease 265
and SOD 127
and tea 127
bioavailability 127
Mania
and catecholamines 42
and lecithin 263
Manic-depressive illness 262–3
and folic acid 263
and glycine 96
and vanadium 194, 263
and vitamin C supplementation 263
Mannosans 63
MAO inhibitor drugs 191
Marasmus 139
Marshmallow 127
Measles 264
and vitamin A 2
and vitamin A supplementation 264
Meat
and breast cancer 222
and osteoporosis 268
Megavitamin therapy 128
Melanin and manganese 127
Melanoma 225
and Gerson diet 225
Melatonin 103, 128, 190
and brain tumours 219
and breast cancer 223
and free radicals 86
and immune function 255
Memory impairment and taurine 207
Menaquinone 113
Menopause 264
and obesity 147
and soya flour 264
and soya products 147, 176

and vitamin E 70
supplements for 315
Menstruation
painful 271–2
painful, supplements for 315
Mental development in children and iron deficiency 261
Mental illness
and nutritional deficiency 143
higher nutritional needs in 315
Mental performance
and ginkgo biloba 207
and iron deficiency 261
and vitamin supplementation 262
Menthol 151
Mercapturic acid 94
Mercury 129
accumulation in kidneys 259
and alkylglycerols 7
sensitivity 130
toxicity, and selenium 172
Metabolic rate 130
and adrenaline 42
Metabolism 130, 285
Metabolites, alcohols and aldehydes as 2
Methaemoglobin 137
Methionine 130–31
and adrenal glands 4
and alcohol consumption 6
and depression 131
and folic acid availability 131
and HIV 204
and homocysteine 102, 131
and hydroxyl radicals 86
and hypochlorite detoxification 60
and parkinsonism 271
diet high in 185
metabolism, and folic acid 81
metabolism, and serine 173
Methyl alcohol and aspartame 13
Methylation and detoxification 59, 60
Methylfolate 82
Methylmalonic acid 144
Methylmethioninesulfonium chloride 192
Methylxanthines 131
and coffee 51
Micronutrients 131
Migraine 243
and allergy 7
and calcium 244
and dietary treatment for children 244
and exclusion diet 213
and feverfew 78
and food intolerance 244
and high-carbohydrate diet 244
and magnesium supplementation 244
and milk intolerance 132
and tartrazine 180

and vitamin D 244
  premenstrual, calcium
    supplementation for 274
  premenstrual, vitamin D
    supplementation for 274
Milk 131
Milk products, fermented, and breast
  cancer 222
Milk thistle 174
Mineral absorption and vitamin D 56
Mineral consumption and bone
  density 268, 269
Mineral deficiencies and
  hyperactivity 252
Mineral water 132
Mineralocorticoids 4
Minerals and vegetarian diet 294
Miscarriage 298
  and alcohol consumption 273
  and diet 297
  and pesticides 153
  and selenium 272
  and smoking 273
  and sperm 297
  and zinc deficiency 213, 272
  habitual, and folic acid deficiency 81
Miso 132
  soup 286
Mitochondrion 72
Molybdenum 132–3
  and sulphation ability 61
Mono diets 183
Monoamine oxidase
  and tyramine 191
  inhibitors 42
Monoamines 41, 133
Monosaccharides 38, 39
Monosodium glutamate 133, 175
  and taurine 181
  and vitamin B_6 21
Monounsaturated fats 76
Mood swings 315
Morning sickness
  and vitamin B_6 20
  supplements for 315
Mosquitoes and B vitamins 307
Motor neurone disease 264–5
  and calcium 36, 264–5
  and carnitine 266
  and magnesium 265
  and manganese 265
  and poor detoxification 58, 60
  and vitamin B_2 266
Motor neurons 136
Mouth ulcers and vitamin A 1
Mouth, cracks 17
Mucilages 63
Mucopolysaccharides 134
  and sulphur 179
Mucus colitis
  and dysbiosis 67
  golden seal for 97

Mucus-dissolving effect of NAC 135
Muesli 134
Multiple allergies and rotation diet
  187
Multiple sclerosis 265
  and glutathione peroxidase 265
  and gluten sensitivity 95
  and iodine 109
  and mercury 130
  and tooth fillings 265
Multivitamin use and cleft palate 213
Muscle contraction and calcium 35
Muscle co-ordination and vitamin B_5
  19
Muscle cramps and calcium 36
Muscle weakness and vitamin B_1 15
Muscular dystrophy 266
  and selenium 266
  and vitamin E 69, 70, 266
Mushroom consumption and
  candidiasis 182
Mutagens 297
Myasthenia gravis and vitamin E 68,
  69
Mycotoxins 134
Myelin sheath 136
  and cholesterol 45
  and copper 53
Myricetin 79
Myristic acid 112

N-acetyl cysteine 55, 135
  and asthma 239
  and bronchitis 216, 239
  and emphysema 239
  and fatigue 228
N-acetyl glucosamine 135
N-acetyl-beta-glucosaminidase 179
  and kidney disease 259
NAD 72, 144
Naphthalene 156–7
Naringenin and detoxification 61
Natural hygienists 166
Natural killer cells and manganese
  127
Natural progesterone 159–60
Naturopathy 135, 166
Nephritis and sodium 175
Nerve and muscle function and
  vitamin E 68
Nerve gases 152
Nerve impulses and calcium 35
Nerve tonic, vervain as 195
Nervous tension and St John's wort
  177
Nervous tissue, calcium deposition in
  265
Neurological disease and gluten
  intolerance 266
Neuron 136
Neurosis and sugar consumption 209
Neuro-toxin, aluminium as 8

Neurotransmitters 136
Niacin see Vitamin B_3
Nickel 136
Nicotinic acid see Vitamin B_3
Nitrates 137
Nitric oxide synthase, inhibition by
  melatonin 128
Nitrites 137
Nitrogen balance 137
Nitrogen oxides 149
Nitrogen retention and BCAAs 30
Nitrosamines 137
Nobiletin 79
Non-Hodgkin lymphoma
  and hamburgers 218
  and vegetables 218
Noradrenaline 4, 41–2, 103, 191
Nori 138
Nucleic acids 138
Numbness in feet and legs, vitamin
  B_{12} 22
Nut consumption and cholesterol
  levels 227
Nutrient density 138
Nutrients 138
Nutritional deficiencies 138–43
  allergy as cause of 8
  and chronic illness 201
  and immune function 255, 288
  and mutagens 297
  causes 141–3
  in the chemically sensitive 61–2
Nutritional stress 289
Nutritional therapy 143

Oat bran as slimming aid 286
Obesity
  and birth defects 214
  and hypertension 251
  and psoriasis 276
Octacosanol 146
Octothiamine 16
Oedema and vitamin deficiency 139
Oestradiol 146
Oestriol 146
Oestrogen 103, 146–8
  and alfalfa 6
  and antibiotics 147
  and boron 30
  and embolism and magnesium
    deficiency 247
  and intestinal flora 159
  and iodine deficiency 109
  and liver metabolism 147
  and magnesium 126
  and sage 168
  and sperm count 256
  and thrombosis 126
  and tryptophan 190
  and vitamin B_3 18
  and vitamin C 34
  balancers 160

overload 159
  therapy and endometrial cancer
    219
Oestrogen-balancing
  effects of liquorice 122
  effects of soya 176
Oestrone 146
Oleic acid 76, 148
Olestra 148
Oligoantigenic diet 187
Oligosaccharides 38
Olive oil 148
Omega–3 oils and asthma 211
Optic neuritis and vitamin B$_1$ 16
Organ reserves 140
Organic food 148
Organochlorine pesticides 152
Organophosphorus insecticides 152
Ornithine 149
  and body-building 12
Orotates 149
Orthomolecular medicine 149
Osteoarthritis 266–7
  and beta-carotene 266–7
  and folic acid 267
  and glucosamine sulphate 267
  and vitamin C 266–7
  and vitamin E 266–7
Osteocalcin and vitamin K 114
Osteomalacia 139, 140
Osteoporosis 267–9
  and boron 28
  and calcium 36
  and calcium supplementation 268
  and fluoride 80
  and magnesium deficiency 267
  and magnesium supplementation
    268
  and meat consumption 268
  and phosphate excess 155
  and salt consumption 169
  and vitamin D 56
  and vitamin K 113–14
  supplements for 315
Ovaries and testosterone production
    181
Overload of detoxification pathways
    60
Oxalate excretion
  and magnesium supplementation
    259
  and protein consumption 259
  and vitamin B$_6$ supplementation
    259
Oxalates 149
Oxidative phosphorylation 72
  and vanadium 194
Oxidative stress 85
Oxygen metabolism and Siberian
    ginseng 92
Oxygen supply and iron 109
Oxygen uptake and carnitine 40

Oxygen, lack of for energy production
    54
Oxyhaemoglobin 100
Oxytocin 103, 156
Ozone 149
  and vitamin E 69

PABA 150
Palm oil 190
Palmitate 150
Palmitic acid 150
Pancreatic cancer and coffee 51
Pancreatic enzymes 65
Pancreatic insufficiency and
    selenium 171
Pancreatic juices, alkalinity of 153
Pancreatin 150
Pancreatitis 269–70
  and selenium injections 269–70
Pangamic acid 23
Panic attacks 209
  and caffeine 209
  and inositol 210
  supplements for 314
Pantethine 19
Pantothenic acid see Vitamin B$_5$
Papain 150
Papaya 150
Para-aminobenzoic acid see PABA
Paracetamol damage and silymarin
    174
Paracetamol overdose, treatment of
    60, 135
Paranoid delusions and folic acid
    deficiency 81
Parasites and Artemisia annua 12
Parasitic infections
  and malabsorption 142
  and vitamin B$_{12}$ 22
Parathyroid hormone 103, 150
  and phosphate 155
  and toxic metal absorption 265
Parkinson's disease 270–71
  and acetylcholine 3
  and cigarette smoking 270
  and dopamine 42
  and environmental factors 270
  and head trauma 270
  and heavy metal exposure 270
  and iodine 109
  and methionine 131, 271
  and octacosanol 146
  and pesticide use 270
  and poor detoxification 58, 60
  and solvent abuse 271
  and tooth fillings 270
  and tyrosine 191, 271
  and vitamin B$_6$ 21
  and vitamin C supplementation 271
  and vitamin E 69
  and vitamin E supplementation
    271

  and weed-killer 270
  and wood preservatives 270
Parsley 151
Pau D'Arco 117, 151
Pauling, Dr Linus 149
Paw-paw 150
Pectin and cholesterol 46
Pectins 63
Pellagra 139
  and vitamin needs 143
Peppermint 151
Pepsin 64, 65
Peptide bonds 162
Peptides 9
Periodontal disease 271
Periods, heavy and manganese 127
Periods, painful 271–2
  and fish oil 272
  and fish oil supplementation
    272
  and iron 110
  and magnesium supplementation
    272
  and vitamin B$_3$ 18
  supplements for 315
Peristalsis and acetylcholine 3
Pernicious anaemia 22, 139
Peroxidation
  and vitamin E 68
  as source of aldehydes 58
Peroxides 85, 86
Peroxyl radical and melatonin 128
Pesticide poisoning 152–3
Pesticide residues in cod liver oil
    50
Pesticide use and parkinsonism 270
Pesticides 151–3
  and acetylcholine 3
  and breast cancer 222
  and immune function 255
  and immunity 288
pH 153
  of blood 3
Phenylalanine 154, 191
Phenylketonuria 13
Phosphate 155
Phosphate excess and parathyroid
    hormone 155
Phosphatidylcholine 47, 155
Phosphatidylinositol 155
Phosphatidylserine 154–5, 172
Phospholipids 154, 155
  and cell membranes 42
Phosphoric acid 138
  and metabolism 3
Phosphorus 155
  and calcium status 268
Photochemical smog 149
Phylketonuria 154
Phylloquinone 113
Physical stress 289
Phytase 156

Quercetin 79, 80, 165
    and allergy 206
    and prostaglandins 161
    as antioxidant 11
    synthesis by bacteria 165
Quinoa 165

Radiotherapy and alkylglycerols 7
Raffinose 63
Rape seed oil 73
Rare food diet 187
Rationing foods 286
Raw food diet 166, 187
Raynaud's disease 277
    and fish oil supplementation 277
    and Ginkgo biloba 91
Rea, Dr William 21, 60, 61
Reactive oxygen species 86
Reading disability and lead exposure
    261
Ready-made meals 295
Recommended Dietary Allowance 317
Recreational drugs and HIV 203
Red pepper see Capsicum
Reference Nutrient Intake see RNI
Refined carbohydrate
    and blood sugar 182
    and gallstones 242
Refined foods
    and hyperactivity 261
    and IQ 261
Reishi mushroom 166
Research 201
    methodology 201
Restless leg syndrome and iron 110
Retarded growth 139
Retinol 1
Rheumatism and copper 54
Rheumatoid arthritis 277–8
    and copper 54
    and EPA/fish oil 278
    and essential fatty acids 278
    and ginger 91
    and GLA 278
    and gluten sensitivity 95
    and histidine 101
    and low-allergen diet 278
    and polyunsaturated fat 278
    and selenium 278
    and vitamin B₅ 19
Rhodanese 116
Rhubarb and oxalates 149
Riboflavin see Vitamin B₂ 17
Rice bran oil 87
Rickets 140
    and vitamin D 56
RNA 138
RNI 64, 167, 317
Rosaceae 83
Rosemary 167
Rotation diet 187
    and asthma 211

Royal jelly 167
Rutaceae 83
Rutin 79, 80
    and allergy 206
    and bee pollen 24
    and buckwheat 31
    and prostaglandins 161

S-adenosyl methionine 131, 168
    and depression 234
Saccharin 168
Sage 168
Salami and tyramine 7
Salicylates 168
Saliva and calcium 35
Salivary amylase 64
Salmonella infection 84
Salt 169, 175
Salt sensitivity 169
Saturated fat 76
    and gallstones 242
    and high cholesterol 227
    and lung cancer 221
Saw palmetto 169–70
Scalp disease and biotin 26
Scars and vitamin E 69
Schilling test 144
Schizophrenia 278–80
    and B complex vitamin
        deficiencies 279
    and bowel toxins 188
    and coenzyme Q10 279
    and dopamine 42
    and essential fatty acids 77, 279,
        280
    and fish oil supplementation 280
    and folic acid 234, 280
    and gluten sensitivity 95
    and histamine 131
    and methionine 131
    and prenatal nutritional
        deficiencies 279–80
    and tooth fillings 279
    and tyrosine 191
    and vitamin B₃ 18
    and vitamin B₆ 21
    and vitamin C 280
    and zinc deficiency in pregnancy
        279
    drugs and choline 47
    drugs and vitamin E 69
School performance and iron 110
Schussler, Wilhelm 189
Scurvy 140, 170
    'rebound' 34
Seaweed
    and iodine 109
    and vitamin B₁₂ 22
Secondary plant metabolites 170–71
Secretin 65
Seizures and vitamin B₆ deficiency
    240

Selenium 171–2
    and acne 202
    and Aids 205
    and anxiety 209
    and asthma 210, 211
    and birth defects 213
    and bladder cancer prevention 217
    and cancer prevention 216, 217
    and creatinine clearance 259
    and depression 209, 233
    and epilepsy 240
    and free radicals 86, 299–300
    and hepatitis 250
    and HIV 203
    and hydroxyl radicals 86
    and hypothyroidism 254
    and immune function 255, 288
    and kidney function 259
    and liver cancer 219
    and LRNI 64
    and lung cancer prevention 217
    and mercury 130
    and miscarriage 272
    and muscular dystrophy 266
    and rheumatoid arthritis 278
    and thyroid hormone 171
    and thyroid hormone activation
        189
    and vegetarian diet 294
    deficiency, and atherosclerosis
        248
    deficiency, and heart disease
        247–8
    injections, and pancreatitis 269–70
    soil levels 171
    supplementation, and
        atherosclerosis 249
    supplementation, and sperm
        motility 257
Senility 206, 302–3
    and calcium 36
    and vitamin B₁ 15
Sensitivity to light and zinc
    deficiency 199
Serenoa repens 169–70
Serine 172
Serotonin 173
    and depression 190–91
    and tryptophan 190
Sex drive in women and testosterone
    181
Sex hormones and adrenal glands 4
Shark cartilage 173
Shark liver oil 7
Sheep dip, health effects on farmers
    153
Shiitake mushrooms 173
Shingles and vitamin E 69
Short-chain fatty acids from dietary
    fibre 63
Shoyu sauce 174
Sickle cell anaemia